Progress
in
Drug Metabolism

Volume 3

Progress in Drug Metabolism

Volume 3

Edited by

J. W. Bridges

*Institute of Industrial and Environmental Health and Safety,
University of Surrey*

L. F. Chasseaud

*Department of Metabolism and Pharmacokinetics,
Huntingdon Research Centre*

A Wiley—Interscience Publication

JOHN WILEY & SONS
CHICHESTER · NEW YORK · BRISBANE · TORONTO

Library of Congress Catalog Card Number 75-19446

ISBN 0 471 99711 0

Printed in Great Britain by John Wright & Sons Ltd, at the Stonebridge Press, Bristol

Contributors to Volume 3

S. Brechbühler   *Ciba–Geigy AG, Basel, Switzerland*

G. T. Brooks   *Agricultural Research Council, Unit of Invertebrate Chemistry and Physiology, University of Sussex, Brighton, Sussex*

I. C. Calder   *School of Chemistry, University of Melbourne, Victoria, Australia*

J. P. Dubois   *Ciba–Geigy AG, Basel, Switzerland*

D. H. Hutson   *Shell Toxicology Laboratory (Tunstall), Sittingbourne Research Centre, Sittingbourne, Kent*

F. Oesch   *Institute of Pharmacology, University of Mainz, Mainz, West Germany*

G. B. Quistad   *Biochemistry Department, Zoecon Corporation, Palo Alto, California, USA*

W. Riess   *Ciba–Geigy AG, Basel, Switzerland*

D. A. Schooley   *Biochemistry Department, Zoecon Corporation, Palo Alto, California, USA*

Preface

The two recent major advances in instrumentation useful to workers in drug metabolism have been those connected with mass spectrometry and liquid chromatography. Mass spectrometry was reviewed in Volume 1 and the use of stable isotopes in mass spectrometry in Volume 2. Liquid chromatography and its applications are now covered in the present volume.

The thinking behind the analytical needs of drug metabolism has received scant attention in the literature. Because of the heavy commitment of those working in drug metabolism to analysis, an examination of the principles underlying assay selection is included in the present volume.

As illustrated by this volume, reviews in this series are not confined to subjects connected with only pharmaceuticals. The term 'drug metabolism' is used in this series to encompass all classes of compounds and their fate in any biological system *in vivo* or *in vitro*.

Epoxides as potentially toxic intermediates in the metabolism of many compounds were discussed in Volume 1. This theme is developed in the present volume through a review on epoxide hydratase.

J. W. BRIDGES
L. F. CHASSEAUD

High-pressure, high-resolution liquid chromatography and its application to pesticide analysis and biochemistry

D. A. Schooley and G. B. Quistad

INTRODUCTION

The development of liquid chromatography has been characterized by two periods of dormancy. This technique is generally acknowledged to have been discovered by Tswett, who in 1903–6 separated plant pigments by liquid column chromatography with calcium carbonate and other adsorbents. As discussed by Ettre and Horvath (1975) in an historical review, chemists of Tswett's era felt that his 'chromatographic analysis' was unsuited for preparative work, in an

1

era when preparative isolation was accomplished by extraction, distillation, or crystallization. Column adsorption chromatography saw little use in the ensuing decades, but in 1931, Kuhn, Winterstein, and Lederer triggered a popularization of the technique with a preparative isolation of xanthophylls by bed development in a column. The technique was soon widely adopted; modifications were made such as the extension from bed development to elution chromatography (Reichstein and Van Euw, 1938). The popularity of column chromatography in the 1930s inspired the development of liquid–liquid partition chromatography (Martin and Synge, 1941), paper chromatography (Consden, Gordon, and Martin, 1944), reversed-phase chromatography (Howard and Martin, 1950), and gas–liquid chromatography (James and Martin, 1951).

However, further development of adsorption chromatography was relatively modest from the late 30s until about 1968–9, when several firms introduced 'high pressure liquid chromatographs' as integral units. Probably the rapid maturation of gas–liquid chromatography (g.l.c.) as a tool for qualitative and quantitative analysis, and the rapid popularization of thin-layer chromatography (t.l.c.), contributed to the neglect of technological advances in column liquid chromatography during the 50s and early 60s. It remains curious that this oldest of chromatographic techniques was the slowest to mature.

The renaissance in liquid chromatography (l.c.) has been accepted most eagerly by researchers in biochemistry, natural products chemistry, pharmaceuticals (reviewed by Wheals and Jane, 1977), pesticide chemistry, and related areas where the chemicals of interest are frequently too non-volatile or unstable for g.l.c. separation. The early dogma that liquid chromatography would not be useful for preparative purposes has been clearly refuted, and its superiority in this respect over g.l.c. is becoming widely recognized. Rapid improvements have been made in l.c. instrumentation—especially in pumping systems, injectors, and columns—so that rapid analyses can be made with high resolution. Detection of samples by l.c. remains more of a problem than in g.l.c., especially with respect to the lack of a high-sensitivity, 'universal' detector (like the hydrogen flame ionization detector in g.l.c.) and also with respect to the relatively immature technology of most types of selective, high-sensitivity l.c. detectors. The latter factor may explain why adoption of modern l.c. for detection and quantitation of pesticide residues has been comparatively slow.

Nevertheless, liquid chromatography is playing a rapidly increasing role in pesticide analysis. Prior to presenting an overview of applications of modern l.c. to pesticide analysis (metabolism studies, residue analysis, and formulations), we shall present a general discussion of this technique, especially those facets most relevant to these applications. A number of texts are available (Snyder and Kirkland, 1974; Brown, 1973; Perry *et al*, 1972; Kirkland, 1971a) which discuss in detail, theory, instrumentation, and general applications of the various modes of liquid chromatography. We present a condensed, largely non-mathematical discussion of chromatographic theory, with comparisons between g.l.c. and l.c., since basic understanding of theory is essential for efficient use of l.c. methods. We discuss apparatus only in general terms, because of previous coverage and the rapid evolution of commercial instruments. Because of the importance of specific, sensitive detectors in pesticide analysis, special emphasis is given to this subject. Exact conditions for analysis of over 220 pesticides are presented in tabular form, and general discussion of preferred techniques for l.c. analysis of pesticides is arranged according to structural classification. Residue analysis of pesticides was reviewed by Horgan (1973) and Moye (1975), so our emphasis in this area is on subsequent work. Reviews of l.c. applications to multiresidue analysis have been presented by Sidwell (1977) and Ishii (1976, in Japanese). We have attempted as thorough a literature coverage as possible until January 1978. We have not reviewed use of classical column chromatography for clean-up of pesticide residues or as a purification technique in synthetic chemistry.

Finally, there is no standard abbreviation for this technique. Most widely used is h.p.l.c. which can represent a choice between high pressure l.c., high performance l.c., or perhaps even high price l.c.! Also used are high resolution liquid chromatography, h.r.l.c.; high efficiency l.c., h.e.l.c.; and high speed l.c., h.s.l.c. In the authors' opinions, resolution, efficiency, and speed are more evocative of the results obtained with this method than 'pressure' or 'performance'. To compromise, we shall use l.c. (the abbreviation favoured by Snyder and Kirkland, 1974) and allow the readers to append prefixes of their choice if desired.

THEORY

In this section chromatographic theory is reviewed briefly. For newcomers to this field, supplementary discussion can be found in the texts referenced previously.

Band Broadening and Column Efficiency

Column efficiency is determined according to the theoretical plate model advanced by Martin and Synge (1941). Thus, the column is imagined to consist of discrete regions termed theoretical plates, each of which corresponds to a single step of a counter-current distribution apparatus (or a separatory funnel). When the number of theoretical plates (N) is sufficiently large, the band shape of a discrete species of retarded solutes moving through a chromatography column should approximate a Gaussian distribution. The value of N can be determined from the retention volume (V_R) and the bandwidth ($w = 4\sigma$) as shown in figure 1. This model requires the unrealistic assumption that a chromatographic system consists of discrete regions. Actually, in moving through a chromatographic bed, a solute is either adsorbed to the support and stationary, or in solution and moving with the velocity of the mobile phase until it is next adsorbed. Such motion corresponds to a 'random walk' mathematical model. Statistical analysis of a sharp band of solute molecules so moving through a column also reveals that the molecules will gradually assume a Gaussian distribution, with the band broadening as migration increases.

Such models assume instantaneous equilibrium of solute between mobile and stationary phase, and ignore rates of diffusion, mobile phase velocity, packing

4

particle size, and other factors. Consideration of the dynamics of the chromatographic process is necessary to describe quantitatively the parameters that
contribute to band spreading in chromatography. The first comprehensive
theory to relate these parameters was provided by van Deemter *et al* (1956).
Data on which their theoretical interpretations were based were derived from
g.l.c., due to convenience of measurement at that time. Studies of the effect of
changes in mobile phase velocity on the height equivalent to a theoretical plate,
H (= number of plates N/column height in mm), revealed curves that are

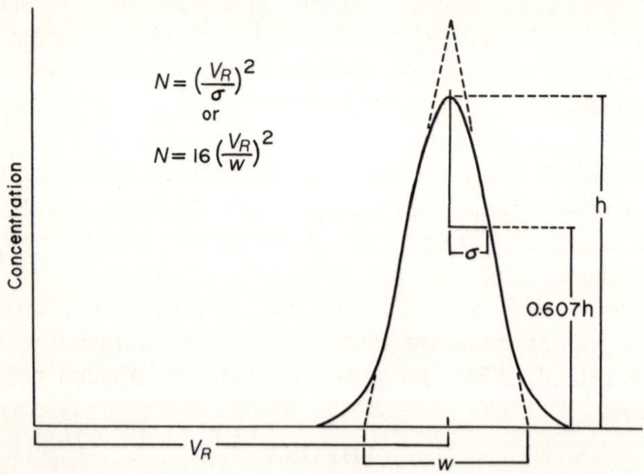

Figure 1 Definition of parameters and equations used in determining the efficiency
of a chromatographic column. An idealized chromatographic peak is Gaussian and the
peak width (w) is equal to four standard deviations (4σ). These parameters are measured
by (a) determining peak width at $0.607h$ to obtain 2σ, or (b) drawing tangents at the
inflection points ($0.607h$) to obtain w. Measurement of peak width at halfheight gives
$2\sigma \times \sqrt{(2 \ln 2)}$, requiring use of a different formula: $N = 5.54\,(V_R/\text{halfheight width})^2$.
From Schooley and Nakanishi (1973), reproduced by permission of Academic Press

roughly hyperbolic with a pronounced decrease in efficiency (increase in H)
found below certain values of the carrier velocity (figure 2). The optimum carrier
velocity for minimum H (maximum efficiency) and the curve shape are quite
dependent on the type of carrier gas, so their consideration is thus important for
achieving maximum efficiency in g.l.c. The van Deemter theory is summarized
in equation (1).

$$(A) \qquad (B) \qquad (C)$$

$$H = 2\lambda d_\mathrm{p} + \frac{2\gamma D_\mathrm{m}}{v} + \frac{\omega d_\mathrm{p}{}^2}{D_\mathrm{m}}\,v \qquad (1)$$

where d_p is the average particle diameter of packing, D_m the diffusivity of sample
in the mobile phase, v the mobile phase velocity, and λ, γ, ω are constants of
order unity, characteristic of the type of packing and bed structure. Equation (1)
consists of three terms. The first (A) is the contribution of eddy diffusion, or
diffusion due to solute molecules moving, not in a straight line, but around and
under particles, and is generally considered to be independent of mobile phase

velocity. The second factor (*B*) causing band broadening is axial (or longitudinal) diffusion, the tendency of solute to diffuse away from band centre with time, and is inversely proportional to solvent velocity. The last term (*C*) is the resistance of sample to mass transfer and is proportional to mobile phase velocity. 'Mass transfer' is an expression of the time spent by solute molecules diffusing into or out of the support and/or bound to specific sites in adsorption chromatography. While the above equation is somewhat oversimplified, it

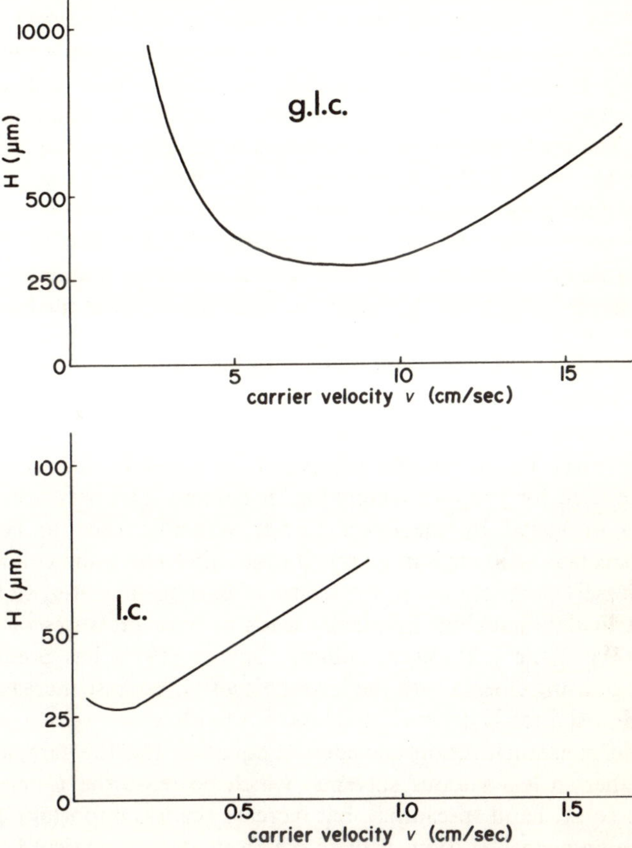

Figure 2 Approximation of curves obtained for the dependency of theoretical plate height (*H*) on carrier velocity (*v*) for g.l.c. (upper) and l.c. (lower). Note that the axes are 10-fold exaggerated below because of the lower values of *H* and *v* in l.c.

nevertheless provides valuable insight into the factors controlling band broadening, so that we may understand how to maximize efficiency.

The most important differences between the techniques of l.c. and g.l.c. are attributable to the difference in properties of liquids and gases. As pointed out by Giddings (1965), the most crucial distinction is that gases show almost no attraction for solute molecules, whereas liquid mobile phases can interact with solutes by several mechanisms. Thus, in l.c., *selectivity* is determined both by

6

mobile phase and stationary phase, while in g.l.c. only the stationary phase is of importance. Differences in column *efficiency* between l.c. and g.l.c. arise because diffusivity of solute is 10^4–10^5 times slower in liquids than gases, and viscosities of liquids are $\sim 10^2$ higher than those of gases. Returning to the van Deemter equation, we see that the enormously lower solute diffusivity in l.c. will make the axial transfer term (B) of very little consequence. Since this term is inversely proportional to solvent velocity, van Deemter-type plots for l.c. show less tendency for 'optimum' carrier velocities than in g.l.c., for only at inconveniently slow carrier velocities is an increase in H (decrease in N) noted (figure 2). The mass transfer term (C) is proportional to mobile phase velocity, but inversely proportional to solute diffusivity. To obtain high efficiency in l.c., mobile phase velocity must be lower than in g.l.c. to accommodate the lower diffusivity. The far lower sample diffusivities in l.c. diminish the importance of the B term, but increase the importance of the C term, when compared to g.l.c.

Decreasing the packing particle diameter will not only decrease band broadening due to eddy diffusion (A), but especially band broadening due to mass transfer (C) which is dependent on the square of particle diameter. Thus, there has been a steady trend towards smaller l.c. packings with the current technology represented by 'microparticulate' packings in the 5–10 μm range. While it is theoretically desirable to use small diameter packings in g.l.c., it is not generally feasible to use packings smaller than 125–150 μm (100–120 mesh), as otherwise column back pressure becomes excessive.

The high viscosity of liquids compared to gases ($\sim 100\times$) immediately suggests the need for proportionately higher column inlet pressures in l.c. This situation is mitigated by the lower carrier velocities used in l.c. (typically ~ 0.25 cm/s versus ~ 10 cm/s in g.l.c.). On the other hand, the column permeability is inversely proportional to the *square* of particle diameter, so that the use of microparticulate packings frequently leads to back pressures of 30–200 atm (~ 500–3,000 psi) for a 25–30 cm column. Snyder (1971) has pointed out the desirability of using eluents with the lowest viscosity, because increased viscosity causes an almost directly proportional loss in N (with carrier velocity and column identity held constant). Again considering equation (1), the sample diffusivity (D_m) is higher in less viscous solvents, which decrease the C term (a major contributor to l.c. band spreading), but increase the less important B term.

The preceding considerations explain why a modern analytical l.c. column is shorter, packed with smaller particles, and eluted more slowly than a g.l.c. column. Since H for a properly packed 10 μm silica l.c. column may approach 0.02 mm ($= 2d_p$), a 25 cm analytical column can exhibit 10,000 plates. In contrast, an efficiently packed g.l.c. column will on occasion show $H = 0.3$ mm, requiring a 300 cm column to produce 10,000 plates.

Retention

Retention in l.c. is measured by a parameter termed the capacity factor (k'), defined as the ratio of the amount of solute in the stationary phase (N_s) to the amount of solute in the mobile phase (N_m). Larger values of k' indicate more of the solute to be in the stationary phase, and hence more strongly retained. Equation (2) shows that k' is also equal to the thermodynamic equilibrium distribution coefficient, K, times the ratio of the volume of stationary

$$k' = \frac{N_s}{N_m} = K\frac{V_s}{V_m} \tag{2}$$

phase (V_s) to the volume of mobile phase (V_m) in the column (more commonly termed the void volume, V_0). From other relationships, it can be shown that

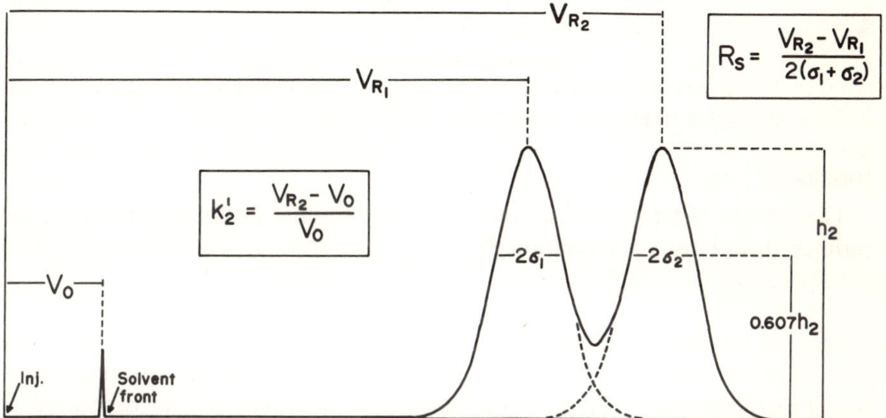

Figure 3 Parameters used for measuring (a) retention (capacity factor, k') and (b) resolution (R_s). Measurement of column void volume (V_0) is usually obtained with an unretained solute. While some texts recommend measurement of w for R_s determination, measurement of 2σ is easier for partially overlapping peaks

k' is related to the experimentally observed V_0 and the retention volume (V_R) of the solute peaks as shown in equation (3) and figure 3.

$$k' = \frac{V_R - V_0}{V_0} \tag{3}$$

It is occasionally of interest to compare R_f values observed on t.l.c. to k' values obtained for the same solutes on l.c. (Table 1). The relationship between k' and R_f is given by the expressions in equations (4).

$$k' = \frac{1 - R_f}{R_f}; \quad R_f = \frac{1}{k' + 1} \tag{4}$$

Strictly speaking, such a transformation is valid only if adsorbent of identical structure and activity is used for both the l.c. and t.l.c. experiments. These equations may nevertheless provide a means of extrapolating from existing t.l.c. data for choice of an approximate solvent system for l.c. analysis of an unfamiliar solute. For a systematic study of this problem, see Hara (1977). The recent introduction of alkyl-bonded (C_{18}) reversed-phase t.l.c. plates will be valuable for scouting solvent systems for reversed-phase l.c.

Table 1 Comparison of R_f and k'

R_f	k'
1	0
0·75	0·333
0·5	1·0
0·4	1·5
0·333*	2·0
0·2	4
0·1	9
0	∞

*Snyder (1968) has shown that an R_f of $\frac{1}{3}$ gives optimum resolution (valid for single bed development in t.l.c. only).

Resolution

The relative retention (α) of two chromatographic peaks is defined as the ratio of their k' values (equation 5).

$$\alpha = k_2'/k_1' \tag{5}$$

When $\alpha = 1\cdot1$ or less, the resolution of peaks is fairly difficult on l.c., requiring 2,000–5,000 theoretical plates (depending on how complete the resolution must be). The quantitative value of resolution (R_s) is defined as the difference in retention volumes of two peaks divided by half the sum of their band widths (4σ) (equation 6).

$$R_s = \frac{V_{R2} - V_{R1}}{2\sigma_2 + 2\sigma_1} \simeq \frac{V_{R2} - V_{R1}}{4\sigma} \tag{6}$$

From equation (6) and other relationships, a general equation (7) can be derived which expresses resolution in terms of selectivity (I), capacity factor (II) and efficiency (III) (values of k' and N are measured for the slower eluting component).

$$\qquad\quad (I) \qquad\quad (II) \quad\ (III)$$

$$R_s = \frac{1}{4}\left(\frac{\alpha - 1}{\alpha}\right)\left(\frac{k'}{1+k'}\right)(\sqrt{N}) \tag{7}$$

Equation (7) provides insight into the factors controlling resolution, and therefore which parameters should be altered to improve a separation.

The first step in developing a separation is to find a proper k' value (i.e. to optimize the solvent polarity). The retention term in equation (7) shows that as k' goes to zero, so does resolution. There is also little point in choosing excessively long k' values (> 10). While it is important to choose an efficient column, term (III) of equation (7) shows that resolution increases only with the square root of N. For a given column, N is maximized by choosing low viscosity solvents or heating the column to reduce the viscosity. Other approaches to increase N are to use a column with packing of smaller d_p (equation 1) or to increase column length by adding series-connected columns. The latter approach may frequently be a last resort, since quadrupling column length is required to double resolution. For trace analyses, highly efficient columns are desired because they produce sharper peaks of higher amplitude, enhancing detectability.

The selectivity term (I) of equation (7) is characteristic of the column packing and solvent combination. Usually the most direct way of improving a difficult l.c. separation is to choose either a different solvent mixture or column, analogous to changing the stationary phase in g.l.c. The ability of various solvents to interact with solutes *via* different mechanisms—dispersion, dipole interaction, or hydrogen bonding (either proton donors or acceptors)—provides many possibilities for altering α.

MODES OF LIQUID CHROMATOGRAPHY

Classically, four modes of l.c. are recognized, based on the mechanism of separation. Liquid–solid chromatography (l.s.c.) is historically the oldest technique, with separations based on the selective adsorption of samples by a solid from the mobile phase. Commonly used adsorbents are silica, alumina, magnesium silicate, and occasionally others such as charcoal.

Liquid–liquid or partition chromatography (l.l.c.) is similar to l.s.c. except that the solid support is coated with a liquid stationary phase which is immiscible with the mobile phase. It is necessary to presaturate the mobile phase with stationary phase to retard the dissolution of the stationary phase from the column, and to control carefully the temperature of the system. Usually a precolumn is inserted between the pump and injector to assure that the eluent is presaturated with stationary phase.

In both l.s.c. and l.l.c, it is rare that a pure solvent is used as the mobile phase. Usually, mixed solvents must be used to adjust the solvent strength to the proper level. It may frequently be difficult to decide if a separation is purely adsorptive or purely partitioning; in many cases a mixture of processes may be occurring. This is especially true if the eluent contains appreciable amounts of polar components such as water, acids, glycols, or alcohols, which are strongly bound by supports such as silica or alumina.

Both l.l.c. and l.s.c. can be further subdivided into 'normal' and reversed-phase categories, according to the nomenclature of Howard and Martin (1950). 'Normal' phase consists of a polar stationary phase or adsorbent, and reversed-phase (r.p.) utilizes a non-polar stationary phase or support (silica coated with paraffin oil; charcoal) eluted with a polar solvent usually containing water. In r.p. chromatography, hydrophilic ('more polar') substances elute first, and stronger solvents (leading to faster elution) are less polar. Due to the reversal of polarity considerations, it is usually desirable to speak of solvent strength rather than polarity.

Currently the most popular sorbents for l.c. are modified silicas with functionality chemically bonded to surface silanol groups. The most frequently used of these sorbents are those with bonded alkyl functionality, usually C_{18}, employed in the reversed-phase mode. These supports pose a problem of nomenclature because there is considerable controversy whether they function by an adsorption (l.s.c.) or partition (l.l.c.) mechanism. In a recent review, Horvath and Melander (1977) have argued that the partition mechanism is unlikely, as the layer of bonded hydrocarbon is only a monolayer thick and subject to translational and rotational constraints. Colin and Guiochon (1977) reviewed in detail the various retention mechanism theories, and concurred with the opinion of Pryde (1974) that 'it seems a little irrelevant to argue whether the mechanism is by partition or adsorption for neither term is strictly applicable'. The latter suggested the term liquid–solid-partition chromatography, although bonded reversed-phase chromatography seems as descriptive. Recent data of Scott and Kucera (1977) show that the hydrocarbon chains of several r.p. sorbents (C_2, C_8, and C_{18}) associate with the organic component of the eluent, forming a monolayer which is *not* displaced by the sample. From this they conclude that the sample most likely interacts with the monolayer of solvent and not with the hydrocarbon chain.

Gel chromatography, also termed exclusion chromatography or gel-permeation chromatography (g.p.c.), is used to separate on the basis of molecular weight. Theoretical treatment of gel chromatography is different from that presented earlier in this review for l.l.c. and l.s.c. since there is no true 'retention' mechanism. The separation is controlled by the column packing, not by the solvent (in the absence of unwanted adsorptive interactions). The synthetic gel packings contain a large volume of pores which imbibe solvent and admit small molecules easily, medium-sized ones with more difficulty, and larger ones not at all. By controlling pore size, the molecular weight range for which a gel is effective is altered. A solute of molecular weight (or size) such that it is totally excluded from the pores elutes at the exclusion volume (V_0), whereas a small solute which is free to totally permeate the pores elutes at V_t. The quantity of solvent held within the pores (V_i) is equal to ($V_t - V_0$). As V_0 and V_i are frequently nearly the same, the number of peaks separable on a given gel is rather small. Nevertheless, the technique has been indispensable in polymer and protein chemistry for analytical and preparative purposes. For researchers in pesticide and natural products chemistry, g.p.c. can be the easiest way of separating low molecular weight substances of interest from triglyceride and other higher molecular weight components.

Ion-exchange chromatography has a multitude of applications in biochemistry and inorganic chemistry. In fact, Snyder and Kirkland (1974) assert that probably more separations are currently achieved by ion-exchange than any other l.c. mode. Supports are usually cross-linked polystyrene beads functionalized to contain cationic or anionic sites, although in other applications functionalized silicas or gel permeation materials such as Sephadex are used. The mobile phase is usually an aqueous buffer containing a counter ion with the same charge as the sample ion, and separation is achieved by the competition of these ions for the oppositely charged ionic group on the support. In addition to the ionic mechanism of separation, it is not uncommon to find a tendency towards reversed-phase-type interactions between organic species in aqueous solutions and the polystyrene-based ion-exchange supports. Ion-exchange Sephadex gels used in biochemistry may show mixtures of ion-exchange and molecular exclusion mechanisms.

Recently the technique of ion-pair chromatography was developed by Schill and coworkers (reviewed by Gloor and Johnson, 1977, and by Schill *et al*, 1977) as an alternative to ion-exchange chromatography. Originally the technique consisted of coating an ionic organic compound onto a support such as silica or cellulose. Ionic organic species of opposite charge may then interact by forming ion-pairs with the reagent with varying degrees of both ionic affinity and lipophilicity. More recently the popular bonded-phase l.c. columns have been used for reversed-phase ion-pair chromatography, with ion-pairing reagents dissolved in the mobile phase. This modification has the advantage that both ionized and neutral components may be separated under the same conditions. The technique has also been termed soap chromatography, when alkyl sulphonates or sulphates are used as the ion-pairing reagent for separation of cationic organic species. Many factors can be altered to control retention, such as the type and size of counter ion, its concentration, mobile phase pH, and organic modifier type and concentration. Scott and Kucera (1977) have investigated the importance of wetting of the bonded-r.p. packings by the mobile phase on ion-pair chromatographic retention. With high water content where the *hydrophobic* column surface is non-wetted, the ionic reagent was found to be adsorbed to the column with concomitant increase in retention of counter-ionic species. When the hydrophobic packing was wetted (moderate to high organic modifier content), the ionic reagent was totally in the mobile phase, and counter-ionic species showed decreased retention. It is not yet clear if this will be true of all ion-pairing reagents.

Thus, in addition to the four classically recognized modes of l.c., two newer variants deserve separate classification due to their distinctiveness and utility: bonded-phase l.c. and ion-pair l.c. Bonded-r.p. l.c. has already proved to be extremely useful in pesticide metabolism studies, and ion-pair l.c. has great promise of further advancing this field in facilitating isolation of polar, ionic conjugates.

PACKINGS AND COLUMNS

An extremely comprehensive review of this subject was published recently (Majors, 1977), including specifications of over 110 types of l.c. packings and/or prepacked columns.

Types of Column Packings

Following the introduction of commercial liquid chromatographs in the late 1960s, porous layer beads (or pellicular adsorbents) were developed to provide more efficient columns. The porous layer beads consist of 30–40 μm glass beads chemically treated to provide a surface deposit of silica or other adsorbent, and provide much higher efficiency than similarly sized totally porous adsorbents because of better mass transfer of adsorbed solute. Good columns of these materials can be readily dry-packed, but the lower surface area compared to porous adsorbents leads to substantially lower capacity for sample.

Reduction of particle size also improves mass transfer sufficiently so that totally porous packings can be used. Small porous packings in the 5–10 μm range were introduced in the early 1970s and are generally referred to as microparticulate packings. Production of efficient microparticulate columns requires special slurry packing techniques generally using high pressures. Commercially available prepacked columns are usually only 25 or 30 cm in length, longer columns being more difficult to pack. The principal limitation of microparticles is in fact the difficulty of reproducibly packing efficient, durable columns. The most common internal diameter (i.d.) for analytical columns is 0·4–0·46 cm, as such columns are more efficient than with 0·2–0·3 cm i.d. Use of smaller bore columns is frequently desirable, however, with trace analysis work to improve limits of detection. Microparticulate columns provide better efficiency and much higher sample capacity than those packed with pellicular materials and have consequently displaced the latter in most applications. Since column permeability is proportional to the square of particle diameter, a column of 10 μm microparticles requires 16 times the back pressure of one of 40 μm porous layer beads of equivalent length.

Silica constitutes by far the most popular material, not only as a microparticulate adsorbent and as a support in l.l.c., but also as a support for chemical functionalization to bonded-r.p. and ion-exchange packings. Both spherical and irregular silicas are available, each with certain slight advantages claimed over the other. The principal disadvantage of silica-based packings is that mobile phase pH must not exceed 7–8, or the column performance will degrade due to dissolution of packing.

In order to ensure reliable analyses, it is essential that retention data are as reproducible as possible. We have observed large differences in retentivity between nominally identical prepacked columns of silica gel of different lots, which could not be compensated by adjusting the water content. Such variations are at present by no means uncommon. In order to achieve reproducible results with a given column, the experimenter must control the water content of the silica column and therefore of the solvent. Water is necessary to moderate the active sites of silica so that linear capacity of sample and column efficiency are optimized. It is more convenient to add a small amount of a polar constituent such as methanol or isopropanol to a solvent mixture as moderator than to control the water content. Ample data (Kirkland, 1973a; Engelhardt, 1977; Thomas *et al*, 1977) exist to show, however, that attempts to replace water with alcohols lead to lower efficiencies and, in certain cases, distorted and abnormal peak shapes. Because of difficulty of determining the optimum solvent water content for each instance, Snyder (1968) recommends that eluents routinely be 50% water saturated as a reasonable expedient.

Selectivity of silicas varies considerably with surface area, pore size, and other parameters. Figure 4 shows the difference in selectivity of separation of DDT and related substances on three silica gels of identical structure differing only in pore widths (4, 6, and 10 nm). Such differences can be exploited to advantage.

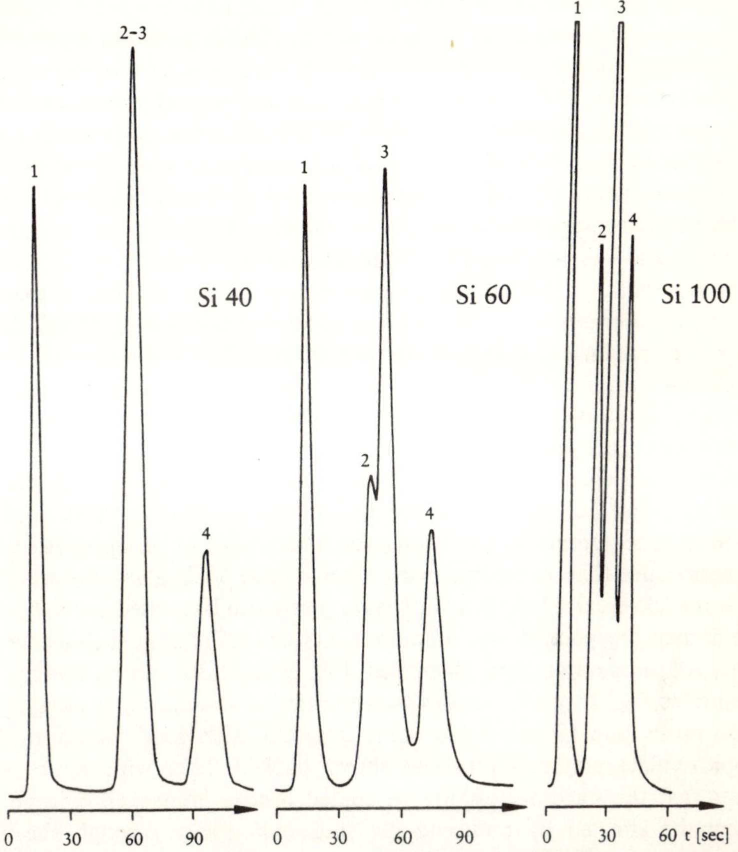

Figure 4 Differences in selectivity of three silicas with nominally identical structure, but with different pore widths (4, 6, and 10 nm). Separation of DDT and its degradation products: *p,p'*-DDE (1), 4,4'-DDM (2), *o,p'*-DDT (3), and *p,p'*-DDT (4). The three columns were accurately adjusted to the same activity by means of a precolumn, and eluted with *n*-heptane at 2·0 ml/min under identical conditions. Reproduced by permission of Dr F. Eisenbeiss and E. Merck, Darmstadt

Alumina has been used far less extensively as an l.c. adsorbent than silica, although it is known to have selectivity advantages for certain classes of compounds. It appears that water content is more difficult to control with alumina. A moisture control system has been described (Boehme and Engelhardt, 1977) for alumina l.c. to circumvent this problem. Alumina is more stable at alkaline pH than silica.

Bonded-phase packings utilize silica as the support. Functionality is attached *via* the silanol hydroxy groups, usually by reaction with an alkylchlorosilane or alkylmethoxysilane to give an alkyl group attached with a hydrolytically stable siloxane bond. The most widely used packings, usually including 'C_{18}' or 'ODS' in their trade names, are prepared from octadecyltrichlorosilane. Reaction of silica gels with alkyltrichlorosilanes under anhydrous conditions yields a monolayer of bonded alkyl residues, while in the presence of some water the trichlorosilane will also polymerize on the support to give a cross-linked material. Scott and Kucera (1977) compared the behaviour of several commercial reversed-phase packings when eluted with non-polar solvents (normal-phase conditions), and concluded that two of these packings contained a large proportion of underivatized silanol groups due to the observed silica-like behaviour. Synthesis of bonded-phase supports is clearly a complicated process requiring much experience, and has been reviewed (Grushka, 1974; Pryde, 1974; Cox, 1977).

Reproducibility in bonded-phase chromatography is far better than is the case with silica or alumina. The mechanism of separation is different, the active sites of silica are largely removed, and the mobile phase is very polar. However, prepacked r.p. columns seem to have shorter useful lives than the corresponding microparticulate silica columns, especially with regard to gradual settling of the bed structure accompanied by loss of efficiency.

Liquid–liquid chromatography has become far less popular with the advent of bonded-phase l.c. because of the greater experimental convenience of the latter technique. Optimizing k' values and selectivity in l.l.c. appears to require more experience than is the case with other modes. Pellicular supports are convenient for 'classical' l.l.c., as a stationary phase can be coated onto the support which is then dry-packed into a column. Leitch (1971) used such a method for analysis of methomyl, and discussed the precautions necessary for highly reproducible, highly precise results with an internal standard l.l.c. assay. Column life was more than 12 months in continuous use with good precision. Because microparticulate columns must be slurry packed, l.l.c. with these packings requires that the stationary phase be coated onto a prepacked column *in situ*. This can be effected by pumping the stationary phase through the column, followed by the mobile phase.

Gel chromatography packings are all-important in determining the nature of separation achieved. Many gels with large pores for separation of high molecular weight biochemicals are so soft that they cannot be considered as modern l.c. packings, as they can tolerate only gravity flow. Gels for lower molecular weight ranges can usually be more rigid because of smaller pore size, and so can tolerate higher pressures. These gels are usually polystyrene beads, although vinyl acetate polymers, silica, and some of the more rigid cross-linked dextran and poly-acrylamide gels are also used. Microparticulate packings have also been introduced for g.p.c. to improve efficiency (reviewed by Vivilecchia *et al*, 1977).

Just as instrumentation for ion-exchange chromatography antedates that for other modes of l.c., the use of 10 μm microparticulate, spherical ion-exchange resins was common well before microparticulate l.s.c. packings were widely used. Despite this early use of microparticulate supports, pellicular ion-exchange resins have been introduced and still find many applications. This is attributable to their higher permeabilities, good mass transfer properties, and their resistance to swelling in the eluent. Microparticulate resins are typically styrene–divinyl-benzene copolymers with ionic functionality, and usually swell to some extent in the eluent, making them somewhat less desirable than pellicular resins in certain gradient elution applications. The low sample capacity of pellicular ion-exchange packings is a frequent liability.

Care of Columns

Prepacked microparticulate columns are expensive and may have very short useful lives if mistreated. Control of mobile phase pH is especially important for silica-based packings, as already mentioned. Recently the use of guard columns has been recommended by column producers (Whatman and others). Typically a guard column will be $4–6 \times 0.2$ cm in size and dry-packed with an appropriate pellicular support of the same type as the $25–30 \times 0.4$ cm micro-particulate column (i.e. reversed-phase or silica). The frits of the guard column trap particulate matter, and the pellicular support retains impurities which would otherwise stick to the top of the analytical column. As both frits and pellicular support are easily and inexpensively replaced, use of guard columns is strongly recommended. Their use has little or no effect on column efficiency for solutes of reasonable k' value. Frequently a column bed structure will settle slightly on prolonged use, causing a void which results in loss of efficiency and tailing. This can be rectified on occasion by opening the top of the column and filling the void with 40 μm glass beads (Whatman) or a pellicular support similar to the existing column packing. Filtering of mobile phase through fluoropolymer membrane filters has been recommended to protect the check valves of certain types of pumping systems.

INSTRUMENTATION

A recent article by McNair and Chandler (1976) reviews various models of integrated liquid chromatographs from 19 manufacturers. Instrument quality, sophistication, and price vary considerably. In the early 1970s, construction of custom liquid chromatographs from selected commercial components was rather popular. Due to increases in quality of commercial instrumentation (with frequently little or no increase in cost) this practice is now less popular.

Mobile Phase Pumping Systems

The ideal l.c. pumping system should provide a pulseless flow of solvent for detector baseline stability; a constant, accurate flow rate for good reproduci-bility between analyses; and should be amenable to use with both isocratic (fixed solvent composition) elution and gradient elution. Also, the pump should be able to use an unlimited solvent supply and allow rapid solvent changeover.

The cheapest, simplest, and perhaps most reliable pumps are of the pneumatic amplifier type. While gas-pressurized solvent holding coils are cheaper, they are hardly worthy of consideration by the serious chromatographer. Pneumatic amplifiers are essentially pulseless, but suffer from the disadvantage of being constant pressure devices, rather than delivering a constant flow. Thus changes in system back pressure, resulting from the plugging of a column inlet frit or eluent viscosity change during a gradient, can cause the flow to change. Devices are available which monitor and control flow to some extent.

Constant flow pumps are usually more expensive and complicated than pneumatic amplifiers. One type, motor-driven syringe pumps, provide constant, pulseless flow, but the fixed solvent capacity in the syringe reservoir makes extended running and solvent changeover difficult. Small-volume, reciprocating pumps deliver a constant, but inherently pulsating, flow of solvent. Considerable ingenuity has been devoted to modifying these pumps to produce a less pulsating flow. Hydraulic and mechanical pulse-damping systems have been employed, but use of multiple-headed pumps with out-of-phase pistons is currently the most widespread method of controlling pulsation. Some of these devices incorporate transducers to monitor flow and alter the pump speed *via* a feedback circuit to further suppress residual pulsation, and for greater accuracy.

Capability for solvent gradient elution is usually an accessory. With pneumatic amplifier pumps, the second solvent is retained in a holding coil pressurized by the pump and is mixed with the weaker solvent using solenoid valves and a programmer. Until recently, all gradient elution systems utilizing small volume reciprocating pumps required the use of two separate pumps and a controlling programmer. Such systems are quite costly. However, a new system (Spectra-Physics, Bakalyar *et al*, 1977) utilizes a single small-volume reciprocating pump equipped with a microprocessor-controlled mixing valve on the pump inlet, which allows use of even ternary solvent gradients. This advance renders use of ternary solvent systems in isocratic elution much easier as well.

Injectors

In early commercial liquid chromatographs, syringe injection through a septum was rather common. Due to higher back pressures and the corrosive effects of solvents, septum life is normally far shorter in l.c. than in g.l.c. With the advent of good sample loop injector valves, together with a trend toward higher column back pressures, septum injection is far less common today. Most loop injectors are six-port switching valves or variants thereof. The sample loop is of fixed size but usually changeable. Repcatability of injection volume is far better than that achievable with a syringe. Certain loop injectors can be filled with a syringe when this feature is desired for convenience.

A major difference between g.l.c. and l.c. is that comparatively large injection volumes are well tolerated in l.c., provided the injection solvent is not stronger than the eluent. Ideally, the injection solvent should be weaker than the eluent, in which case sample will be retained as a sharp zone at the column head until all injection solvent has passed into the column. This factor may be quite useful for trace analysis of environmental samples.

Data Processing

Many laboratories find it desirable to equip liquid chromatographs with electronic digital integrators, especially if analyses are quantitative and repetitive. With the recent proliferation of microprocessor technology, it has become possible to incorporate the digital integrator into the instrument and to use the microprocessor to control instrument parameters such as flow rate, recorder attenuation, and gradient composition. At least three firms have introduced such instruments where all commands are entered electronically.

Detectors

As mentioned earlier, the greatest problem in liquid chromatography is still the shortcomings of various detection devices. The lack of a sensitive, 'universal' detector is particularly acute. Therefore more discussion of this phase of the instrumentation than others is warranted.

The *differential refractometric* (or refractive index; hence, r.i.) detector is 'universal' in response, but has low sensitivity (~ 1 µg for analytical columns), is very sensitive to flow and temperature variations, and cannot be used with gradient elution. The prime utility of the r.i. detector is in gel-permeation chromatography, preparative work, and where alternative detectors are not suitable. It is not well suited for trace analysis and has seen infrequent use in pesticide research.

The fixed-wavelength *ultraviolet (u.v.) absorbance detector* is the most commonly used. Such units incorporate a 254 nm low pressure mercury lamp; many have the capability of using a medium pressure mercury lamp to monitor at certain longer wavelengths (such as 280, 313, 334, 366, 405, 436, and/or 546 nm) with the use of accessory filters. These detectors are sensitive, cheap, and relatively unaffected by flow and temperature fluctuations. They do limit the choice of mobile phases to those with reasonable spectral clarity at the appropriate wavelength. Detection limits of 1–10 ng are routine for a modern u.v. detector with a sample of moderate extinction coefficient ($\varepsilon \sim 10^4$).

Variable wavelength u.v./visible absorption detectors commonly utilize as a light source the monochromator from a low-cost ultraviolet/visible spectrophotometer. These units are considerably more expensive than a fixed-wavelength u.v. detector, but the increased versatility is obvious. The signal-to-noise ratio of the best of these units is currently nearly an order of magnitude worse at 254 nm than a high quality fixed-wavelength detector. Consequently there are still cogent reasons, aside from price, for selecting a fixed-wavelength unit if the sample to be measured has a reasonable extinction coefficient at 254 nm. While specialized applications may require near u.v. and visible wavelengths for detection, the majority of published applications with these detectors have utilized low u.v. wavelengths (205–220 nm). In this spectral range, nearly all organic molecules have some absorption, such as saturated esters and even sugars. There are corresponding restrictions on solvent choice and purity. If the signal-to-noise ratio of these detectors can be improved, they will probably be the most desired detectors for average analyses.

Fluorimetric detectors are both highly sensitive and selective. The best units are based on spectrofluorimeters; the excitation wavelength is provided by a monochromator and the emission wavelength is selected with either a monochromator or filters. The inherent sensitivity of the fluorescence process is so high that detection of low picogram quantities is possible in some cases. If the desired component is fluorescent, this is clearly the detector of choice for trace analysis of environmental samples. Derivatization of non-fluorescent samples with fluorescent 'tags' is another promising application for high sensitivity analysis. For example, Frei *et al* (1974) hydrolysed N-methylcarbamate insecticides to their phenolic precursors, then formed the dansyl esters with 1-dimethyl-aminonaphthalene-5-sulphonyl chloride. These moderately fluorescent derivatives were separated on liquid–liquid chromatography prior to detection.

Transport detectors use a moving wire, belt, disc, or other transport system to remove a fraction of the l.c. column effluent. The solvent is evaporated in a furnace, hopefully leaving the sample on the transport device, which is then heated more strongly in oxygen to convert the sample to CO_2, which is swept through a catalyst bed with hydrogen and reduced to methane. The methane passes through a g.l.c. flame ionization detector (f.i.d.). Consequently these devices are also called flame ionization detectors. It can be appreciated from the above that such detectors are mechanically complex and therefore quite expensive. The units have the virtue of placing few restrictions on choice of solvent and are usable with gradients, but have suffered from limitations in sensitivity and reliability. Several variants of this unit have been offered commercially, and all but one have been discontinued.

An *alkali flame ionization detector* for l.c. has been described (Slais and Krejci, 1974). Like the f.i.d., this device is a transport mechanism equipped with a modified g.l.c. detector. The detector was selective for halogenated organics (2,000 times greater response than for a hydrocarbon), but sensitivity was extremely poor.

Electron capture detectors (e.c.d.) are of such great importance in g.l.c. analysis of pesticides that there has been an obvious interest in their application to l.c. The earliest such unit was a modified transport detector in which the vaporized sample was passed through an e.c.d. unit. However, Willmott and Dolphin (1974) found that under certain conditions the l.c. column effluent can be vaporized and passed directly through an e.c.d. They used silica l.c. with hexane eluent to separate organochlorine insecticides, and were able to detect 40 pg of aldrin. This sensitivity is about 100 times that of the transport detector-based e.c.d. The surprising tolerance of the detector for large volumes of hexane vapour may be related to the usual procedure of incorporating 5–10% methane into carrier gas in g.l.c./c.c.d. A commercial unit based on the work of Willmott and Dolphin is available (Pye Unicam).

Another g.l.c. detector that has been modified for l.c. use is the *Coulson electrolytic conductivity detector* (c.e.c.d.). Dolan and Seiber (1977) used reversed-phase l.c. at low flow rates (0·5 ml/min maximum) to separate chlorinated pesticides. The l.c. column effluent was vaporized in a furnace, then passed into a quartz pyrolysis tube (700–900 °C) with hydrogen gas. The HCl resulting from chlorinated samples was detected conductometrically. The detector was found to be selective for organochlorine compounds with respect to hydrocarbons, but somewhat less so than a g.l.c./c.e.c.d. The sensitivity was rather poor with a minimum detectable quantity of 5–50 ng for lindane.

The *amperometric (polarographic) detector* is one of the more recent l.c. detectors to be introduced commercially. Only one firm is currently offering this detector (Bioanalytical Systems). Publications with experimental prototypes show extremely high sensitivity for certain classes of compounds. The detector cells contain electrodes which can be set at a constant potential difference, and electrolytic oxidation (or reduction) of substrate is manifest as a current. The mobile phase must have appreciable conductivity, suggesting applications in ion-exchange and certain reversed-phase systems. Koen *et al* (1970) were able to analyse parathion and methyl parathion in plant extracts using a dropping mercury electrode (nitro group reduction); their detection limits of $<0·1$ ppm (1 ng detectable) could doubtless be improved with modern high-efficiency columns. Kissinger *et al* (1973) were able to separate and detect catecholamines at picogram levels using an improved amperometric cell set for oxidation. While these devices are affected both by temperature and flow rate, their selectivity and high sensitivity make them, according to Kirkland (1974), one of the most promising detectors for trace analysis.

Coupled *liquid chromatography–mass spectrometry* has resulted from the logic that whatever is good for g.l.c. must also be good for l.c. While coupling of a gas chromatograph to a mass spectrometer is technically formidable, it appears simple compared to 'interfacing' a liquid chromatograph and an m.s. To illustrate the inherent difficulty, the mobile phase must be vaporized and solvent vapour and sample separated prior to introduction into the ion source. A usual mobile phase flow rate of 1 ml/min would correspond to the following quantities of vapour at 20 °C and 1 atm: water, 1,330 ml/min; methanol, 590 ml/min; hexane, 180 ml/min. Nevertheless, a number of successful applications of this technique have been published (Arpino *et al*, 1974; McFadden *et al*, 1977, and references cited therein), and an l.c./m.s. interface is now commercially available (Finnigan). The latter device utilizes a belt transport system for solvent removal *in vacuo*, prior to flash vaporization of the sample from the belt adjacent to an aperture leading to the ion source. Another approach (Arpino *et al*, 1974) is to introduce a small fraction ($\sim 1\%$) of the column effluent into the ion chamber directly, with the m.s. operating in the chemical ionization mode and utilizing the solvent vapour as reagent gas. These techniques have been used for acquisition of full mass spectra, and also for operation in the selected ion monitoring mode (multiple ion detection, mass fragmentography). The selectivity and sensitivity of the latter technique with g.l.c. separation are becoming widely known; the sensitivity with l.c. separation is frequently in the subnanogram range. This is unquestionably the most expensive l.c. detector by more than an order of magnitude!

Radioactivity monitors have not been widely used in l.c. despite the obvious utility of such devices in the life sciences, in pesticide biochemistry in particular. The reasons for this are twofold. The simple alternative of fraction collection of l.c. column effluent, with subsequent liquid scintillation counting, is easy but tedious, and allows detection of very small quantities of weak β-emitters which are most important in biochemical studies. Continuous flow monitoring of l.c. eluents for weak β-emitters has generally required scintillation detector cells which have low counting efficiency, excessive cell volumes leading to severe peak broadening, or both. High counting efficiencies can be obtained in homogeneous systems (Hunt, 1968; Reeve and Crozier, 1977), where a liquid scintilation solution is mixed with the column effluent prior to counting, but preparative isolation of labelled products is not feasible with this approach. Heterogeneous systems utilize a flow cell packed with scintillator crystals or beads (glass doped with inorganic salts), allowing collection of unchanged sample but with lower efficiency than in homogeneous systems (Byrne, 1971; Snyder and Kirkland, 1974). Improvements in sensitivity of commercially available heterogeneous systems have apparently been made, although the authors have no personal experience with these units. Clearly continuous flow monitoring has substantial time-saving advantages over collection of fractions which must be radioassayed subsequently.

In summary, a variety of l.c. detectors are available with varying degrees of selectivity and sensitivity. No single type of detector can be relied on to the exclusion of others; the choice depends on the sample type to be analysed and the limits of detectability required. The above listing is not all-inclusive; we have not discussed certain detectors with more limited utility which have not as yet seen use in pesticide separations (e.g. infrared absorbance and conductivity detectors). The most successful l.c. detectors appear to be those which have no counterpart in g.l.c., such as the u.v. absorbance, fluorimetric, and (potentially) amperometric detectors. Adaptation of g.l.c. detectors to l.c., such as the f.i.d., c.e.c.d., and (to some extent) the electron capture detector, has been more difficult due to their non-compatibility with liquid mobile phases.

DERIVATIZATION

Derivatization is often used in g.l.c. to enhance volatility or to prevent sample decomposition on the column. Such is not the case with l.c., and in fact l.c. is now replacing g.l.c. for many such analyses. On the other hand, derivatization may be required in l.c. to allow detection where the sample has no inherent functionality eliciting detector response, or where the lower detection limits of a highly sensitive, specific detector may be desired.

This topic is further divided into precolumn and postcolumn derivatization techniques. The former methods have been reviewed by Ross (1977), while both approaches were reviewed by Lawrence and Frei (1976). The 'precolumn' methods involve formation of a derivative by a high-yield chemical reaction prior to injection. It is desirable to use reagents and conditions that generate as few by-products as possible to avoid the frequent necessity of clean-up by t.l.c. or other methods, prior to l.c. analysis. Representative examples from the literature include the conversion of carbonyl compounds to their highly u.v.-active 2,4-dinitrophenylhydrazones (Papa and Turner, 1972; Selim and Cook, 1978); conversion of fatty acids to u.v.-active phenacyl esters (Borch, 1975), *p*-bromophenacyl esters (Durst *et al*, 1975), or *p*-nitrobenzyl esters (Grushka *et al*, 1975); conversion of alcohols (such as hexachlorophene) to the strongly u.v.-active *p*-methoxybenzoates (Porcaro and Shubiak, 1972); and dansylation of phenols (Cassidy *et al*, 1974), organophosphates (Lawrence *et al*, 1976) and carbamates (Frei *et al*, 1974) to give fluorescent phenolic esters of 5-dimethyl-aminonaphthalene-1-sulphonic acid. Fluorimetric derivatization for pesticide residue analysis has been reviewed (Lawrence and Frei, 1974).

In postcolumn derivatization (also termed reaction detection), the l.c. column effluent is mixed with a constant flow of reagent solution and after appropriate treatment (heating, etc.) passed through a detector. A classic, important example is amino acid analysis by ion-exchange employing the first widely used high pressure liquid chromatograph, the automatic amino acid analyser (Spackman *et al*, 1958). In early units, the reagent was ninhydrin, and the coloured product was detected photometrically at 570 nm. More recently, detection limits have been lowered by use of the reaction of primary amino acids with either fluorescamine or *o*-phthalaldehyde, followed by fluorimetric detection.

Carbonyl compounds have been determined also by postcolumn derivatization to their 2,4-dinitrophenylhydrazones (Deelder and Hendricks, 1973). As the reaction is not instantaneous, the column eluent, mixed with derivatizing reagent supplied by a separate metering pump, is passed through a long tube. In order to prevent peak broadening during the long residence time in the tube, the liquid stream is segmented with gas bubbles, which are subsequently removed with a debubbler immediately before photometric detection. Singer *et al* (1977) have developed a nitrosamide-specific detector based on the Griess reagent. The colour reaction depends on liberation of nitrite ion from nitrosamides, nitrosocarbamates, or alkyl nitrites at 90 °C under acidic conditions. Subsequent reaction of nitrous acid with sulphanilic acid gives a diazonium salt, which couples with naphthylethylenediamine to generate a purple dye, detected at 550 nm. Again, the reaction is sufficiently slow (3 minutes) to require air segmentation of the fluid. While not particularly sensitive (0·5 nmol), the process is extraordinarily specific; even simple N-nitrosoamines do not interfere. Several applications for analysis of nitrosocarbamates were described, such as nitrosocarbaryl. The method may be useful for environmental analysis.

Fine *et al* (1976) have described the use of a so-called thermal energy analyser coupled to an l.c. for analysis of non-volatile N-nitrosoamines in foodstuffs. This detector uses a heated furnace containing tungsten oxide to convert catalytically N-nitroso compounds to the nitrosyl radical, which reacts with added ozone to

22

generate excited NO_2. The excited NO_2 emits photons in the near infrared, which are detected photometrically. This reaction detector was first applied in g.l.c. separations; unfortunately Fine *et al* (1976) did not give details of adapting the unit for l.c. use. The method appears to be highly sensitive and specific, allowing analysis of non-volatile N-nitroso compounds in crude extracts of foodstuffs with detection limits of 10 ppb.

Moye and Wade (1976, see also Moye, 1975) devised an ingenious enzymic reaction detector for acetylcholinesterase inhibitors. The reversed-phase l.c. column eluent was mixed with aqueous acetylcholinesterase enzyme (from housefly heads or bovine erythrocytes), segmented with air bubbles, and heated to 40 °C. Then the non-fluorescing substrate N-methylindoxyl acetate was metered in, and hydrolysed by the enzyme to the fluorescent N-methyl-indoxyl. Thus, a fluorescent baseline is produced, but in the presence of an enzyme inhibitor, fluorescence is inhibited. Samples of N-methylcarbamate and organophosphate pesticides were detected as negative peaks. With a low efficiency column, detection limits ranged from 0·2 ng for carbofuran to 800 ng for fonofos. The method would appear to be extremely specific. Ramsteiner and Hörmann (1975) briefly described a conceptually similar system for analysis of cholinesterase inhibitors. A buffered mixture of acetylthiocholine and 5,5'-dithiobis-(2-nitrobenzoic acid) (DTNB) was metered into a premix of column effluent and cholinesterase. The enzyme cleaves acetylthiocholine to thiocholine, which generates a yellow colour with the sulphydryl reagent DTNB. Detection at 420 nm gives an absorbance baseline which is decreased by enzyme inhibitors. Detection limits for dicrotophos and CGA 18809 were about 20 ng.

Dozens of specific colour reagents are known in the literature, but go largely ignored in this era of instrumentation. The above examples of the coupling of instrumentation and colour reactions suggest the great potential that exists for development of further specific detection devices.

APPLICATIONS

Gel Permeation Chromatography for Lipid Removal for Residue Analysis

Stalling *et al* (1972) evaluated four g.p.c. gels (Bio-Beads S-X2, S-X4, and S-X8, and Sephadex LH-20) eluted with different solvents for removal of lipids from pesticide residue samples. The best combination was Bio-Beads S-X2 eluted with cyclohexane, which gave 99·5% removal of fish lipids from a lower molecular weight zone containing chlorinated hydrocarbon insecticides, malathion, parathion, and polychlorinated biphenyls (PCB's). Using a column 23–27 cm × 2·5 cm i.d., up to 500 mg of lipid could be separated (figure 5) in about 1 hour with less than 0·5% of the mass included in the pesticide fraction. Recoveries of pesticides ranged from 95% to 100%. Samples could be analysed directly after clean-up by g.l.c./e.c.d. Extracts of channel catfish were cleaned up by g.p.c. or by standard acetonitrile/petroleum ether partitioning plus florisil chromatography, and analysed by g.l.c./e.c.d. for comparison. Virtually identical values were obtained for residues of a number of pesticides, but the g.p.c. method was easier and used less solvent.

Tindle and Stalling (1972) subsequently described an automated apparatus for performing these separations, which could accommodate 23 samples. Griffitt and Craun (1974) evaluated this system, and found it to be more efficient than acetonitrile partitioning for clean-up and to provide better recoveries. They also observed appreciable differences in elution patterns for various pesticides with parathion, methyl parathion, and several other compounds eluting substantially slower than most chlorinated hydrocarbons. This suggests the superposition of g.p.c. and affinity effects. Johnson *et al* (1976) reported use of a commercial automated g.p.c. unit (Analytical Biochemistry Laboratories) for clean-up of animal and plant extracts. They utilized Stalling's improved system

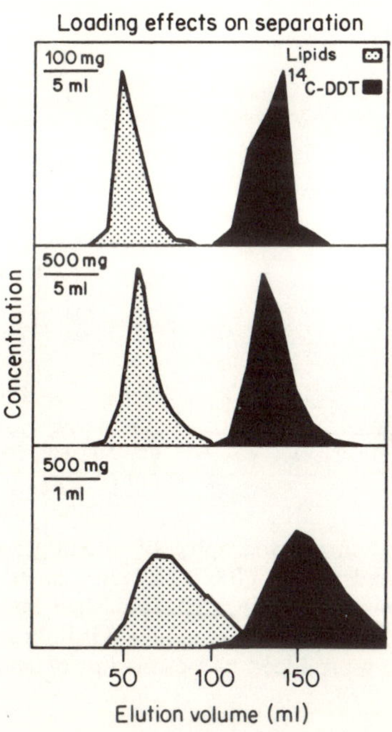

Figure 5 Separation of lipid–pesticide mixtures with Bio-Beads S-X2 eluted with cyclohexane: effects of sample volume and lipid concentration. From Stalling *et al* (1972), reproduced by permission of the Association of Official Analytical Chemists

(Bio-Beads S-X3 eluted with toluene–ethyl acetate, 1 : 3) which allows larger samples (1·5 g) and faster elution (30 minutes). Elution data for PCB's and about 30 pesticides revealed only slight differences in elution volumes, indicating that a g.p.c. retention mechanism is operating with minor affinity effects. Clean-up was evaluated by g.l.c. analysis using both electron capture and flame photometric detectors. Chicken and turkey fat and fish lipid were efficiently cleaned up by g.p.c. alone, while plant extracts and soapstock required an additional florisil chromatography. A commercial unit with the improved Bio-Beads S-X3 column was successfully used for clean-up of chicken tissue extracts for toxaphene analysis (Bush *et al*, 1978).

Kuehl and Leonard (1978) used Bio-Beads S-X2 eluted with cyclohexane–dichloromethane (1 : 1), and found substantial retention of more polar organics such as pentachlorophenol and *p*-chlorophenol. The retentivity was advantageous for identification of xenobiotics in fish tissues by g.l.c.–m.s. analysis of several more retained fractions.

Quistad *et al* (1974) used g.p.c. in isolating [5-^{14}C]methoprene and metabolites from plant tissue (figure 6). The column was $100 \times 1\cdot27$ cm Bio-Beads S-X2 eluted with dichloromethane. Chlorophyll and many related plant pigments were removed, greatly simplifying subsequent t.l.c. purification.

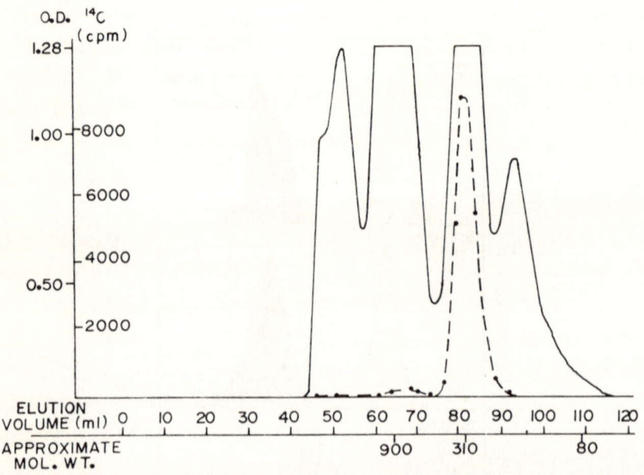

Figure 6 Gel permeation chromatography of methoprene from metabolism by alfalfa. Column is Bio-Beads S-X2 ($100 \times 1\cdot27$ cm) eluted with dichloromethane; radioactivity (counts per minute) is indicated by dashed line (– – –); u.v. absorbance at 254 nm [1·28 absorbance units full scale (a.u.f.s.)] is indicated by a solid line (——). From Quistad *et al* (1974), reproduced by permission of American Chemical Society

In all above applications, soft gels were used which swell greatly in the eluents. While the efficiency of such columns (in terms if N) is not high, good separations are obtained because the volume of solvent in the pores (V_i) is large compared to V_0. In conventional rigid gels which swell less, but tolerate higher pressure, V_i is smaller with respect to V_0, so that longer columns are needed to effect a separation than with softer gels. Recent advances in microparticulate g.p.c. packings have allowed rapid, efficient separations with short columns. Currently these columns are quite expensive ($500 for a $30 \times 0\cdot8$ cm prepacked column) and have reduced sample capacity compared to the 2·5 cm bore columns discussed above. Accordingly, we are not aware of published reports of their use for pesticide residue clean-up. Such columns have been used to advantage for isolation of metabolites of methabenzthiazuron (Mittelstaedt *et al*, 1977) and trifluralin (Heck *et al*, 1977).

Insecticides

DDT, chlorinated hydrocarbons

DDT and chlorinated hydrocarbons were much studied in the early development of modern liquid chromatography. As the field usage of polychlorinated pesticides has greatly decreased in recent years, so also has the l.c. literature for these compounds. Using more recent technology, good separations of DDT (and analogues) from mixtures of chlorinated hydrocarbons have been reported on Spherosil (Vermont *et al*, 1975) and β,β'-oxydipropionitrile impregnated silica (Majors, 1973; Viricel and Lemar, 1976).

Residue analysis. Several groups have reported residue methods for organochlorine pesticides in fat. Hoogeveen *et al* (1976) and Dolphin *et al* (1976) used an automated l.c. apparatus with a precolumn (5 μm Partisil) to retain milk fat. A series of switching valves allowed the pesticides to pass through an analytical column of Partisil for resolution and subsequent detection by e.c. Contaminating fat was then simply backflushed from the precolumn to renovate the system. Desirable features included ability to inject substantial volumes (up to several hundred microlitres) and a limit of detection of $\sim 0{\cdot}1$ ppm for DDT, DDE, lindane, and dieldrin. Rohleder *et al* (1976) also separated a variety of organochlorines on microparticulate silica (Merckosorb SI 60, 10 μm) by first eluting with hexane and then with acetone to remove adsorbed triglyceride. Larose (1974) described a residue method for lindane in water samples and fish extracts. Lindane was eluted from a Corasil II column with hexane which is not a strong enough solvent to elute the major contaminants (fats and oils) which are retained on the column. Zimmerli and Marek (1975) used Porasil A eluted with hexane–methylene chloride (9 : 1) to separate organochlorine pesticides from up to 50 mg of lipid prior to analysis by g.l.c. Dolan and Seiber (1977) used Vydac 201 TP reversed-phase to analyse aldrin and dieldrin at 0·1 ppm in water and lettuce. An important factor in their l.c. system was a Coulson electrolytic conductivity (chlorine-selective) detector which was particularly useful for those chlorinated hydrocarbon pesticides which are not amenable to u.v. detection (e.g. mirex, heptachlor, aldrin, dieldrin, and endrin). An l.c. residue method for dicofol in carrots at 0·1 ppm utilizing a MicroPak Si-10 column and u.v. detection was described by Pflugmacher and Ebing (1975).

Environmental degradation. Feil *et al* (1975) used l.c. on Permaphase ODS to examine the metabolites of *o,p'*-DDT in chicken excreta. Hydroxylated and methoxylated *o,p'*-DDT, -DDA, and -DDE were isolated for structural verification with mixtures of acetonitrile–water. Yost and Miller (1976) used Porasil A to follow the relative photolability rates of N-(α-trichloromethylbenzyl) anilines (DDT analogues).

PCB's

Although polychlorinated biphenyls (PCB's) are not pesticides, they are ubiquitous environmental pollutants and often coelute with trace amounts of pesticide residues. Several papers have discussed the resolution of PCB's from DDT (Eisenbeiss and Sieper, 1973; Fishbein, 1974; Aitzetmüller, 1975) and other chlorinated hydrocarbons (Rohleder *et al*, 1976; Hoogeveen, 1976). Aitzetmüller (1975) concluded that given the lower sensitivity of available l.c. detectors, l.c. will not replace g.l.c. as a final determination step for PCB's in trace residue analysis. However, l.c. is advantageous for clean-up prior to g.l.c. or for analysis of larger amounts of PCB's or DDT. A comprehensive review of PCB analysis is available elsewhere (Krull, 1977). Pacco and Mukherji (1977) described separation of PCB's from a polymeric matrix by g.p.c. using μStyragel columns. Several groups have reported excellent resolution of PCB mixtures (Brinkman *et al*, 1976a, b; Hanai and Walton, 1977; Krupcik *et al*, 1977). Analyses of polybrominated biphenyls are also available (Kok *et al*, 1977; Hass *et al*, 1978).

Organophosphorus insecticides

Although u.v. detection is suitable for many organophosphates, a variety of other detectors have also been used, including flame ionization (Szalontai, 1976), cholinesterase inhibition (Ramsteiner and Hörmann, 1975; Moye and Wade, 1976), Coulson electrolytic conductivity (Dolan and Seiber, 1977), polarographic (Koen *et al*, 1970), and fluorimetric (Lawrence *et al*, 1976). A versatile solvent system consisting of various alcohols in hexane was used by Szalontai (1976) to resolve efficiently 23 organophosphates on silica (6–8 μm). Microparticulate silica (LiChrosorb SI 60, 5 μm) also resolves the *cis–trans* isomers of several chlorovinyl phosphates (figure 7, Self *et al*, 1975).

Residue analysis. Older applications of l.c. to organophosphate analysis have been adequately reviewed by Moye (1975). In one such method Koen *et al* (1970) could detect parathion and methyl parathion in lettuce with a polarographic detector, at 0·03 and 0·1 ppm, respectively. Henry *et al* (1971) concluded that l.c. was 'an ideal method' for the analysis of Abate™ (temephos) and other thermally unstable compounds. Their method could detect 1 ng of Abate™ and was useful for residues in salt marsh ponds (water and organic matter) and mosquito larvae.

A general discussion of fluorigenic labelling as applied to residue analysis of organophosphate pesticides has been provided by Lawrence *et al* (1976). Hydrolysis of certain organophosphates (30–40 minutes) gave phenols which could be dansylated (90 minutes) for ultimate fluorimetric detection. Several compounds could be measured at a 5–10 ng limit of detection which allowed determination of fenthion at 0·02 ppm in water samples.

Paschal *et al* (1977) detailed an l.c. method for determination of methyl and ethyl parathion at the ppb level in runoff water using variable wavelength detection. Trace residues were preconcentrated by a factor of 100 with XAD-2

Table 2 LC conditions for DDT and analogues*

Compound	Mobile phase	Detector	Column	Reference
DDT	I. heptane : isoPrOH (70 : 30)	UV	Permaphase ETH	59, 141
	II. isooctane	UV	33% ODPN on MicroPak	144
	III. hexane	RI	Corasil I and II	140
	IV. hexane	RI	Alumina N18, Act. II, III	51
	V. hexane	UV	Spherosil XOA 400 (10–20 μm, coated with ODPN, 100 : 120)	245
p,p'- and *o,p'*-	VI. hexane	UV 254, 210	Perisorb A	49, 59
(also DDE)	VII. hexane	UV	LiChrosorb SI 60 (10 μm) and Merck Alox-T (10 μm)	195
(also DDE)	VIII. hexane	EC	Partisil (5 and 10 μm)	43, 81
p,p'- and *o,p'*- (also *p,p'*- and *o,p'*-DDE	IX. hexane	UV 254, 205	LiChrosorb SI 60 (5 μm)	15
p,p'-	X. hexane	EC, UV	Spherisorb S10W (10 μm)	255
p,p'- and *o,p'*-	XI. isooctane	UV	10% ODPN on Porasil 60	253
p,p'- (also *p,p'*-DDE)	XII. hexane : CH$_2$Cl$_2$ (9 : 1)	UV, glc	Porasil A	262
p,p'- and *o,p'*-	XIII. cyclohexane	—	Bio-Beads S-X2	68
p,p'- and *o,p'*- (also *p,p'*-DDE)	XIV. toluene : EtOAc (1 : 3)	glc fract.	Bio-Beads S-X3	98
(also DDE)	XV. CHCl$_3$, cyclohexane, hexane, MeOH, toluene, CH$_2$Cl$_2$, THF, EtOH	radio. count fract.	Bio-Beads S-X2, S-X4, S-X8, Sephadex LH-20	227, 238
p,p'- and *o,p'*- (also *p,p'*-DDE)	XVI. 29 and 50% aq. MeOH or EtOH	UV	Vydac RP	206
	XVII. isooctane (satd with ODPN)	UV	25% ODPN on LiChrosorb SI 60 (5 μm)	248

* See Appendix for an explanation of the abbreviations and layout used in this and subsequent Tables.

Table 2 (*cont.*)

Compound	Mobile phase	Detector	Column	Reference
(also DDE)	XVIII. pet. ether	RI	Corasil II	130, 155
p,p'- and o,p'- (also DDE)	XIX. light petroleum	UV 235	LiChrosorb SI 60 (10 μm)	1
p,p'-	XX. MeCN : H_2O (1 : 1)	UV 235	Partisil ODS	166
	XXI. pet. ether + 20% benzene	flame ioniz.	silica gel L 50/71	47
p,p'- and o,p'- (also p,p'-DDE, p,p'-DDA, Dichlorobenzophenone)	XXII. MeOH : H_2O (80 : 20)	UV, CEC	Vydac 201 TP RP	42
p,p'- (also p,p'-DDE)	XXIII. CH_2Cl_2, CH_2Cl_2 : cyclohexane mixtures	UV	Bio-Beads S-X2	124
	XXIV. 90% MeCN or EtOH in H_2O, 70 °C	UV	pyrocarbon–silica	73
	XXV. 80 or 100% MeCN in H_2O, 55 °C	UV	graphitized carbon	73
3-Hydroxy-o,p'-DDT and -DDA; 4-hydroxy-3-methoxy-o,p'-DDT, -DDA, and -DDE	XXVI. MeCN : H_2O (1 : 1, 1 : 3)	UV	Permaphase ODS	57
Chlorobenzilate	XXVII. MeCN : H_2O (25–75 : 75–25 grad.)	UV 220	LiChrosorb RP-18	213
Dicofol (Kelthane™)	XXVIII. hexane XXIX. CH_2Cl_2 (also XIII, XXII)	UV UV	MicroPak Si-10 silica gel (10 μm)	169 30 42, 68

Compound		Reference (conditions)	Detection	Support/column	Ref.
Ethylan (Perthane™)	Et—⬡—CH(—⬡—Et)—CH—Cl Cl	XIII, XXII	—	—	42, 68
Methoxychlor	MeO—⬡—CH(—⬡—OMe)—CCl₃	XXX. isooctane	UV	4% ODPN on Anakrom A (160–170 mesh)	107
		XXXI. hexane	UV	0·5% ODPN on CSP support	110
		(also II, IV, V, XIII–XVII, XX, XXII, XXVII)	—	—	42, 51, 68, 98, 144, 166, 206, 213, 227, 238, 245, 248
Monodechloromethoxychlor		XXX, XXXI	—	—	107, 110
TDE (DDD)	Cl—⬡—CH(—⬡—Cl)—CH—Cl Cl	I–III, VII–IX, XI–XVI, XXII	—	—	15, 42, 43, 59, 68, 81, 98, 140, 141, 144, 195, 206, 227, 238, 253, 262
N-(α-Trichloromethyl-*p*-methoxybenzyl)-*p*-methoxyaniline	MeO—⬡—NCH(—⬡—OMe)—CCl₃	XXXII. isopropyl ether : hexane (1 : 1) (also five photoproducts)	UV	Porasil A	152

Table 2 (*cont.*)

Compound	Mobile phase	Detector	Column	Reference
N-(α-Trichloromethylbenzyl) anilines	XXXII.	—	—	259
R—⟨NHCH—OR′ with CCl$_3$⟩				
PCB's—polychlorinated biphenyls (Cl's, Cl's)	XXXIII. MeCN : H$_2$O (90 : 10)	UV 205	LiChrosorb RP-18	213
	XXXIV. pentane	UV 254, 205	Pragosil (5 μm silica)	122
	XXXV. dry hexane	UV 205	LiChrosorb SI 60 (5 μm)	14
	XXXVI. MeOH : H$_2$O (55 : 45)	UV	Permaphase ODS	260
	XXXVII. MeOH : H$_2$O (20 : 80) to (75 : 25) grad.	UV	Permaphase ODS (37 μm)	112
	XXXVIII. CHCl$_3$	UV	μStyragel	164
	XXXIX. MeOH : H$_2$O (60 : 40), (30 : 70) to (100 : 0) grad.	UV	Permaphase ODS	28
	(also VI–X, XIV–XVI, XIX, XXIII, XXIV)	—	—	1, 15, 49, 59, 73, 81, 98, 124, 195, 206, 227, 238, 255

Table 3 LC conditions for cyclodienes and chlorinated hydrocarbons

Compound	Mobile phase	Detector	Column	Reference
Aldrin	I. isooctane	UV	10% ODPN on Porasil 60	253
	II. hexane	UV	Spherosil XOA 400 (10–20 μm, coated with ODPN, 100 : 120)	245
	III. hexane	RI	Alumina N18, Act II, III	51
	IV. hexane	UV	Merckosorb SI 60 (10 μm) and Merck Alox-T (10 μm)	195
	V. hexane	RI	Corasil I and II	140
	VI. hexane	EC UV 230	Spherisorb SIOW (10 μm)	255
	VII. hexane	UV 254, 205	LiChrosorb SI 60 (5 μm)	15
	VIII. pentane	UV, ms	Durapak/Carbowax 400 on Porasil	150
	IX. isooctane	UV	33% ODPN on MicroPak	144
	X. cyclohexane	—	Bio-Beads S-X2	68
	XI. toluene : EtOAc (1 : 3)	glc fract.	Bio-Beads S-X3	98
	XII. MeOH : H$_2$O (80 : 20)	UV, CEC	Vydac 201 TP RP	42
	XIII. 90% MeCN or EtOH in H$_2$O, 70 °C	UV	pyrocarbon–silica	73
	XIV. 80% or 100% MeCN in H$_2$O, 55 °C	UV	graphitized carbon	73
	XV. isooctane (satd with ODPN)	UV	25% ODPN on LiChrosorb SI 60 (5 μm)	248

Table 3 (*cont.*)

Compound	Mobile phase	Detector	Column	Reference
Chlordane 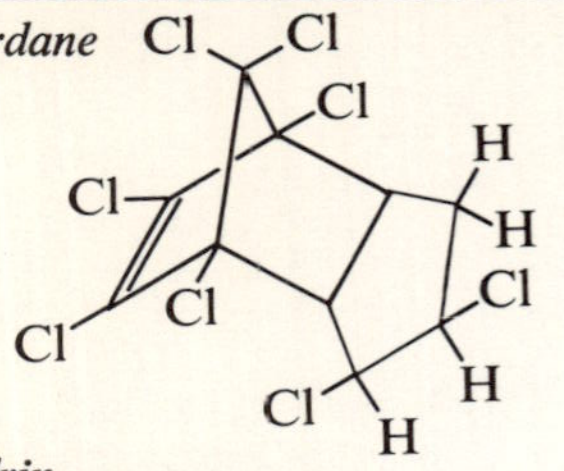	XVI. CH_2Cl_2; CH_2Cl_2 : cyclohexane mixtures	UV	Bio-Beads S-X2	124
	XVII. $CHCl_3$, cyclohexane, hexane, MeOH, toluene, CH_2Cl_2, THF, EtOH (also IV, X, XI)	radio. count, glc fract.	Bio-Beads S-X2, S-X4, S-X8, Sephadex LH-20	227, 238 68, 98, 195
Dieldrin 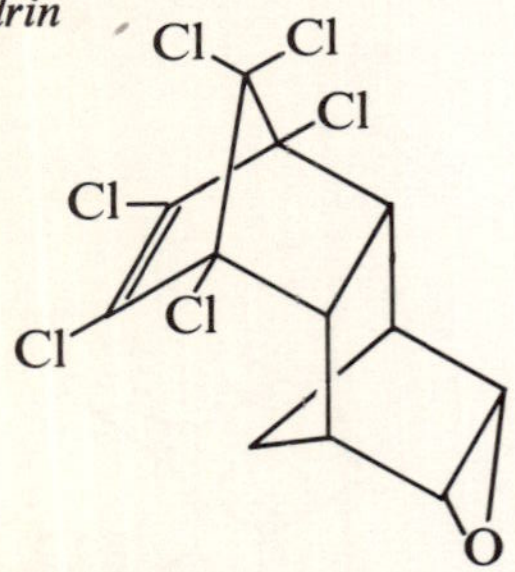	XVIII. hexane : CH_2Cl_2 (9:1)	UV, glc	Porasil A	262
	XIX. heptane : isoPrOH (70 : 30)	UV	Permaphase ETH	59, 141
	XX. hexane	EC	Partisil (5 and 10 µm)	43, 81
	XXI. 29 and 50% aq. MeOH or EtOH (also II–IV, VI, IX–XII, XV, XVII)	UV	Vydac RP	206 42,51, 68, 98, 144, 195, 227, 238, 245, 248, 255
Photodieldrin	X			68
Endosulfan (Thiodan™) 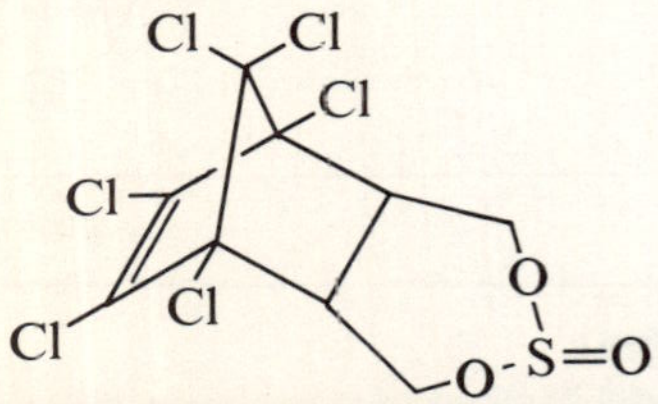	X (also endosulfan sulphate)			68

Endrin 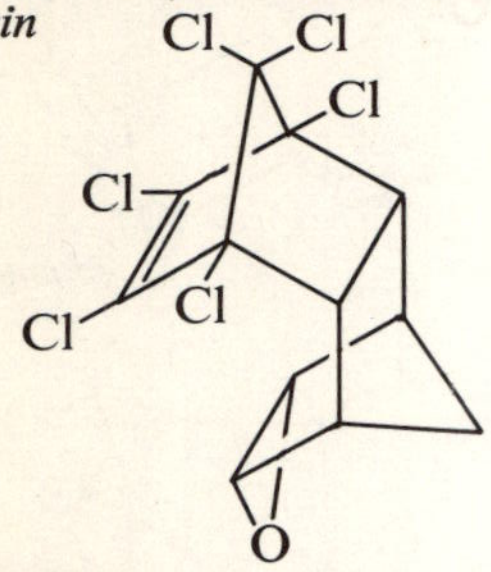	XXII. pet. ether	RI	Corasil II	130
	XXIII. light pet. + 20% benzene	flame ioniz.	silica gel L 50/71	47
	XXIV. MeCN : H_2O (25–75 : 75–25) (also I-III, V, VI, X-XII, XVII, XVIII)	UV 220	LiChrosorb RP-18	213 42, 51, 68, 98, 140, 227, 238, 245, 253, 255, 262
Heptachlor 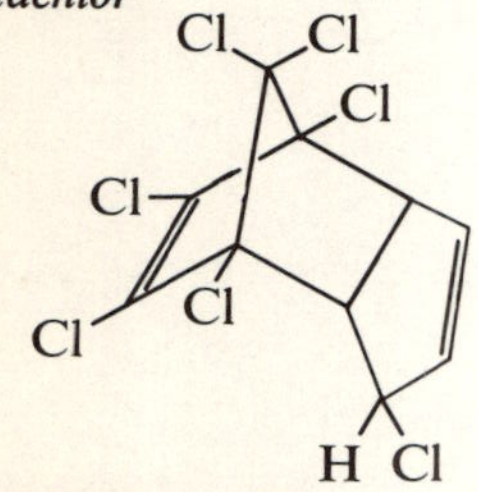	I–IV, VI, VII, X–XII, XVII			15, 42, 51, 68, 98, 195, 238, 245, 253, 255
Heptachlor epoxide	X–XII, XXI			42, 68, 98, 206
Isodrin 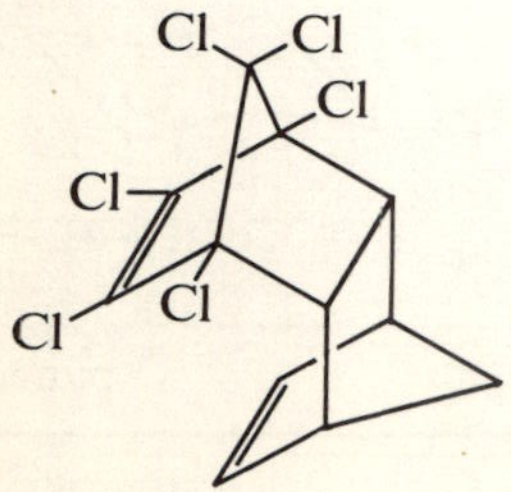	IV			195

Table 3 (*cont.*)

Compound	Mobile phase	Detector	Column	Reference
Lindane (γ-HCH, γ-BHC) 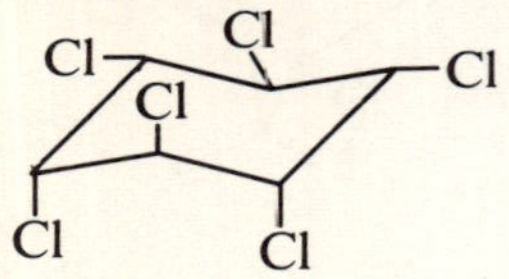	XXV. 15% EtOH in EtOAc (also I, III–VI, X–XII, XVII, XVIII, XX, XXII, XXIII)	UV	Spherisorb CN	213 42, 43, 47, 51, 68, 81, 98, 130, 140, 155, 195, 227, 238, 253, 255, 262
α-BHC	X, XI, XVIII, XX, XXII			43, 68, 81, 98, 130, 155, 262
β-BHC	X, XVIII, XX			43, 68, 81, 262
δ-BHC	X			68
Mirex 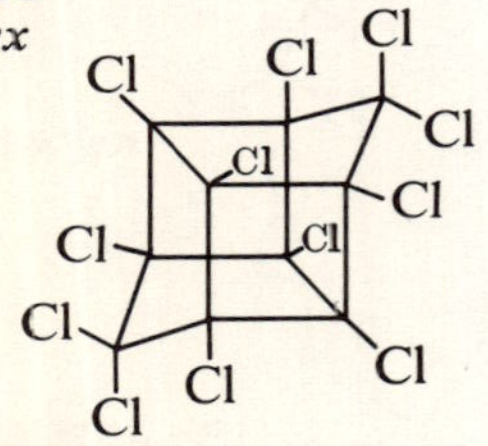	IX-XII			42, 68, 98, 144
Toxaphene 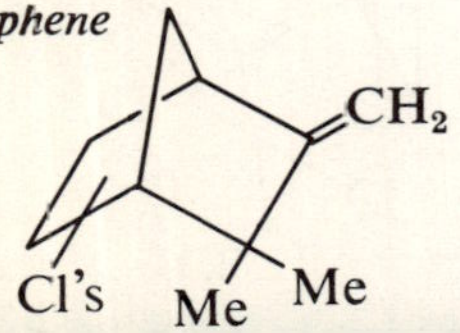	XI			19, 98

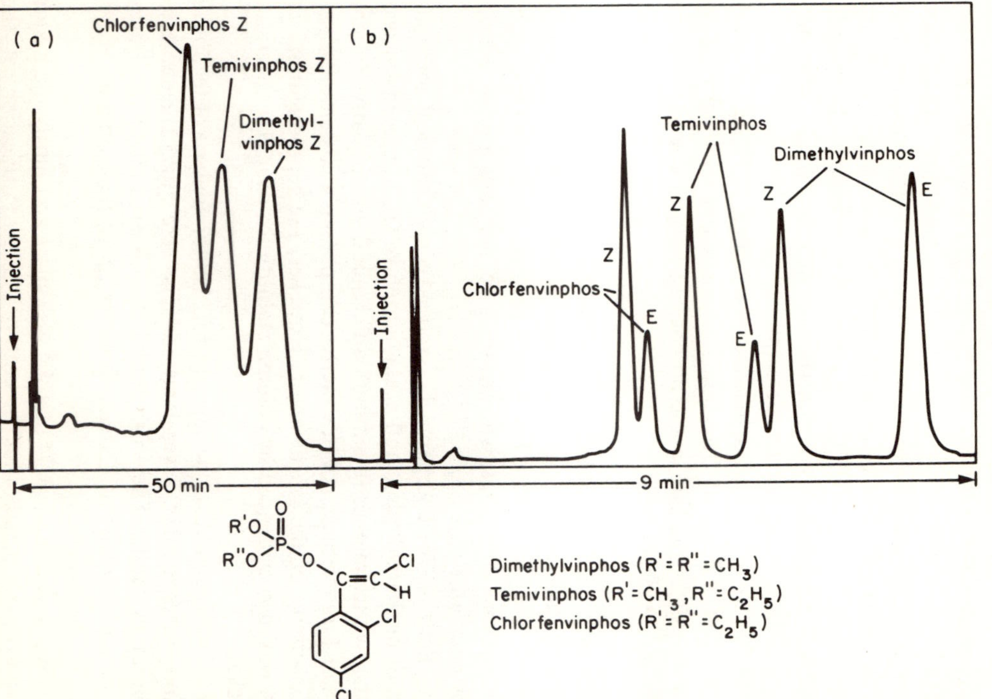

Figure 7 Comparison of separation of organophosphate pesticides by liquid chromatography with different column packings: (a) Porasil A (37–75 μm), 1000 × 2 mm i.d. column eluted with diethyl ether–hexane (4 : 6) at 0·92 ml/min; and (b) LiChrosorb SI 60 (5 μm), 100 × 4·5 mm i.d. column eluted with 2-propanol–hexane (1 : 99) at 2·73 ml/min; u.v. detection at 254 nm. From Self *et al* (1975), reproduced by permission of the Chemical Society

macroreticular resin. Of 21 different pesticide residues which could interfere in certain field situations, only fonofos coeluted with parathion. By simply monitoring u.v. absorbance at 280 nm instead of 270 nm the interference was overcome. L.c. analysis circumvented the problems in parathion determination by t.l.c. (slow, difficult to quantify) and g.l.c. (thermal lability).

Kvalvag *et al* (1977a, b) reported a method for parathion, paraoxon, and azinphosmethyl oxon residues in soil dust and on orange leaves. Different u.v. wavelengths were chosen for reversed- and normal-phase applications since polar solvents produced a bathochromic (red) shift in maximum absorbance. Kvalvag *et al* (1977b) also used a colorimetric detector which was described in greater detail by Ott (1977). The colorimetric detector was specific for nitro-aromatics but was 4-fold less sensitive (100 ng versus 25 ng) than u.v. absorbance. Ott (1977) also concluded that a colorimetric l.c. detector would offer less quantitative reproducibility than an u.v. detector.

Bowman *et al* (1978) used l.c. in trace analysis of etrimfos, as well as its oxon and hydrolysis product. Limits of detection in corn and alfalfa were about 0·5 ppm with an u.v. detector, but in the absence of natural coextractives as little as 0·05 ppm was evident.

Formulations. L.c. was used by Zehner and Simonaitis (1977) to determine pirimiphos methyl in formulations and by Jackson (1976, 1977) for methyl parathion. As Zehner and Simonaitis (1977) demonstrated, l.c. is often useful for direct analysis of aqueous emulsions, whereas for g.l.c. methods a prior extraction procedure is mandatory.

Lubkowitz and Petit (1976) compared l.c. and g.l.c. as analytical methods for formulations of methamidophos and acetamidophos. Good agreement was found between the two techniques (maximum difference 2%). A relatively poor limit of detection of 1 μg for these non-u.v.-active compounds also demonstrates the inherent insensitivity of the r.i. detector. However, the reproducibility of their l.c. method was also evidenced by column stability for over 200 injections of either insecticide.

Marshall *et al* (1974) found l.c. to be superior to g.l.c. for analysis of technical grade fenitrothion. In particular, several bis-adducts were quite amenable to l.c., but were thermally labile. They also found the upper limit of the linear dynamic range for u.v. response at 280 nm to be 95 μg for fenitrothion.

Metabolism. Zulalian and Blinn (1977) used l.c. to isolate and purify the major aglycone of mephosfolan metabolites in cotton plants. Purification of the dehydro-hydroxymethyl aglycone with Zorbax SIL allowed structural identification by standard spectral methods.

Carbamates

Dorough and Thorstenson (1975) presented a review of carbamate insecticide analysis, including usage of l.c. A more comprehensive treatment of carbamate analysis by l.c. was given by Sparacino and Hines (1976). The following conclusions were presented by the latter authors:

1. As a group, thermal lability precludes direct analysis of carbamates by g.l.c.
2. Except for carbaryl, methomyl, and Mobam^{TM}, the λ_{max} of each of 30 carbamates studied lies in the region 190–210 nm with $\varepsilon > 9,000$. The ε at λ_{max} can be as much as 2–3 orders of magnitude larger than the corresponding ε's at 254 and 280 nm.
3. Reversed-phase l.c. gave generally superior results compared to normal phase packings. Acetonitrile–water mixtures gave the best overall results because of greater u.v. clarity in the 195–220 nm region and increased resolution due to lower viscosity compared to methanol–water.

An example of the efficient resolution of carbamates on μBondapak C_{18} is shown in figure 8.

Carbamates have been used as probes to explore several aspects of l.c. technology. Kikta and Stange (1977) noted that diurnal variations in temperature of 12 °C were typical in their laboratory during summer months which resulted in peak height variations of $\pm 6\%$ for carbofuran. In order to improve quantitative precision and accuracy for trace analysis they used phenones (acylbenzenes) as internal standards. These authors project that such phenones would be useful in at least 90% of all current l.c. systems. McFadden et al (1976) used carbaryl and propoxur to examine a mass spectrometer as a l.c. detector. The detection limit for carbaryl was only 1 ng by m.s., a sensitivity not much better than u.v. although specificity should be enhanced. Kikta et al (1977) experienced difficulty in separating carbofuran from its corresponding 7-benzofuranol at ambient temperature. However, a rather dramatic resolution of these two components occurred by elevating the column temperature to 70 °C. The analysis of carbamates with fluorimetric enzyme inhibition presented by Moye and Wade (1976) has already been discussed herein.

Residue analysis. Frei et al (1974) analysed methiocarb and carbofuran in soil and water samples by hydrolysis, dansylation, and fluorimetric detection. Hosler (1974) used an octadecyl-coated Sil-X-II column to follow the photolysis and hydrolysis of mexacarbate. In addition to a comprehensive comparison of the l.c. properties of 17 carbamate and urea pesticides, Aten and Bourke (1977) applied their methodology to methiocarb analysis in Brussels sprouts.

Lawrence and coworkers also demonstrated the utility of *direct analysis* of carbamates in field residue samples, i.e. usage of l.c. without chemical derivatization as the final detection step. From the work of Lawrence and Leduc (1977), it is evident that carbofuran residues at the 0·1 ppm level in carrots, potatoes, turnips, cabbage, and corn are detectable by l.c. Lawrence (1977) also presented l.c. chromatograms for 0·1 ppm residues of mexacarbate, aminocarb, propoxur, swep, Mobam^{TM}, and carbaryl in potatoes, wheat, corn, and cabbage (figures 9 and 10). Lawrence et al (1977) and Lawrence and Leduc (1977) noticed a remarkable difference in u.v. sensitivity of carbofuran, 3-hydroxycarbofuran, and 3-ketocarbofuran at 254 nm versus 280 nm, which is vividly

Table 4 LC conditions for organophosphorus insecticides

Compound	Mobile phase	Detector	Column	Reference
Acephate (Acetamidophos, Orthene™) 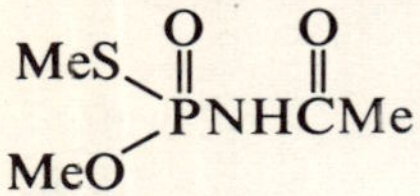	I. MeOH : H$_2$O (10 : 90)	RI	μBondapak C$_{18}$	142
Azinphos ethyl R = Et 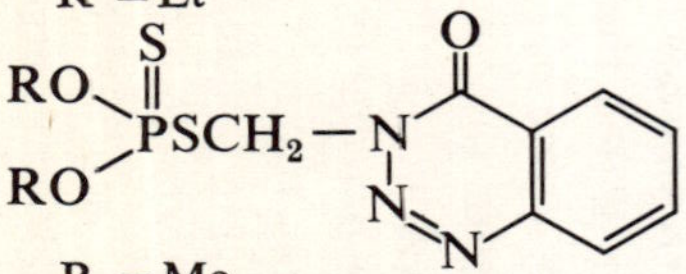	II. MeCN : H$_2$O (50 : 50)	UV 285	Partisil ODS	166
	III. MeCN : H$_2$O (25–75 : 75–25 grad.)	UV 220	LiChrosorb RP-18	213
R = Me *Azinphos methyl* (Guthion™)	IV. 29 and 50% aq. MeOH or EtOH	UV	Vydac RP	206
	V. 2% PrOH in hexane	flame ioniz.	silica gel (6 μm)	232
	VI. MeOH : H$_2$O (80 : 20)	UV, CEC	Vydac 201 TP RP	42
(also Azinphos methyl oxon)	VII. MeCN : H$_2$O (20 : 80) (also III)	UV 285	μBondapak C$_{18}$	126 213
Carbophenothion (Trithion™)	VIII. cyclohexane (also V)	—	Bio-Beads S-X2	68 232
Chlorfenvinphos 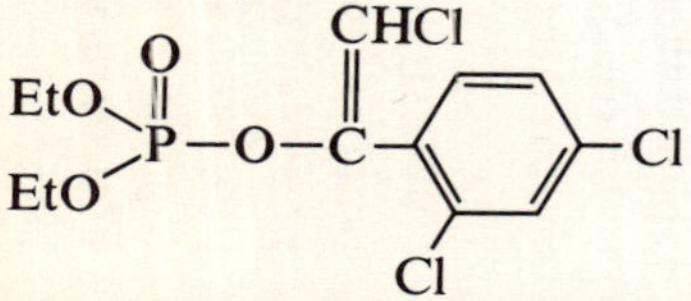	IX. ether : hexane (4 : 6)	UV	Porasil A (37–75 μm)	208
	X. isoPrOH : hexane (1 : 99)	UV	LiChrosorb SI 60 (5 μm)	208

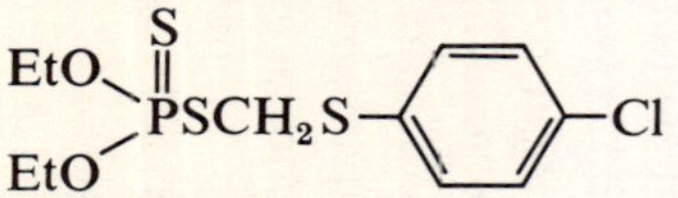

Compound		Eluent	Detection	Column	Ref.
Chlorpyrifos (Dursban™)		XI. 0–50% MeOH in H_2O, 20% aq. EtOH; 20% aq. acetone; 0·1 M phosphate buffer, pH 7 [also II (290 nm), VI]	fluor. enz. inhib.	Permaphase ODS, Pellidon, Vydac RP, Durapak Carbowax 400, SCX, SAX	155, 156 42, 166
Crotoxyphos (Ciodrin™) 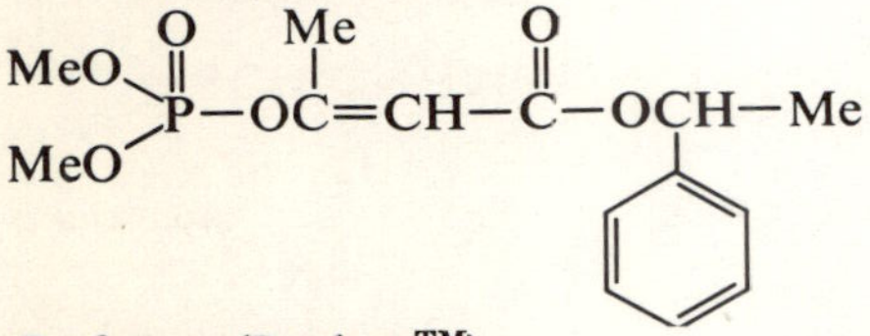		XII. 3% EtOH in hexane	flame ioniz.	silica gel (6 μm)	232
Crufomate (Ruelene™) 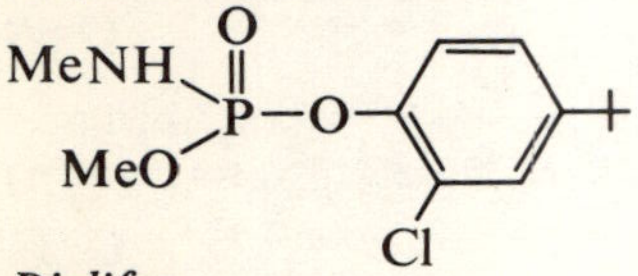		XIII. 10% $CHCl_3$ in hexane (dansyl der.)	fluor.	silica gel (10 μm)	138
		XIV. 5% PrOH in hexane	flame ioniz.	silica gel (6 μm)	232
Dialifos (*Dialifor*) 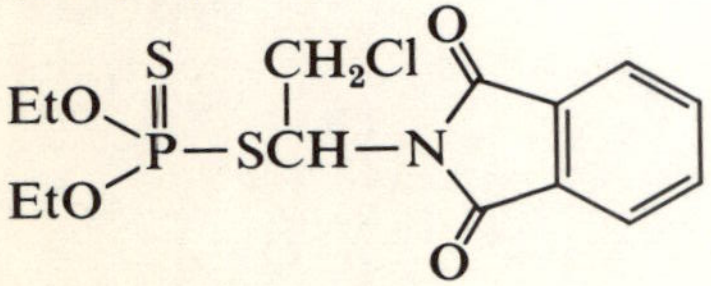		II. (290 nm)			166
Diazinon 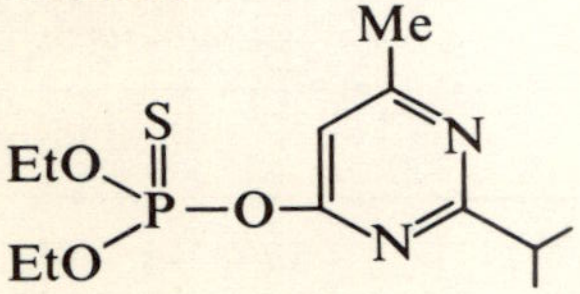		XV. toluene : EtOAc (1 : 3)	glc fract.	Bio-Beads S-X3	98
		XVI. CH_2Cl_2	UV	silica (10 μm)	30
		[also II (245 nm), IV, VIII]			68, 166, 206

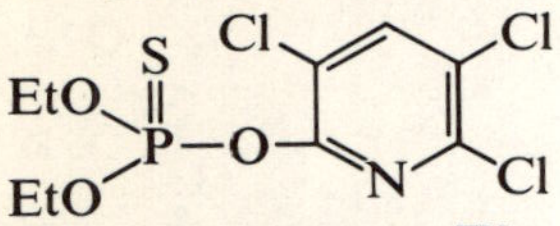

Table 4 (*cont.*)

Compound	Mobile phase	Detector	Column	Reference
Dicapthon	IV			206
Dichlorvos	XVII. 0·5% PrOH in hexane (also XV)	flame ioniz.	silica gel (6 μm)	232 98
Dicrotophos (Carbicron[TM], Bidrin[TM])	XVIII. H_2O	UV 297, ChE inhib.	Permaphase ETH	187
	XIX. 10% EtOH in hexane	flame ioniz.	silica gel (6 μm)	232
Dimethoate	III, XIX			213, 232
Dimethylvinphos	IX, X			208

Disulfoton (Di-Syston™)

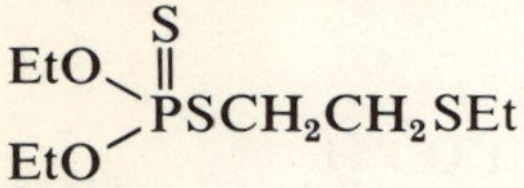

EtO, S
‖
PSCH$_2$CH$_2$SEt
EtO

EPN

(phenyl)(S)(OEt)P—O—C$_6$H$_4$—NO$_2$

Ethion

EtO, S   S, OEt
‖   ‖
PSCH$_2$SP
EtO   OEt

Etrimfos

MeO, S
‖
P—O—(pyrimidine: 2-Et, 6-OEt)
MeO

Fenchlorphos (Ronnel)

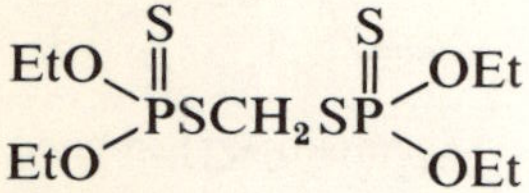

MeO, S
‖
P—O—C$_6$H$_2$Cl$_3$
MeO

Fenitrothion

MeO, S
‖
P—O—C$_6$H$_3$(Me)—NO$_2$
MeO

VI, XV				42, 98
XX. hexane	UV	0·5% ODPN on CSP support		108
XXI. isooctane	UV	10% ODPN on Porasil 60		253
VIII				68
XXII. MeOH : H$_2$O (70 : 30); also etrimfos oxon and 6-ethoxy-2-ethyl-4-hydroxypyrimidine)	UV	μBondapak C$_{18}$		13
XXIII. 1% PrOH in hexane	flame ioniz.	silica gel (6 μm)		232
[also III, VI, VIII, XIII (dansyl der.)]				42, 68, 138, 213
XXIV. EtOAc : hexane (12·5 : 87·5, 30 : 70)	UV 280	Corasil II		147
XXV. EtOAc : hexane (15 : 85, 10 : 90) [also II (265 nm), III, XIII (dansyl der.)]	UV 280	ODPN on Porasil (37–75 μm)		147 138, 166, 213

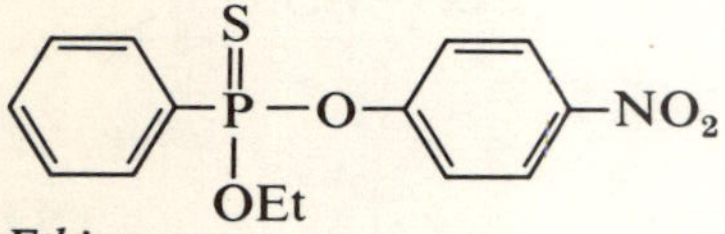

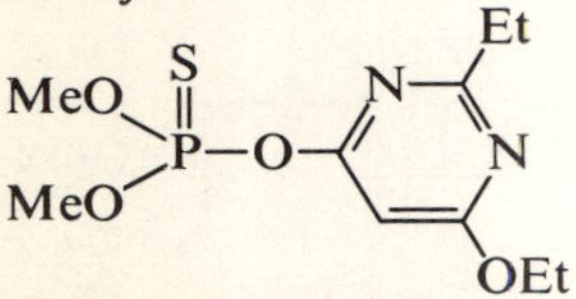

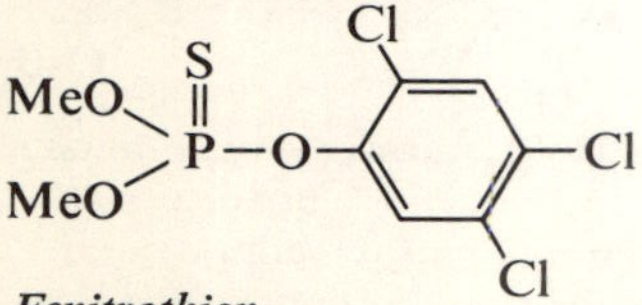

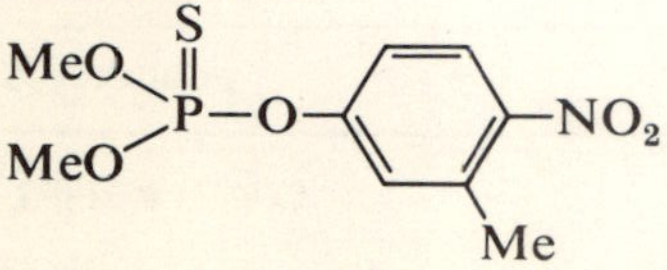

Table 4 (*cont.*)

Compound	Mobile phase	Detector	Column	Reference
bis-Fenitrothion; *S*-Methyl-bis-fenitrothion; 3-Methyl-4-nitrophenol; Fenitrooxon	XXIV, XXV			147
Fensulfothion (Dasanit™)	XV			98
Fenthion	XXVI. 5% MeOH in hexane (dansyl der.) [also XIII (dansyl der.)]	fluor.	0·5% ODPN on Zipax	60 138
Fonofos (Dyfonate™)	II. (240 nm), XI, XIX			155, 156, 232
Malathion	XXVII. CHCl$_3$, cyclohexane, hexane, MeOH, toluene, CH$_2$Cl$_2$, THF, EtOH	glc, radio. count	Bio-Beads S-X2, S-X4, S-X8, Sephadex LH-20	227, 238
	XXVIII. pentane	UV, ms	Durapak Carbowax 400/Porasil	150
	(also IV, V, VIII, XV, XVI)			30, 68, 98, 206, 232
Malaoxon	VIII			68

Compound	Solvent system	Detection	Support / column	Ref.
Mephosfolan (Cytrolane™)	XXIX. CH$_2$Cl$_2$: isoPrOH (95 : 5) (for dehydro-hydroxymethylmephosfolan only)	—	Zorbax-SIL	263
Methamidophos (Monitor™)	I			142
Methyl parathion	XXX. H$_2$O : EtOH : HOAc : NaOH : HCl (60·1 : 38·8 : 0·80 : 0·21 : 0·09) satd with isooctane	polar.	silanized diatomaceous earth (isooctane coated, 10% w/w)	118, 119, 155
	XXXI. MeOH : H$_2$O (40 : 60)	UV	Permaphase ODS	95
	XXXII. CHCl$_3$ (40% H$_2$O satd)	UV	microparticulate silica	96
	[also II (270 nm), III, IV, VI, VIII, XI, XIII (dansyl der.), XV, XVI, XXI, XXIII]			30, 42 68, 98 138, 155, 156, 166, 206, 213, 232, 253
Mevinphos (Phosdrin™)	VI, XIX			42, 232
Monocrotophos (Nuvacron™, Azodrin™)	VI, XVIII, XIX			42, 187, 232

Table 4 (*cont.*)

Compound	Mobile phase	Detector	Column	Reference
Naled MeO₂P—OCHBr—CBrCl₂ (MeO, O)	XII			232
Oxydemeton-methyl (Meta-Systox-R™) MeO₂P—SCH₂CH₂SEt (MeO, O, O)	VI			42
Parathion EtO₂P—O—C₆H₄—NO₂ (EtO, S)	XXXIII. 10–100% MeCN in H₂O grad.	UV 272	Bondapak C₁₈/Corasil (37–50 μm)	125, 163
	XXXIV. 1·5% dioxane in hexane	UV 265	Carbowax 400 on Corasil (37–50 μm)	125
	[also II (270 nm), III, IV, VI, VIII, XI, XV, XXIII, XXVII, XXX]			42, 68, 98, 118, 119, 155, 156, 166, 206, 213, 227, 232, 238
Paraoxon	XXXV. 1·2–22·5% dioxane in hexane	UV 265	Carbowax 400 on Corasil (37–50 μm)	125
	(also III, VI, VIII, XXXIII, XXXIV)			42, 68, 125, 163, 213
p-Nitrophenol	[II (270 nm), XXX]			118, 119, 155, 166

Compound	Conditions	Detection	Support	Ref.
Phenthoate (Cidial[TM]) 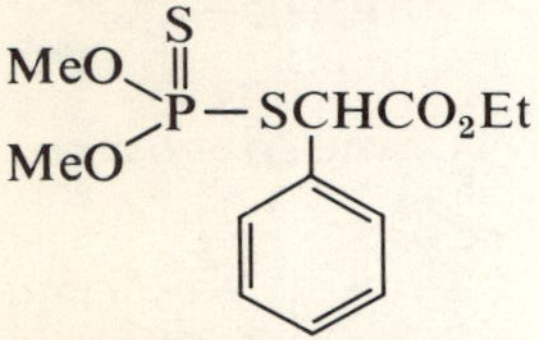	XXXVI. 0·25% PrOH in hexane	flame ioniz.	silica gel (6 μm)	232
Phorate (Thimet[TM]) 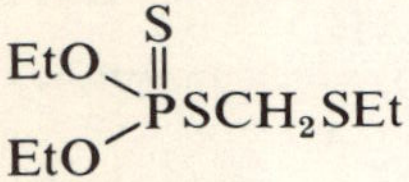	[II (220 nm), V, VIII]			68, 166, 232
Phosalone 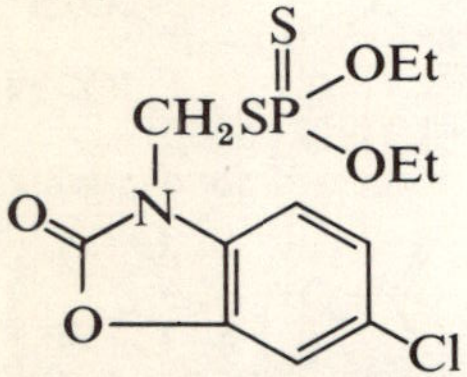	XXXV			232
Phosmet (Imidan[TM], Prolate[TM]) 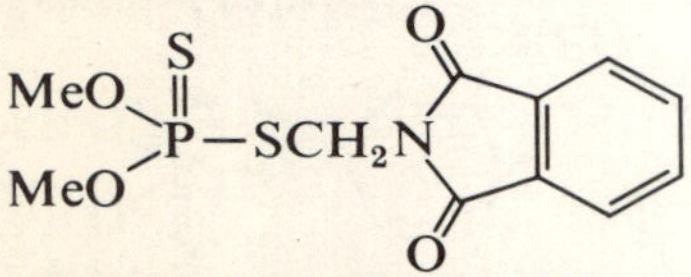	II (230 nm), XXXV			166, 232
Phosphamidon (Dimecron[TM]) 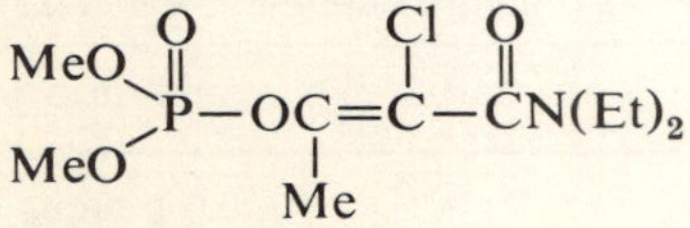	III, XVIII, XIX			187, 213, 232

Table 4 (*cont.*)

Compound	Mobile phase	Detector	Column	Reference
Pirimiphos methyl (Actellic[TM]) 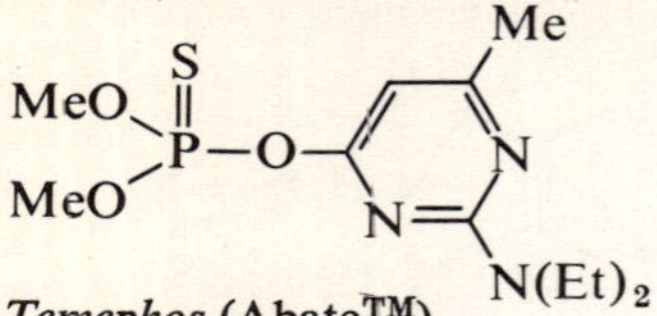	XXXVII. MeOH : H₂O (45 : 55)	UV	Permaphase ODS	261
Temephos (Abate[TM]) 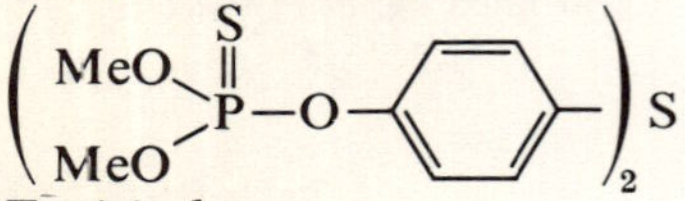	XXXVIII. heptane (also VI)	UV	1 % ODPN on Zipax	79, 112, 155, 201 42
Temivinphos 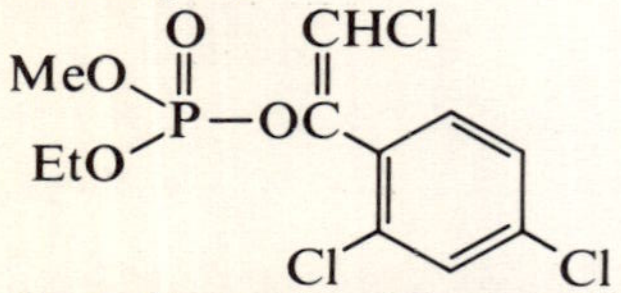	IX, X			208
Tetrachlorvinphos (Gardona[TM]) 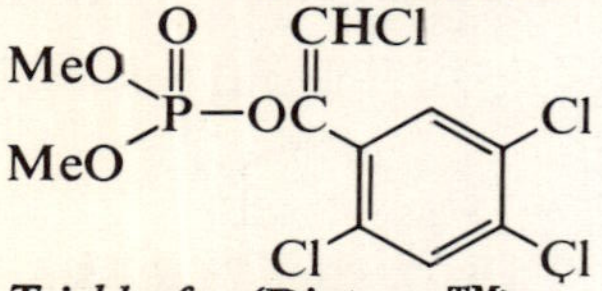	XXXIX. 1·5 and 3·0 % EtOH in hexane	flame ioniz.	silica gel (6 μm)	232
Trichlorfon (Dipterex[TM]) 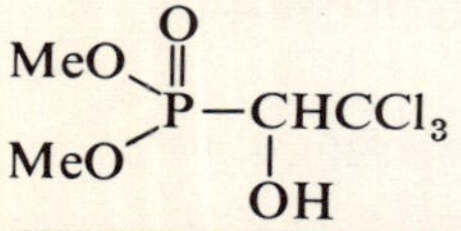	XIX			232

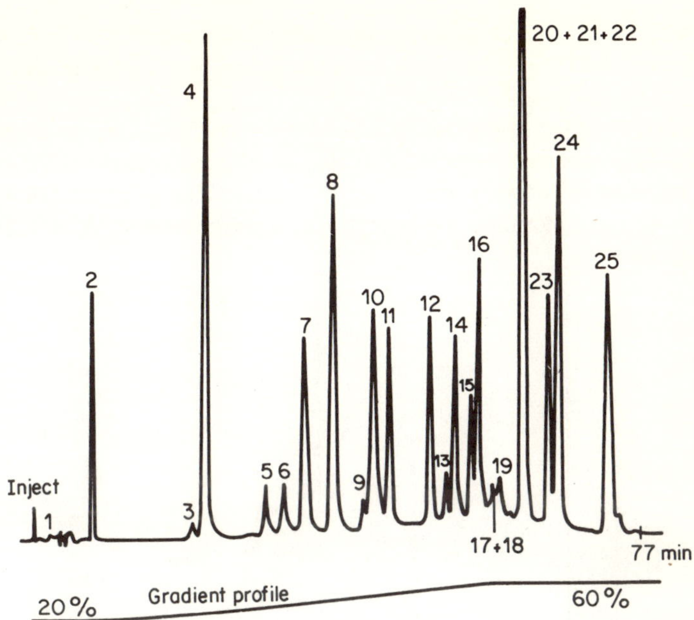

Figure 8 Separation of carbamate pesticides. Column, µBondapak C_{18}; mobile phase, 20–60% acetonitrile in water, concave gradient (60 min); flow rate, 1·0 ml/min; u.v. detection at 220 nm (1·0 a.u.f.s.). Peaks: (1) solvent front, (2) methomyl, (3) aldicarb, (4) isolan, (5) propoxur, (6) carbofuran, (7) Mobam™, (8) carbaryl, (9) Landrin™, (10) propham, (11) carbanolate, (12) methiocarb, (13) mexacarbate, (14) phenmedipham, (15) chlorpropham, (16) EPTC, (17) metalkamate, (18) captafol, (19) barban, (20) cycloate, (21) vernolate, (22) pebulate, (23) butylate, (24) di-allate, (25) tri-allate. From Sparacino and Hines (1976), reproduced by permission of Preston Publications, Inc.

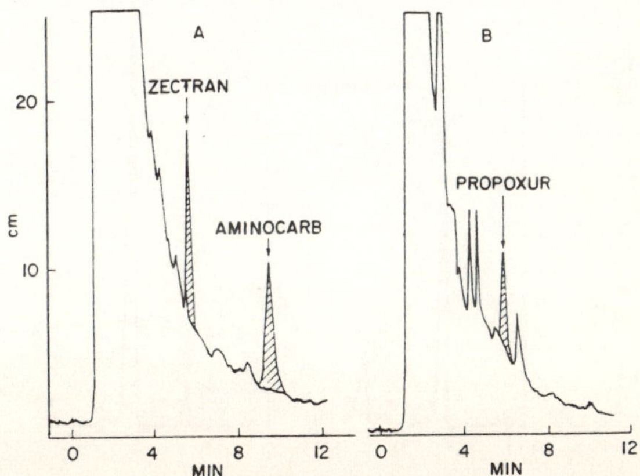

Figure 9 Chromatograms of: (A) Zectran (mexacarbate) and aminocarb in corn (0·1 ppm); 50 mg equiv. of corn injected; (B) propoxur in cabbage (0·1 ppm); 100 mg equiv. of cabbage injected. Column, LiChrosorb SI 60 (5 µm), 250 × 2·8 mm, eluted with 5% 2-propanol in isooctane; both chromatograms, 1·0 ml/min flow rate; u.v. detection, 254 nm, 0·001 a.u.f.s. From Lawrence (1977), reproduced by permission of American Chemical Society

depicted in figure 11. It is evident that wavelength selection for l.c. analysis with u.v. detection is crucial in determination of the actual limit of detection for trace residues.

Fine *et al* (1976) used N-nitroso specific thermal energy detection for analysis of N-nitroso compounds in several foodstuffs. N-Nitrosocarbaryl was detectable in crude extracts of cooked bacon at 0·01 ppm. Thean *et al* (1978) used μBondapak C_{18} to determine methomyl and oxamyl residues in a variety of vegetable crops.

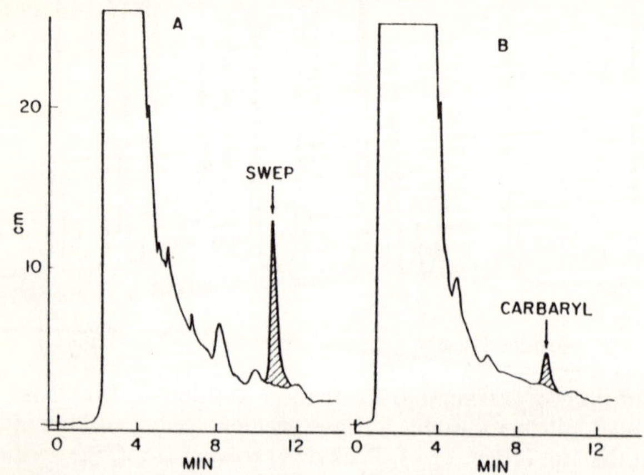

Figure 10   Chromatograms of: (A) swep in potato (0·1 ppm); 10 mg equiv. of potato injected; 0·4 ml/min flow rate; 0·001 a.u.f.s.; (B) carbaryl in wheat (0·1 ppm); 50 mg equiv. of wheat injected; 1·0 ml/min flow rate; 0·002 a.u.f.s. Other conditions same as figure 9. From Lawrence (1977), reproduced by permission of American Chemical Society

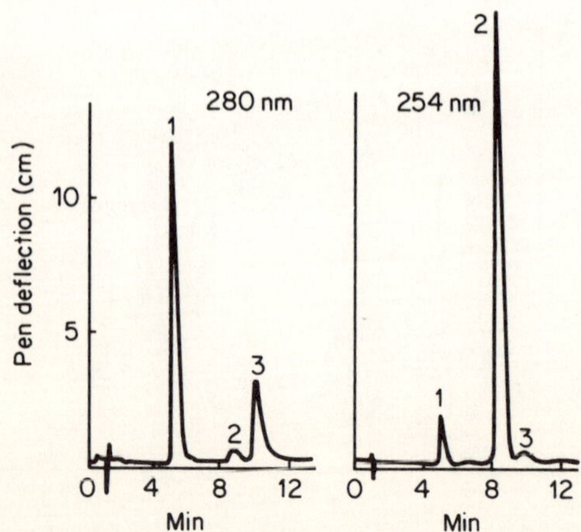

Figure 11   Chromatograms of a mixture of 200 ng of carbofuran (1), 135 ng of 3-ketocarbofuran (2), and 200 ng of 3-hydroxycarbofuran (3) at 254 and 280 nm detection. Sensitivity, 0·01 a.u.f.s. Except for column i.d. (2·2 mm), other conditions same as figure 9. From Lawrence and Leduc (1977), reproduced by permission of American Chemical Society

Table 5 LC conditions for carbamates

Compound	Mobile phase	Detector	Column	Reference
Aldicarb (Temik™)	I. MeCN : H_2O (30–50 : 70–50)	UV	μBondapak C_{18}	155
	II. 20–60% MeCN in H_2O	UV 220	μBondapak C_{18}	225
HC=NOCNHMe (with O above C)	III. 0–50% MeOH in H_2O; 20% aq. EtOH; 20% aq. acetone; 0·1 M phosphate buffer, pH 7	fluor. enz. inhib.	Permaphase ODS; Pellidon; Vydac RP; Durapak; Carbowax 400; SCX; SAX	155, 155
Me—C—Me	IV. MeOH : H_2O (1 : 1, 1 : 2); MeCN; MeOH; isoPrOH; isoPrOH : hexane (1 : 1)	UV	Partisil-10 ODS	4
SMe	V. 1–10% isoPrOH in heptane	UV 220	Si-10, CN-10, NH_2-10	225
(dansyl der.)	VI. benzene : pet. ether (60 : 40)	fluor.	Corasil I	61
(dansyl der.)	VII. hexane : acetone (98 : 2)	fluor.	Corasil I	61
(dansyl der.)	VIII. hexane : EtOH (95 : 5)	fluor.	Porasil (satd with ODPN)	61
(dansyl der.)	IX. hexane : EtOH (95 : 5)	fluor.	Zipax (0·5% ODPN)	61
(also Aldicarb sulphoxide and sulphone)	X. 15–40% MeCN in H_2O	UV 220	μBondapak C_{18}	225
Aminocarb (Matacil™)	XI. 5% isoPrOH in isooctane	UV	LiChrosorb SI 60 (5 μm)	133
	XII. MeOH : H_2O (6 : 94)	UV	Permaphase ODS	46, 155, 237
$(Me)_2N$—ring—OCNHMe (with O above C), Me substituent	(also III and IV)			4, 155, 156
Butacarb (dansyl der.)	VI–IX			60, 61, 134, 155

Table 5 (*cont.*)

Compound	Mobile phase	Detector	Column	Reference
Carbanolate (Banol[TM])	II, VI–IX, XI			61, 133, 225
Carbaryl (Sevin[TM])	XIII. MeCN : H$_2$O (50 : 50)	UV	μC$_{18}$	155
	XIV. MeOH : H$_2$O (80 : 20)	UV, CEC	Vydac 201 TP RP	42
	XV. 20% CHCl$_3$ in isooctane	UV	Carbowax 400 on Porasil	33, 155
	XVI. 29 and 50% aq. MeOH or EtOH	UV	Vydac RP	206
(also α- and β-Naphthol, 2-Naphthol *N*-methylcarbamate)	XVII. hexane : CHCl$_3$ (4 : 1)	UV	Corasil II (37–50 μm)	2
(also α-Naphthol)	XVIII. hexane	UV	1% trimethylene glycol on Zipax	201
	XIX. MeCN : H$_2$O (50 : 50)	UV 280	Partisil ODS	166
	XX. CHCl$_3$: isooctane (25 : 75)	UV 294	Corasil II; μPorasil	21
	XXI. CH$_2$Cl$_2$	UV	silica gel (10 μm)	30
(also α-Naphthol)	XXII. 3% isoPrOH in heptane	UV 220	Si-10, CN-10, NH$_2$-10	225
	XXIII. MeCN : H$_2$O (25–75 : 75–25 grad.)	UV 220	LiChrosorb RP-18	213
	(also I–IX, XI, XII, XV)			4, 33, 46, 61, 133, 155, 156, 225, 237

	XXIV. MeOH : H_2O : 0·07 M phosphate buffer, pH 6·4 (95 : 3 : 2)	fluor.	Hitachi gel 3010	120
(as α-Naphthol)				
α-Naphthol	IV, XII, XV			4, 33, 46, 155, 237
N-Nitrosocarbaryl	XXV. 1–5% acetone in isooctane; 1% isoPrOH in CH_2Cl_2	UV, therm. energy	μPorasil	58
	XXVI. 25–70% PrOH in H_2O grad.	nitro. spec., UV	μBondapak C_{18}	216
	XXVII. pentane	UV, ms	Durapak Carbowax 400/Porasil	150
Carbofuran (Furadan™)	XXVIII. MeCN : H_2O (50 : 50)	UV 270	Partisil ODS	166
	XXIX. 0·5% isoPrOH in heptane	UV 220	Si-10, CN-10, NH_2-10	225
	XXX. MeCN : H_2O (40 : 60)	UV 220	μBondapak C_{18}	225
	XXXI. MeOH : H_2O (1 : 1)	UV 254, 280	μBondapak C_{18}	105
	XXXII. MeCN : H_2O (25 : 75)	UV	μBondapak C_{18}	106, 155
	XXXIII. isoPrOH : isooctane (3–8 : 97–92)	UV 254, 280	LiChrosorb SI 60 (5 μm)	136
	(also I–III, V–IX, XI, XII)			46, 60, 61, 106, 115, 133, 137, 155, 156, 225, 237
3-Hydroxycarbofuran	III, XI, XXIX–XXXI, XXXIII			105, 133, 136, 137, 155, 156, 225
3-Oxocarbofuran	XI, XXXI, XXXIII			105, 133, 136, 137
Carbofuran-7-ol	I, XXXII			105, 106, 155

Table 5 (*cont.*)

Compound	Mobile phase	Detector	Column	Reference
CPMC 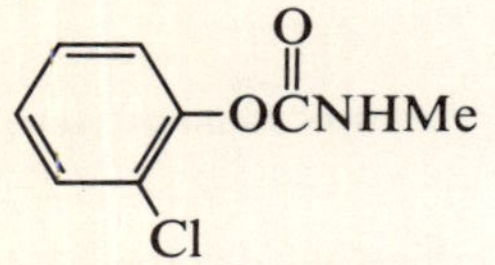	XXXIV. MeOH : H_2O (48 : 52, 56 : 44)	UV 254, 270	MicroPak CH	92
	XXXV. CH_2Cl_2 : hexane, grad. from (5 : 95)	UV	MicroPak NH_2	92
Dimetilan (Snip™) 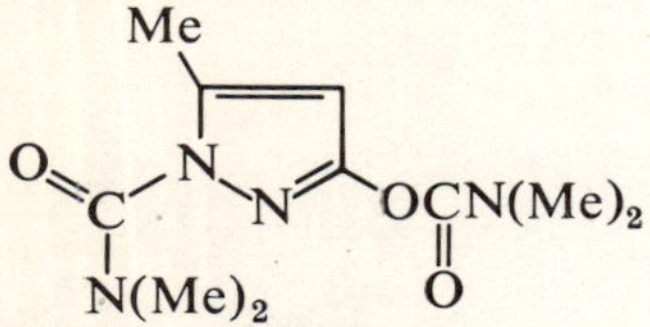	XXXVI. H_2O	UV 297, ChE inhib.	Permaphase ETH	187
Dioxacarb (Elocron™) 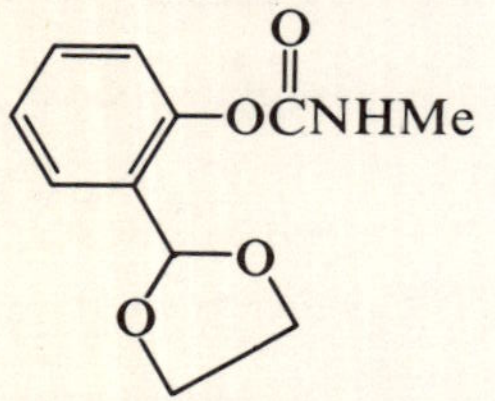	VI-IX, XXXVI			60, 61, 134, 155, 187
Formetanate 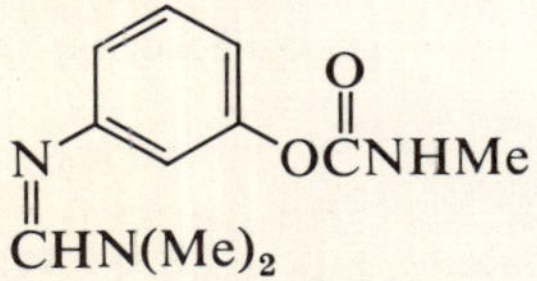	IV			4

| *Formetanate hydrochloride* (Carzol™) | IV, VI–VIII | 60, 61, 134, 155 |
| *Isolan* 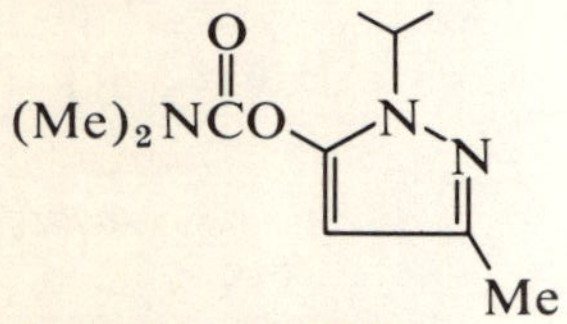 | II | 225 |

(Me)$_2$NCO — pyrazole ring with isopropyl, Me substituents

| *Isoprocarb* (MIPC) 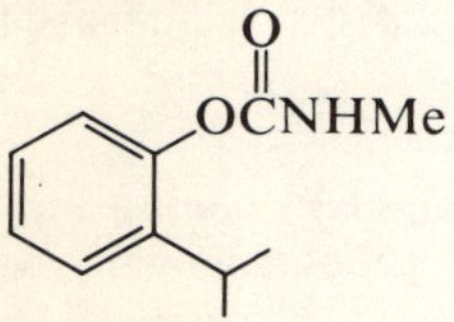 | XXXIV, XXXV | 92 |

| *Landrin*™ 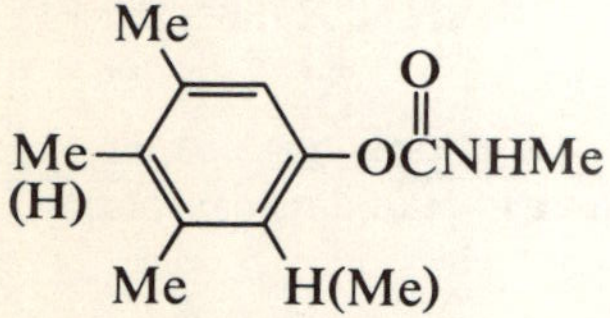 | II, VI–IX, XI, XIII | 46, 61, 133, 155, 225, 237 |

| *N*-Nitrosolandrin | XXVI | 216 |
| *Metalkamate* (Bux,™ Bufencarb) 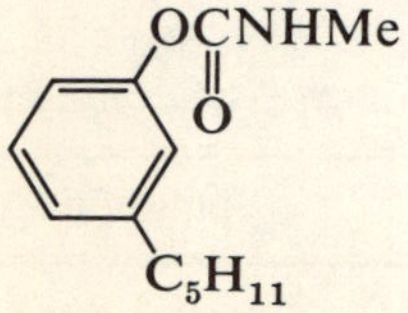 | II, V–IX | 61, 225 |

Table 5 (*cont.*)

Compound	Mobile phase	Detector	Column	Reference
Methiocarb (Mesurol™)	I, II, IV, VI–IX, XI, XII			4, 46, 61, 115, 133, 134, 155, 225, 237
Methiocarb sulphone phenol	IV			4
Methomyl (Lannate™)	XXXVII. 7% $CHCl_3$ in hexane	UV	1% ODPN on Zipax	139
	XXXVIII. isoPrOH : hexane (4 : 96)	UV	Permaphase ETH	155, 237
	XXXIX. MeCN : H_2O buffer (11 : 89)	UV 240	μBondapak C_{18}	235
	(also I, II, IV–IX, XIV)			4, 42, 61, 155, 225
N-Nitrosomethomyl	XXVI.			216, 256
Mexacarbate (Zectran™)	XL. MeOH : H_2O (45 : 55, 15 : 85, 0 : 100) (also 4-dimethylamino-3,5-xylenol)	UV	C_{18} Sil-X-II	84
	(also I–IV, XI)			4, 133, 155, 156, 225
Mobam ™	II, VI–IX, XI			61, 133, 134, 155, 225

MPMC (Meobal™) 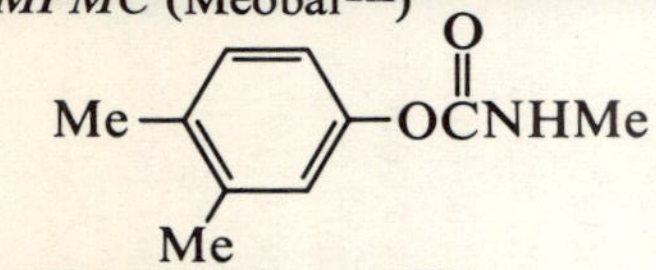	XXXIV, XXXV	92
MTMC (Tsumacide™) 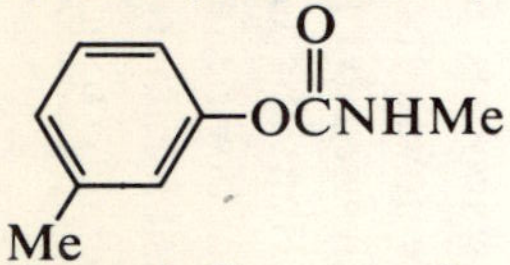	XXXIV (48 : 52 only), XXXV	92
Oxamyl 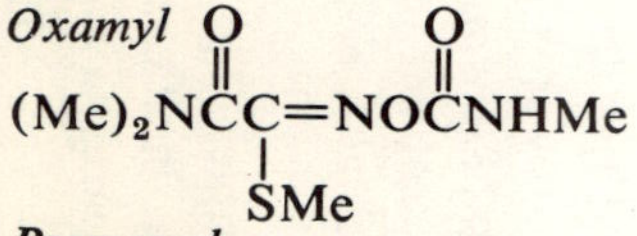	IV, XXXIX	4
Promecarb 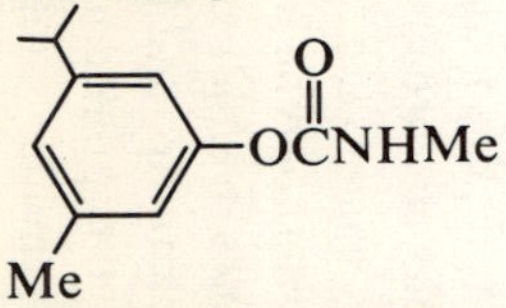	VI–IX	61
Propoxur (Baygon™, PHC) 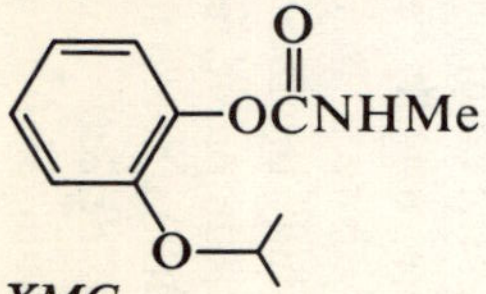	I–III, VI–IX, XI, XXIII, XXVII, XXXII, XXXIV, XXXV	61, 92, 133, 150, 155, 156, 213, 225
XMC 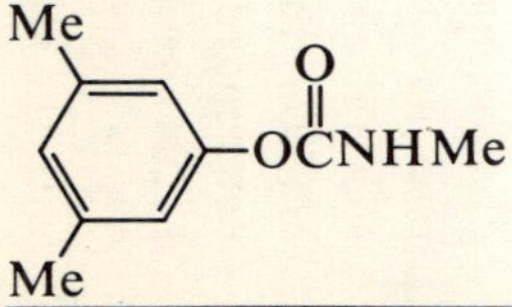	XXXIV (48 : 52 only), XXXV	92

Formulations. Argauer and Warthen (1975) used Corasil II with u.v. detection to determine naphthol and 2-naphthyl N-methylcarbamate impurities in carbaryl formulations. Colvin *et al* (1974) used a Carbowax 400/Porasil column to detect carbaryl by u.v. in pesticide formulations and fertilizers.

Pyrethroids

To date only a few applications have been reported for this class of insecticides. Lam and Grushka (1977) showed good resolution of *cis-* and *trans*-permethrin on silica ($\alpha = 1.7$) and silver aluminosilicate ($\alpha = 1.6$), but not on sodium aluminosilicate ($\alpha = 1$). Using 10 μm silica, Carlstrom (1977) could analyse natural pyrethrins in folpet formulations. Zehner and Simonaitis (1976) resolved *cis-* and *trans*-resmethrin ($\alpha = 1.3$) on octadecyl functionalized Zipax using methanol–water. L.c. on Partisil-5 was useful in separating the *cis-* and *trans*-isomers of cypermethrin ($\alpha = 1.3$, Roberts and Standen, 1977a). The same authors used Partisil-5 to study the metabolites of cypermethrin (*m*-phenoxybenzoic acid and the expected substituted cyclopropanecarboxylic acid) in soil. Several metabolites of WL 41706 from rats and soil were isolated with Partisil-5 and Partisil-5-NH$_2$ columns (Crawford and Hutson, 1977; Roberts and Standen, 1977b).

Insect growth regulators

Much of our own experience has centred around the environmental degradation of methoprene. L.c. has participated prominently in the identification of the 12 metabolites listed in Table 7. Our overall approach in using l.c. for metabolic analysis has been as follows:
1. After extraction, preliminary g.p.c. (e.g. Bio-Beads S-X2) eliminates high molecular weight impurities (if necessary).
2. T.l.c.
3. Derivatization of appropriate t.l.c. zones (if necessary, e.g. acids converted to methyl esters, alcohols benzoylated, etc.).
4. L.c. isolation.

Since we distrust metabolite identifications based only on t.l.c. cochromatography, we rely on the greater resolution of l.c. for structure confirmation by coelution with authentic standards. For routine analyses, reversed-phase packings were used since most of the impurities associated with metabolites tend to be rather polar and, therefore, elute towards the solvent front instead of adhering to the column. For final isolation of new metabolites, normal-phase packings were usually employed because solvent removal for subsequent spectral analysis (e.g. m.s.) is easier. L.c. has also been used by Hammock *et al* (1977) to study the fate of methoprene in houseflies. Hunt and Gilbert (1976) determined methoprene residues in small samples (2 g) of bovine fat using silica l.c. as a penultimate step for clean-up, and l.c. on μPorasil for final quantitation. Their limit of detection of 0·008 ppm compares favourably to g.l.c. methods with the advantage of using a smaller sample.

Diflubenzuron residues have been determined using l.c. by several groups. Schaefer and Dupras (1976, 1977) used MicroPak-CH to quantitate diflubenzuron in water, soil, and vegetation. Their limits of detection were a quite respectable 0·2 ppb in water and 3·8 ppb in soil or vegetation. In manure, diflubenzuron was detectable at 0·25 ppm (Oehler and Holman, 1975) and in milk at 0·1 ppm (Corley *et al*, 1974).

Dorn *et al* (1976) used silica (8 μm) to examine diol and two rearranged allylic alcohols produced from another insect growth regulator (Ro 10-3108) in polluted water.

Miscellaneous compounds active on arthropods

We have employed l.c. extensively in metabolic studies with cycloprate involving plants, rats, dogs, and a cow (Quistad *et al*, 1978a–d). The use of several l.c. systems was essential for the purification of sufficient metabolite mass for structural identification of homologous ω-cyclopropyl fatty acids and a carnitine conjugate of cyclopropanecarboxylic acid.

Several reports have detailed analytical methods for rotenoids. Bushway *et al* (1975b) and Bushway and Hanks (1977) presented both normal- and reversed-phase systems for rotenone with 2 ng sensitivity. Freudenthal *et al* (1977) separated rotenone and five related rotenoids on Zorbax ODS. Moring (1977) analysed root extracts of two plant species for rotenone and three rotenoids using C_{18} reversed-phase l.c. with gradient elution.

Ion-pair chromatography was used by Brown and Sleeman (1977) to determine N,N′-trimethylene-bis-(pyridinium-4-aldoxime) dibromide, a therapeutic reactivator of organophosphate-inhibited cholinesterase. Their mobile phase consisted of 0·01 M 1-heptanesulphonic acid mixed with acetonitrile. U.v. detection at 254 nm achieved a limit of 1 ng.

Analysis of the insecticide synergist, piperonyl butoxide, has been reported in formulations (Bushway *et al*, 1975b) and in cereal crops (Isshiki *et al*, 1977). Phenothiazine has also been analysed in formulations (Byrne, 1976).

Herbicides

Phenoxyalkanoic acids

Eisenbeiss and Sieper (1973) reported a limit of detection of 5 ng for 2,4-D by u.v. at 278 nm and good resolution of 2,4-D, dichlorprop, MCPB, MCPA, and 2,4,5-T. Skelly *et al* (1976, 1977) reported an analytical method for 2,4-D in various formulations using either a reversed-phase microparticulate packing or a strong cation-exchange resin. Esters of 2,4-D could also be analysed by the same method if l.c. were preceded by *in situ* saponification. An important practical observation by Skelly *et al* (1977) was that formulation analysis needed a precolumn to retain original analytical column performance and extend the usable column lifetime from 1 week to 1–2 months of continuous use. Ross *et al* (1977) assayed for N-nitrosodimethylamine with a thermal energy analyser detector in formulations of several phenoxyalkanoic herbicides, including 2,4-D

Table 6 LC conditions for pyrethroids

Compound	Mobile phase	Detector	Column	Reference
Cypermethrin (NRDC-149)	I. 20% CH_2Cl_2 (50% H_2O satd) in pet. ether (also NRDC-159 and 160)	UV, radio. count fract.	Partisil-5 (5 μm)	193
m-Phenoxybenzoic acid	II. 5% EtOH+0·5% HOAc in pet. ether	UV, radio. count fract.	Partisil-5	193
Dichlorovinyl dimethylcyclo-propanecarboxylic acid	III. 1% dioxane+0·1% HOAc in pet. ether	UV, radio. count fract.	Partisil-5	193
Permethrin (*trans* and *cis*)	IV. 0·0017% MeCN in $CHCl_3$: hexane (1 : 53)	UV	silica gel (10 μm); sodium or silver aluminosilicate	127
Pyrethrins	V. MeOH : H_2O (30–100 : 70–0 grad.)	UV	Permaphase ODS	28
	VI. CH_2Cl_2	UV	silica gel (10 μm)	30

Compound	Solvent system	Detection	Column	Ref.
Resmethrin 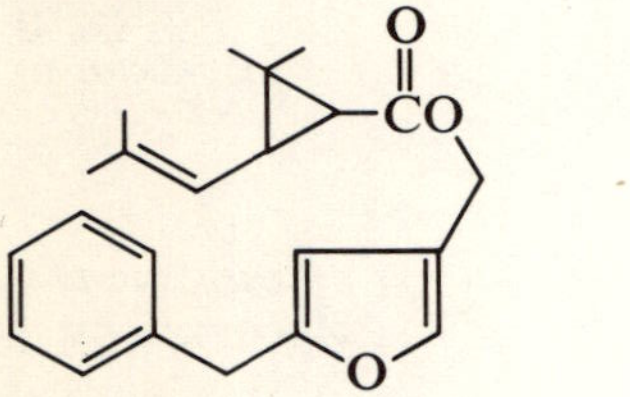	VII. MeOH : H$_2$O (55 : 45, 50 : 50)	UV	Permaphase ODS	260
WL 41706 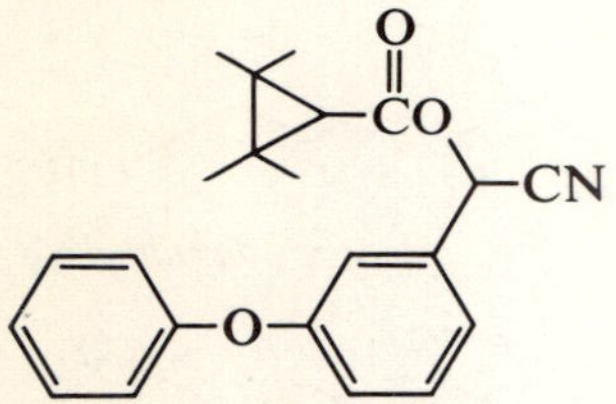	VIII. EtOH : HOAc : pet. ether (10 : 0·1 : 89·9 for 5 μm, 25 : 1 : 74 for 10 μm); for metabolites only: CN→CONH$_2$, *m*-phenoxybenzoic acid, tetramethylcyclopropane-carboxylic acid	radio. monitor	Partisil-5-NH$_2$ (5 μm); Partisil-10-NH$_2$ (10 μm)	194
Tetramethylcyclopropanecarboxylic acid; Hydroxymethyltrimethylcyclo-propanecarboxylic acid	IX. hexane : EtOH : HOAc (98 : 2 : 0·01)	radio. monitor	Partisil-5-NH$_2$	38
Hydroxymethyl-WL 41706	X. hexane : MeOH (97 : 3)	UV, radio. monitor	Partisil-5	38

Table 7 LC conditions for insect growth regulators

Compound	Mobile phase	Detector	Column	Reference
Diflubenzuron (Dimilin™)	MeOH : H_2O (1 : 1)	UV	Permaphase ODS	35, 155
	MeCN : H_2O (57 : 43)	UV	μBondapak C_{18}	159
	MeCN : H_2O (70 : 30)	UV	MicroPak-CH	199
	MeOH : H_2O (60 : 40)	UV	MicroPak-CH	198
Ro 10-3108	3 % MeOH in hexane (for diol and 2 rearranged allylic alcohol metabolites only)	—	silica gel (8 μm)	45
Methoprene (Altosid™)	MeOH : H_2O (75 : 25)	UV	Permaphase ODS	72
	hexane : THF (20 : 1)	UV	Porasil A	90
	hexane : THF (99 : 1)	UV	μPorasil	90
	6·5 % ether in pentane	UV	LiChrosorb SI 60 (10 μm)	202
	4 % ether in pentane	UV	Corasil II	202
	MeOH : H_2O (60 : 40)	UV	Vydac RP	180
	MeOH : H_2O (75 : 25)	UV	Zorbax ODS	181, 182
(also metabolites)	CH_2Cl_2	UV	Bio-Beads S-X2	177, 179
hydroxy-ester	MeOH : H_2O (65 : 35)	UV	Corasil/C_{18}	202, 203
	MeOH : H_2O (60 : 40)	UV	Zorbax ODS	180
	MeOH : H_2O (75 : 25)	UV	Zorbax ODS	181, 182
	MeOH : H_2O (75 : 25)	UV	Permaphase ODS	72
hydroxy-acid				
(free)	MeOH : H_2O (40 : 60)	UV	Corasil/C_{18}	202
(methyl ester)	MeOH : H_2O (60 : 40)	UV	Vydac RP	180

(methyl ester)	MeOH : H_2O (75 : 25)	UV	Vydac RP	181
(methyl ester)	MeOH : H_2O (75 : 25)	UV	Permaphase ODS	72
satd hydroxy-acid (as methyl ester)	MeOH : H_2O (90 : 10)	UV, radio.	Zorbax ODS	181
	ether : pentane (25 : 75)	count	Zorbax SIL	181
methoxy-acid				
(free)	MeOH : H_2O (45 : 55)	UV	Corasil/C_{18}	202
(methyl ester)	MeOH : H_2O (60 : 40)	UV	Vydac RP	180
(methyl ester)	MeOH : H_2O (75 : 25)	UV	Zorbax ODS	181
(methyl ester)	MeOH : H_2O (75 : 25)	UV	Permaphase ODS	72
satd methoxy-acid (as methyl ester)	MeOH : H_2O (90 : 10)	UV, radio.	Zorbax ODS	181
	6·5% ether in pentane	count	Zorbax-SIL	181
satd methoxy-acid + *cholesterol*	5% ether in pentane	radio. count	Zorbax-SIL	181
Methoxycitronellal	10% ether in pentane	radio. count	LiChrosorb SI 60 (10 μm)	177
Hydroxycitronellic acid (methyl ester)	ether : pentane (1 : 1)	RI	LiChrosorb SI 60 (20 μm)	177
Methoxycitronellic acid	grad. 0–100% MeOH in H_2O	radio. count	Poragel PN	202
	30–40% MeOH in H_2O	radio. count	Corasil/C_{18}	202
Natural product metabolites				
Cholesterol	25% ether in pentane	UV	LiChrosorb SI 60	178
Cholesteryl benzoate	0·5% ether in pentane	UV	LiChrosorb SI 60	178
Cholic and deoxycholic acid (benzoylated)	15–30% ether in pentane	UV	LiChrosorb SI 60	178

Table 8 LC conditions for miscellaneous insecticides, acaricides and related compounds

Compound	Mobile phase	Detector	Column	Reference
Azobenzene	I. 29 and 50% aq. MeOH or EtOH	UV	Vydac RP	206
Binapacryl	II. MeCN : H_2O (25–75 : 75–25)	UV 220	LiChrosorb RP-18	213
Chlorbenside	III. cyclohexane (also II)	—	Bio-Beads S-X2	68, 213
Cycloprate (Zardex™)	IV. MeOH : H_2O (90 : 10)	RI	μBondapak C_{18}	183, 184, 185, 186
Metabolites				
14(11cPr) : 0, 16(13cPr) : 0, 18(15cPr) : 0 (as methyl esters)	V. MeOH : H_2O (85–90 : 15–10)	RI	μBondapak C_{18}	183, 184, 185, 186
	VI. ether : hexane (0·5 : 99·5)	RI	Zorbax-SIL	183
8(5cPr) : 0, 10(7cPr) : 0, 12(9cPr) : 0, 14(11cPr) : 0 (as methyl esters)	VII. MeOH : H_2O (80 : 20)	RI	μBondapak C_{18}	185
18(15cPr) : 1 (as methyl ester)	VIII. MeOH : H_2O (87·5 : 12·5)	RI	μBondapak C_{18}	184

Compound	Eluent	Detection	Column	Ref.
CPCA-gly (as *p*-phenylphenacyl ester)	IX. ether : pentane (70 : 30)	UV	Zorbax-SIL	183, 185
	X. MeOH : H_2O (55 : 45)	UV	μBondapak C_{18}	183, 184, 185, 186
CPCA-carnitine	XI. 100% H_2O	RI	μBondapak C_{18}	183, 184, 185, 186
	XII. MeOH	RI, radio. count	Sephadex LH-20	186
CPCA (as *p*-phenylphenacyl ester)	XIII. MeOH : H_2O (70 : 30)	UV	μBondapak C_{18}	183, 184, 185, 186
	XIV. ether : pentane (10 : 90)	UV	Zorbax-SIL	184
Dinocap (Karathane™)	XV. $CHCl_3$: isooctane (25 : 75)	UV 294	Corasil II, μPorasil	21
	XVI. CH_2Cl_2	UV	Silica gel (10 μm)	30

$$H_{17}C_8-\!\!\!\overset{\displaystyle NO_2}{\underset{\displaystyle NO_2}{\bigcirc}}\!\!\!-O\overset{O}{\overset{\|}{C}}-CH=CHMe$$

Compound	Eluent	Detection	Column	Ref.
Ovex (Chlorfenson)	II, III			68, 213

$$Cl-\bigcirc-OSO_2-\bigcirc-Cl$$

Compound	Eluent	Detection	Column	Ref.
Phenothiazine	XVII. MeOH : H_2O (1 : 1)	UV	Vydac RP	26

(Phenothiazine structure: dibenzothiazine, S at top, N–H at bottom)

Compound	Eluent	Detection	Column	Ref.
Piperonyl butoxide	XVIII. EtOH	fluor., UV 290	Hitachi Gel 3010	94
	XIX. MeOH : H_2O (30–100 : 70–0) (also XV, XVI)	UV	Permaphase ODS	28, 21, 30

Table 8 (*cont.*)

Compound	Mobile phase	Detector	Column	Reference
Propargite (Omite™)	XX. MeOH : H$_2$O (80 : 20) (also XVI)	UV, CEC	Vydac 201 TP RP	30, 42 30
Rotenone	XXI. grad. MeOH : H$_2$O : H$_3$PO$_4$ (60 : 39·9 : 0·1) to (85 : 14·9 : 0·1); also deguelin, dehydrorotenone, rotenolone, dehydrodeguelin, tephrosin	UV	Zorbax ODS	62
	XXII. MeOH : H$_2$O (80 : 20, 60 : 40); also 6αβ,12αβ-rotenolone, β-dihydrorotenone, deguelin, dehydrorotenone, tephrosin	UV 280	C$_{18}$ Corasil, μBondapak C$_{18}$	22
	[also XV (35 : 65 too), deguelin, dihydrorotenone, 6αβ,12αβ-rotenolone, tephrosin, XVI]			21, 30
	XXIII. MeCN : H$_2$O (35 : 65 to 100 : 0 grad.); also deguelin, rotenolone, tephrosin	UV	μBondapak C$_{18}$	154

Tetradifon (Tedion™) 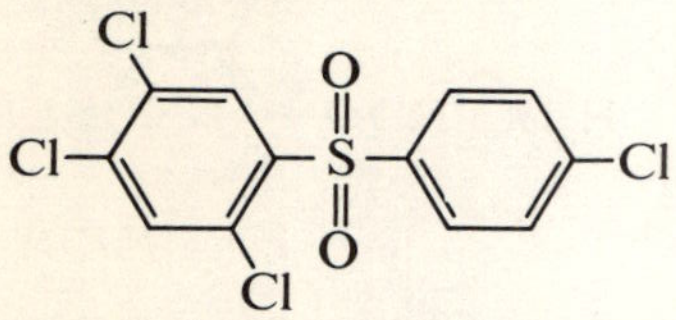	III			68
N,N'-Trimethylene-bis(pyridinium-4-aldoxime) dibromide *TMB-4* 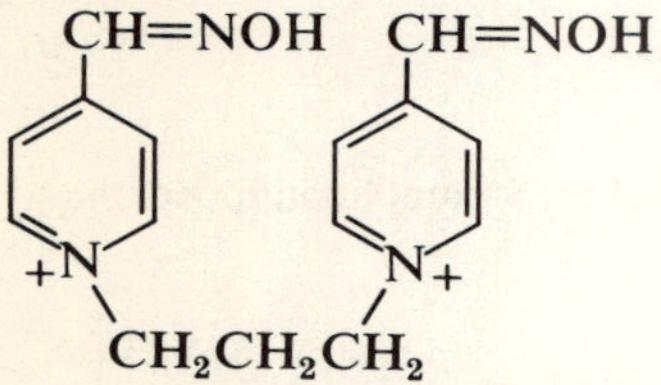	XXIV. MeCN : PIC B-7 (35 : 65)	UV	μBondapak C_{18}	16

Table 9 LC conditions for phenoxyalkanoic acids

Compound	Mobile phase	Detector	Column	Reference
2,4-D	I. hexane : HOAc (92·5 : 7·5)	UV 254, 278	Perisorb A	49, 59
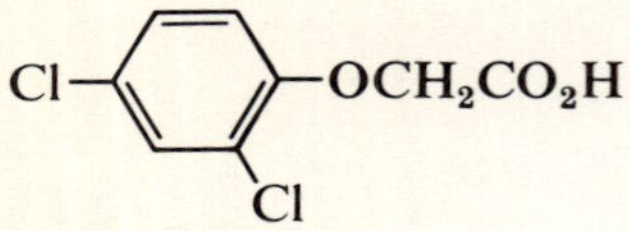 Cl—⬡—OCH₂CO₂H (Cl)	II. 5% isoPrOH in heptane	UV	Permaphase ODS	201
	III. 0·01 M sodium tetraborate + 0·002 M sodium perchlorate	UV 280	Zipax SAX	217
	IV. MeOH : H₂O (80 : 20)	UV, CEC	Vydac 201 TP RP	217
(also Me ester)	V. MeCN : H₂O (20 : 80, pH 3)	UV 280	Partisil ODS (10–25 μm)	218
(also isopropyl, isobutyl, and ethylhexyl esters)	VI. MeOH : H₂O (60 : 40)	UV	Permaphase ODS	201
(as Me, isoPr, Bu, propylene glycol, butoxyethanol, isooctyl, and ethylhexyl esters)	VII. toluene : EtOAc (1 : 3)	glc fract.	Bio-Beads S-X3	98
	VIII. MeCN : H₂O : NH₃ (30 : 70 : 0·6) to (50 : 50 : 0·6)	UV	Spherisorb ODS	213
N-Nitrosodimethylamine (impurity)	IX. CH₂Cl₂ : hexane (1 : 1)	therm. energy, UV	μNH₂	197
Dichlorprop	X. MeCN : H₂O (25–75 : 75–25) (also I)	UV 220	LiChrosorb RP-18	213 49
MCPA 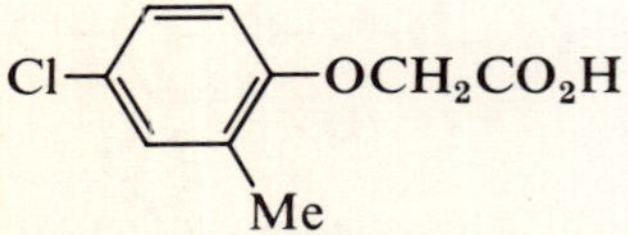	I			49, 59

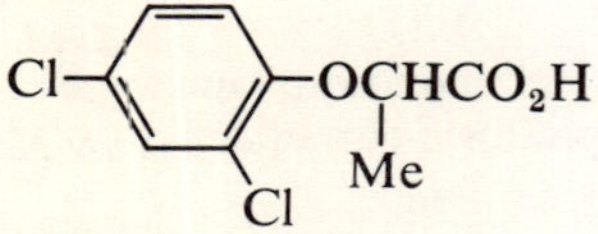

Compound	Method	Ref.
N-Nitrosodimethylamine (impurity)	IX	197
MCPB 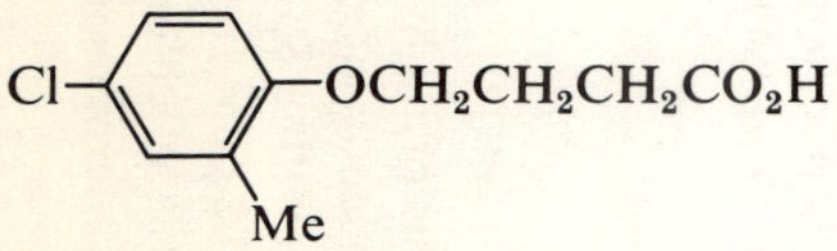	I	49

Cl—⟨benzene ring, Me⟩—$OCH_2CH_2CH_2CO_2H$

| *Silvex* (Fenoprop) 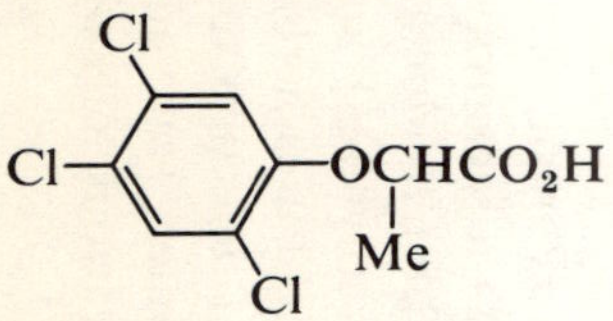 | V, VII (as propylene glycol, methyl esters) | 98, 218 |

Cl, Cl, Cl—⟨benzene ring⟩—$OCHCO_2H$ (Me)

| 2,4,5-*T* 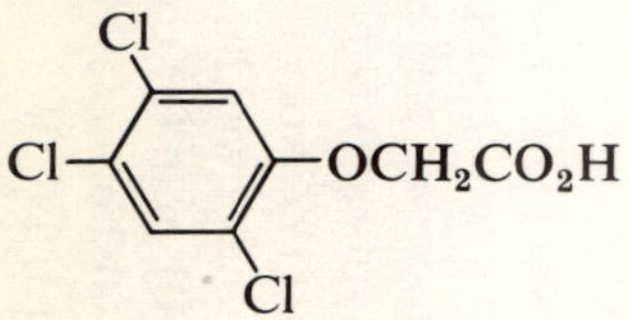 | I, V (as Me ester), VII (as Me, isoPr, Bu, ethylhexyl, isooctyl esters) | 49, 98, 218 |

Cl, Cl, Cl—⟨benzene ring⟩—OCH_2CO_2H

| 2,3,5-*T* | XI. MeCN : H_2O (50 : 50) | UV 250 | Partisil ODS | 166 |
| 2,4,6-*T* | V | | | 218 |

and MCPA. Since N-nitrosodimethylamine is a suspected carcinogen and also present at 0·06% in some herbicides formulated for home use, the utility of this l.c. method is evident.

Triazines

A comprehensive comparison of the relative merits of g.l.c., h.p.l.c., t.l.c., and high-performance t.l.c. was presented by Jork and Roth (1977). The limits of detection for 14 *s*-triazine herbicides by these analytical methods were 0·02–0·03 ng (g.l.c. with alkali flame ionization detection), 1 ng (h.p.l.c. with u.v. detection), 8–13 ng (t.l.c., u.v. detection), and 3–5 ng (h.p.t.l.c., u.v. detection). A comparison of the selectivity of microparticulate silica (Partisil-5) and bonded-phase (NH_2) packings was given by Self *et al* (1975) who showed good resolution of five *s*-triazines on both columns (figure 12). Burkhard and Guth (1976) used l.c. to monitor the acetone-sensitized photodegradation of atrazine, atraton, and ametryne. Hydroxytriazines formed during photolysis were determined directly in aqueous solutions using Sil-X for separation and u.v. detection.

Residue analysis. Byast and coworkers have analysed *s*-triazine residues in water by l.c. Byast (1975) detected as little as 1 ppb of cyanatryn in three environmental water samples. Byast and Cotterill (1975) concluded that l.c. and g.l.c. were equally useful in detection of terbutryne residues in water. The limit for both methods was 1 ppb for a twice-background detector response. Byast (1977) also could detect 0·05 ppm residues of triazines in soil. Fine *et al* (1976) used thermal energy detection for trace analysis of picogram amounts of N-nitrosoatrazine in vodka.

Substituted ureas

Separation of urea herbicides by l.c. is of historical interest as they were the subject of one of the first modern l.c. applications published by Kirkland (Kirkland, 1968; Done *et al*, 1972). L.c. analysis of substituted ureas is especially advantageous because of their inherent thermal instability on g.l.c. analysis. Several groups have demonstrated good separations of urea herbicide mixtures (Gonnet and Rocca, 1975; Pribyl and Herzel, 1976; Subach *et al*, 1976; Aten and Bourke, 1977; Byast, 1977).

Residue analysis. Selim *et al* (1977) used a μPorasil column to detect residues of karbutilate in water, soil, and grasses with a sensitivity limit of 0·01, 0·1, and 0·1 ppm, respectively. L.c. was also useful for residue analysis of its hydrolysis product [N′-(3-hydroxyphenyl)-N,N′-dimethylurea] and demethylated metabolites. Farrington *et al* (1977) resolved eight urea herbicides with a Spherisorb ODS column. They found lower limits of detection to be 0·2 ppm for wheat, 0·2 ppm for soil, and 0·01 ppm for river water. Trace quantities of chlortoluron were assayed at the 0·1–0·2 ppm level in various soils with a Merckosorb SI 60 column (Smith and Lord, 1975).

L.c. is quite applicable to analysis of urea herbicides in food crops. Lawrence (1976b) found 3 ng sensitivity for linuron in cabbage and wheat. Lawrence (1976a) also used a silica (5 μm) column for direct analysis of seven substituted ureas. All these herbicides were easily detectable at 0·1 ppm in cabbage, corn, potatoes, turnips, and wheat. In some cases even 0·005 ppm could be detected,

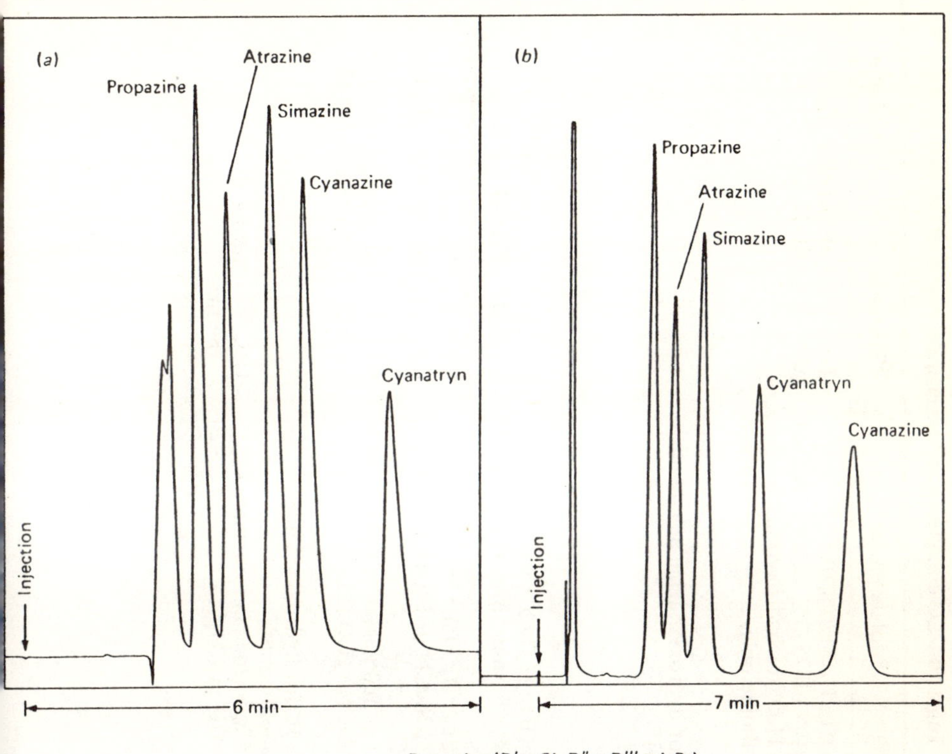

Figure 12 Comparison of selectivity obtained with microparticulate silica and bonded-phase packings in the separation of *s*-triazines: (a) Partisil 5 (5 μm), 100 × 4·5 mm i.d. column, eluted with ether–hexane–methanol (79 : 20 : 1) at 0·9 ml/min; and (b) bonded phase (NH₂), 5 μm, same column and mobile phase except flow rate of 2·3 ml/min, u.v. detection at 230 nm. From Self *et al* (1975), reproduced by permission of the Chemical Society

depending on the food crop and herbicide. Lawrence concluded that l.c. complements g.l.c. in many respects for direct pesticide analysis using the same clean-up procedures for both detection systems.

Formulations and metabolism. Kennedy (1977) used l.c. on μBondapak C₁₈ as a rapid, selective method to monitor the manufacturing process for tebuthiuron.

Table 10 LC conditions for *s*-triazines

Compound	Mobile phase	Detector	Column	Reference
Ametryn	I. MeOH : H$_2$O (70 : 30)	UV	μBondapak C$_{18}$	99
	II. MeCN + 0·75–2% of both HCO$_2$H and H$_2$O (for hydroxytriazine metabolite only)	UV	Sil-X	18
Atraton	I, II (for hydroxytriazine metabolite only)			18, 99
Atrazine	III. MeOH : H$_2$O (20 : 80)	UV 220	C$_{18}$ Sil-X-II	24
	IV. ether : hexane : MeOH (79 : 20 : 1)	UV 230	Partisil 5 (5 μm), 3-aminopropyl silica	208
	V. MeCN : H$_2$O (50 : 50)	UV 265	Partisil ODS	166
	VI. 90% MeCN or EtOH in H$_2$O, 70 °C	UV	pyrocarbon–silica	73
	VII. 80 or 100% MeCN in H$_2$O, 55 °C	UV	graphitized carbon	73
	VIII. MeCN : H$_2$O (25–75 : 75–25 grad.)	UV 220	LiChrosorb RP-18	213
	[also I, II (for hydroxytriazine metabolite only)]			18, 99
N-Nitrosoatrazine	IX. 1–5% acetone in isooctane, 1% isoPrOH in CH$_2$Cl$_2$	UV, therm. energy	μPorasil	58
Desmetryn (X = SMe, R$_1$ = R$_3$ = H, R$_2$ = isoPr, R$_4$ = Me)	I			99

Compound	Method	Detection	Column	Ref.
Chlorazine (X = Cl, R_1 = R_2 = R_3 = R_4 = Et)	I			99
Cyanatryn (X = SMe, R_1 = R_3 = H, R_2 = Et, R_3 = C(Me)$_2$CN)	X. MeOH : H$_2$O (12·5 : 87·5) (also III, IV)	UV	Permaphase ETH	23 24, 208
Cyanazine (X = Cl, R_1 = R_3 = H, R_2 = Et, R_4 = C(Me)$_2$CN)	IV			208
Ipazine (X = Cl, R_1 = H, R_2 = isoPr, R_3 = R_4 = Et)	I			99
Norazine (X = Cl, R_1 = R_3 = H, R_2 = isoPr, R_4 = Me)	I			99
Prometon (X = OMe, R_1 = R_3 = H, R_2 = R_4 = isoPr)	I			99
Prometryn (X = SMe, R_1 = R_3 = H, R_2 = R_4 = isoPr)	I			99
Propazine (X = Cl, R_1 = R_3 = H, R_2 = R_4 = isoPr)	I, IV			99, 208
Simazine (X = Cl, R_1 = R_3 = H, R_2 = R_4 = Et)	I, III, IV			24, 99, 208
Simeton (X = OMe, R_1 = R_3 = H, R_2 = R_4 = Et)	I			99
Simetryn (X = SMe, R_1 = R_3 = H, R_2 = R_4 = Et)	I			99
Terbutryne (X = SMe, R_1 = R_3 = H, R_2 = tertBu, R_4 = Et)	XI. MeOH : H$_2$O (20 : 80) (also III at 227 nm)	UV	Permaphase ETH	25 24
Trietazine (X = Cl, R_1 = H, R_2 = R_3 = R_4 = Et)	I			99

72

L.c. analysis was not prone to interference problems as were encountered with g.l.c. analysis of the trifluoroacetyl derivative. Sidwell and Ruzicka (1976) compared a LiChrosorb SI 60 column with a C_{18}-bonded silica column in the determination of phenylurea herbicides and production impurities. The resolution of ten such substituted ureas is shown in figure 13.

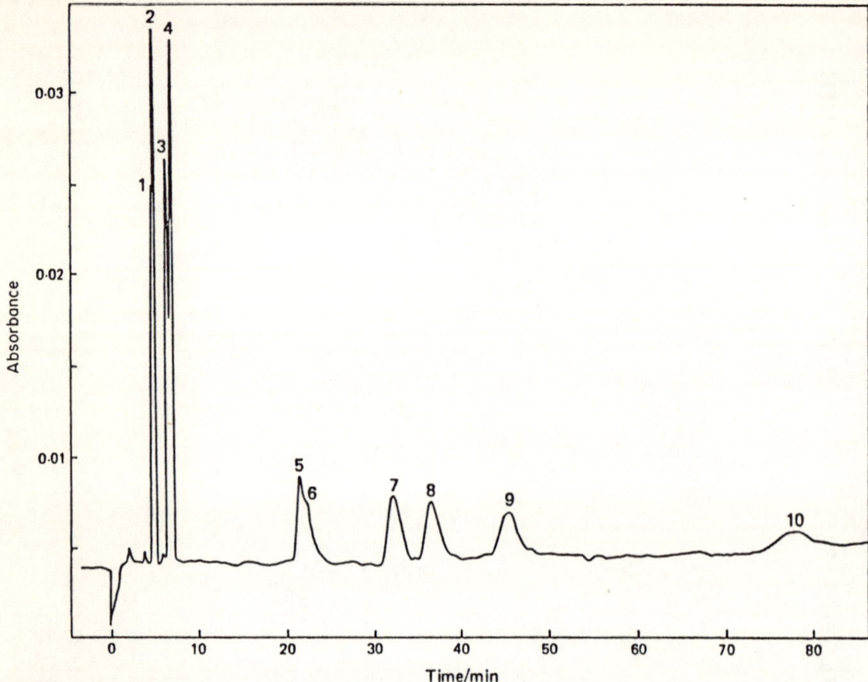

Figure 13 Separation of urea herbicides on a microparticulate (5 μm) silica column: (1) chlorbromuron, (2) linuron, (3) monolinuron, (4) metobromuron, (5) methabenzthiazuron, (6) diuron, (7) chlortoluron, (8) monuron, (9) chloroxuron, and (10) metoxuron. Mobile phase, dichloromethane at a flow rate of 1·2 ml/min. From Sidwell and Ruzicka (1976), reproduced by permission of the Chemical Society

Mittelstaedt *et al* (1977) used a combination of l.c. techniques to follow the fate of methabenzthiazuron in soil. The major demethylated metabolite was first isolated by g.p.c. on μStyragel, then further concentrated and purified with μBondapak and μPorasil columns. Comparative l.c. behaviour of several other potential metabolites was presented.

Dinitroanilines

Formulations. Kennedy (1977) found that reversed-phase l.c. on μBondapak C_{18} provided the best separation for oryzalin and its suspected chemical impurities from manufacturing processes. Kennedy's l.c. method was also useful for trifluralin and ethalfluralin. Ross *et al* (1977) detected N-nitrosodipropylamine impurities in trifluralin formulations with a thermal energy analyser after l.c. separation on a μNH$_2$ column.

Metabolism. Kearney *et al* (1974, 1976) reported the effective use of l.c. to monitor the persistence and metabolism of seven dinitroaniline herbicides in soil. Using Permaphase ODS eluted with methanol–water mixtures, a variety of dealkylated and imidazole metabolites were separated with good resolution. L.c. was particularly useful in metabolite purification prior to m.s. analysis as also demonstrated by Golab *et al* (1975) in studying the fate of oryzalin in soil and plants. Heck *et al* (1977) studied the metabolism of trifluralin in rats with the aid of l.c. Extracts of fat, liver, faeces, and plasma were initially subjected to clean-up via g.p.c. on μStyragel. Heck *et al* (1977) found microparticulate g.p.c. to be more efficient than conventional g.p.c. on Bio-Beads or Sephadex LH-20 gels. Subsequent purification of trifluralin metabolites on μBondapak C_{18} allowed quantitation by field ionization m.s.

Uracils and thiocarbamates

The resolution of substituted uracils by reversed-phase l.c. on C_{18} Sil-X-I was reported by Byast (1977). Lawrence (1976b) could detect terbacil at 0·2 ppm in corn and potatoes with u.v. detection sensitive to as little as 10 ng.

Sparacino and Hines (1976) explored a variety of columns and solvent compositions for thiocarbamate analysis. The resolution of thiocarbamate herbicides from carbamate insecticides is depicted in figure 8.

Acylanilines and N-phenylcarbamates

The most actively studied compounds in these groups are propham and chlorpropham. A relative comparison of the l.c. behaviour on μBondapak C_{18} for these N-phenylcarbamates (carbanilates) is shown in figure 8 (Sparacino and Hines, 1976). A residue method for chlorpropham in onions at 0·05 ppm has been reported (Katayama, 1976). The photolysis of chlorpropham and formation of its major aqueous photoproduct, isopropyl 3-hydroxycarbanilate, was followed using Zorbax ODS (Guzik, 1978).

Workers at the U.S.D.A. laboratory in Fargo, N.D., have repeatedly used l.c. as an integral tool in their metabolic studies. Still and Rusness (1977) used several l.c. systems to characterize polar metabolites of chlorpropham in oats, including S-cysteinyl-hydroxychlorpropham, 4-O-glucosylchlorpropham, and methoxychlorpropham disulphide. Paulson *et al* (1973) used Permaphase ETH to resolve goat urine metabolites of propham; thus, a sulphate ester of 2-hydroxyaniline and an unknown conjugate of 4-hydroxyaniline were identified. Still and Mansager (1975) characterized 2- and 4-acetoxypropham as alfalfa metabolites (after acetylation).

Lawrence (1976b) presented a residue method using LiChrosorb SI 60 for benzoylprop-ethyl in corn. The limit of detection was 0·2 ppm or 10 ng.

Miscellaneous herbicides

Formulations. Skelly *et al* (1976) reported the results of a collaborative study of picloram analysis with Zipax SAX. Betker *et al* (1976) used l.c. to compare the

Table 11 LC conditions for substituted ureas

Compound	Mobile phase	Detector	Column	Reference
Chlorbromuron	I. isoPrOH : isooctane (20 : 80, 10 : 90)	UV	LiChrosorb SI 60 (5 μm)	131
	II. MeOH : H_2O (1 : 1, 1 : 2); MeCN; MeOH; isoPrOH; isoPrOH : hexane (1 : 1)	UV	Partisil-10 ODS	4
	III. CH_2Cl_2	UV 240, 245	LiChrosorb SI 60 (5 μm)	214
	IV. MeOH : H_2O : NH_3 (60 : 40 : 0·6)	UV 240	Spherisorb ODS	54, 213
	V. MeOH : H_2O (60 : 40)	UV 240, 245	C_{18} on LiChrosorb SI 60	214
	VI. MeOH : H_2O (65 : 35)	UV 240, 245	C_{18} on LiChrosorb SI 60	214
Chloroxuron	VII. MeCN : H_2O (25–75 : 75–25 grad.)	UV 220	LiChrosorb RP-18	213
	VIII. 1 % MeOH in CH_2Cl_2	UV 240, 245	LiChrosorb SI 60 (5 μm)	214
	IX. MeOH : H_2O (70 : 30)	UV 240, 245	C_{18} on LiChrosorb SI 60	214
	(also I, III, IV)			54, 131, 213, 214
Chlortoluron	X. 15–20 % MeOH in H_2O	UV 215	C_{18} Sil-X-II	24
	XI. 15 % isoPrOH in hexane	UV 240	Merckosorb SI 60 (10 μm)	220
	XII. 0·5–0·6 % MeOH in CH_2Cl_2	UV 240, 245	LiChrosorb SI 60 (5 μm)	214
	(also III, IV, VI, VIII)			54, 213, 214
Demethylchlortoluron	VIII, X			24, 214
Didemethylchlortoluron	X			24
3-Chloro-4-methylaniline; 1,3-Bis(3-chloro-4-methylphenyl)urea; 3-(4-Methylphenyl)-1,1-dimethylurea	VIII			214

Compound	Conditions	Detection	Column	Ref.
Diuron	XIII. butyl ether	UV	1 % ODPN on Zipax	44
	XIV. butyl ether	UV	4 % ODPN on Gas Chrom P	107
	XV. hexane : CH_2Cl_2 : EtOH (20 : 79 : 1)	UV 247	LiChrosorb SI 60	174
	XVI. butyl ether	UV	1 % ODPN on CSP support	108
	XVII. CH_2Cl_2 (H_2O satd); CH_2Cl_2 : isoPrOH (98·5 : 1·5)	UV	LiChrosorb SI 60 (5 μm)	67
	XVIII. 1 % dioxane in hexane; MeOH : H_2O (35 : 65)	UV	Permaphase ETH	112
	XIX. acetone : hexane (50 : 50) (also I–VI, XII)	UV	LiChrosorb SI 60 (5 μm)	131
				4, 54, 131, 213, 214
Fenuron	I, XIII–XVI, XVIII (1 % dioxane in hexane only)			44, 107, 108, 112, 131, 174
Fluormeturon	XX. MeCN : H_2O (80–10 : 20–90 grad.); also other trifluorotolylureas (also I, II)	UV	Bondapak C_{18}/Corasil (37–50 μm)	231
				4, 131
Isoproturon	XXI. CH_2Cl_2 : isoPrOH (85 : 15) +1 % HOAc	UV	LiChrosorb SI 60 (5 μm)	67
	[also XVII, X (20 % only, 240 nm)]			24, 67
Mono- and didemethylisoproturon	XXI			67

Table 11 (*cont.*)

Compound	Mobile phase	Detector	Column	Reference
Karbutilate (Tandex™)	XXII. 5% THF in heptane	UV	1% ODPN on Zipax	201
	XXIII. 3% EtOH in ethylene chloride	UV	μPorasil	210
m-Aminophenol	XXII			201
Didemethylkarbutilate	XXIV. 7% EtOH in ethylene chloride	UV	μPorasil	210
N′-(3-Hydroxyphenyl)-N,N-dimethylurea	XXV. EtOH : MeCN : ethylene chloride (3 : 10 : 87) (also XXIII)	UV	μPorasil	210
N′-(3-Hydroxyphenyl)-N-methylurea	XXV			210
Demethylkarbutilate	XXIII			210
Linuron	XXVI. acetone : hexane (15 : 85)	UV	LiChrosorb SI 60 (5 μm)	210
	XXVII. MeOH : H₂O (35 : 65)	UV	Permaphase ETH	131
	XXVIII. 10% isoPrOH in isooctane	UV	LiChrosorb SI 60 (5 μm)	112
				132
(dansyl der.)	XXIX. 5% MeOH in hexane [also I (5 : 95 too), II–VI, X (20% only, 250 nm), XII–XIV, XVI, XVII]	fluor.	0·5% ODPN on Zipax	60 4, 24, 44, 54, 67, 107, 108, 131, 213, 214
3,4-Dichloroaniline; 1,3-Bis(3,4-dichlorophenyl)urea; Methyl 3,4-Dichlorophenylcarbamate	III			214

Compound	Solvent / conditions	Detection	Column	Ref.
Methabenzthiazuron	XXX. CHCl$_3$	UV	μStyragel	153
	XXXI. 15–100% MeCN in H$_2$O	UV	μBondapak C$_{18}$	153
	XXXII. CHCl$_3$	UV	μPorasil	153
	[also III, VI, X (20% only, 225 nm), XII, XV]			24, 174, 214
Demethyl metabolite	XXX, XXXI, XXXII			153
2-Aminobenzthiazole; 7-hydroxy metabolite	XXXI, XXXII			153
Metobromuron	III–V, XV			54, 174, 213, 214
Metoxuron	III, V, VIII, XII			214
3-Chloro-4- methoxyaniline; 1,3-Bis(3-chloro-4-methoxyphenyl) urea; 3-(4-Methoxyphenyl)-1,1-dimethylurea; N-Dimethylmetoxuron	VIII			214
Monolinuron	III–V			213, 214
Monuron	I–V, VIII, X (20% only, 250 nm) XII–XIX			4, 24, 44, 54, 67, 107, 108, 112, 131, 174, 213, 214

Table 11 (*cont.*)

Compound	Mobile phase	Detector	Column	Reference
4-Chloroaniline	VIII, XV			174, 214
1,3-Bis(4-chlorophenyl)urea	VIII			214
Neburon	XVII, XVIII			67, 112
Phenobenzuron	XVII			67
Tebuthiuron	XXXIII. MeCN : H_2O (55 : 45); MeCN : MeOH : H_2O (30 : 28 : 42)	UV	μBondapak C_{18}	104
	XXXIV. 1% MeOH in butyl chloride	UV	μBondapak CN	104

Table 12 LC conditions for dinitroanilines

Compound	Mobile phase	Detector	Column	Reference
Dibutalin (Butralin)	I. MeOH : H_2O (50 : 50) (also N-debutyldibutalin, denitrodibutalin)	UV	Permaphase ODS	103
	II. MeOH : H_2O (60 : 40) (also 4-*tert*-butyl-2,6-dinitroaniline with MeOH : H_2O (40 : 60)	UV	Permaphase ODS	102
Dinitramine	I (also deethyl- and dideethyl-dinitramine, imidazole metabolites with MeOH : H_2O, 30 : 70)			103
Ethalfluralin	III. MeCN : MeOH : H_2O (30 : 28 : 42)	UV	μBondapak C_{18}	104

Table 12 (*cont.*)

Compound	Mobile phase	Detector	Column	Reference
Fluchloralin 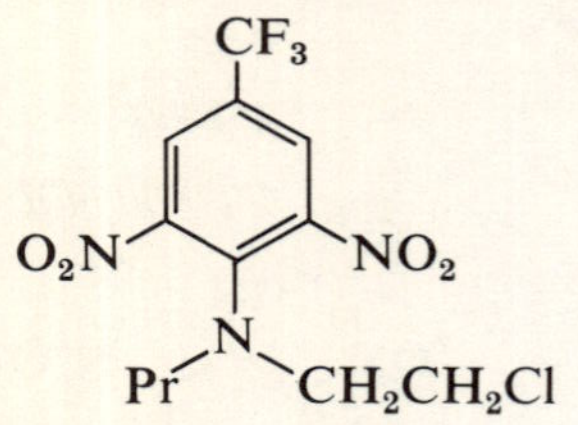	I (also depropylfluchloralin)			103
Chlornidine 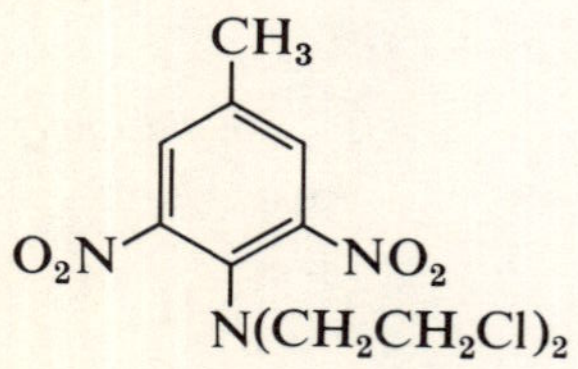	I (also didechloroethylchlornidine)			103
Oryzalin 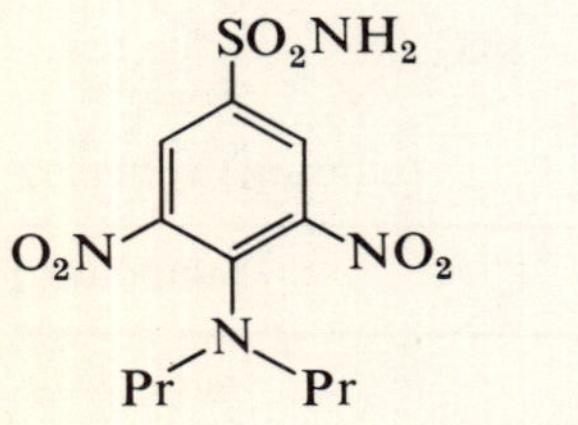	IV. MeCN : H_2O (55 : 45); MeCN : MeOH : H_2O (30 : 28 : 42) (also depropyloryzalin)	UV	μBondapak C_{18}	104
	V. heptane : isoPrOH (95 : 5); (also depropyloryzalin; 3,5-dinitro-N,N-dipropylsulphanilic acid; several benzimidazoles)			66

Compound					
Profluralin	I (also depropylprofluralin)				103
Trifluralin (Treflan™)	VI. 29 and 50% aq. MeOH or EtOH		UV	Vydac RP	206
	VII. MeCN : H_2O (50 : 50)		UV 270	Partisil ODS	166
	VIII. THF		UV 254, 280	μStyragel	78
	IX. MeOH : H_2O (70 : 30)		UV 254, 280	μBondapak C_{18}	78
	X. MeOH : H_2O (80 : 20) [also I (trifluralin, depropyl- and didepropyltrifluralin) and III]		UV CEC	Vydac 201 TP RP	42 103, 104
Imidazole metabolites	XI. MeOH : H_2O (35–40 : 65–60)		UV	Permaphase ODS	103
N-Nitrosodipropylamine impurity	XII. CH_2Cl_2 : hexane (1 : 1)		therm. energy, UV	μNH$_2$	197

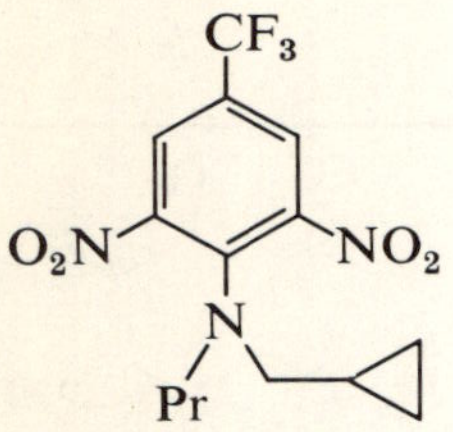

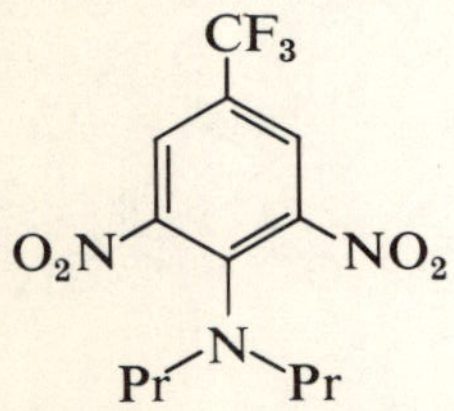

Table 13 LC conditions for substituted uracils

Compound	Mobile phase	Detector	Column	Reference
Lenacil	I. MeOH : H$_2$O (20 : 80)	UV 270	C$_{18}$ Sil-X-II	24
Terbacil	II. 20% isoPrOH in isooctane	UV	LiChrosorb SI 60 (5 μm)	132
	III. MeOH : H$_2$O (10 : 90)	UV 280	C$_{18}$ Sil-X-II	24
Bromacil	III			24

Table 14 LC conditions for thiocarbamates

Compound	Mobile phase	Detector	Column	Reference
Butylate	I. MeCN : H_2O (50 : 50)	UV 220	μBondapak C_{18}	225
	II. 10–30% MeCN in H_2O	UV 220	Permaphase ETH	225
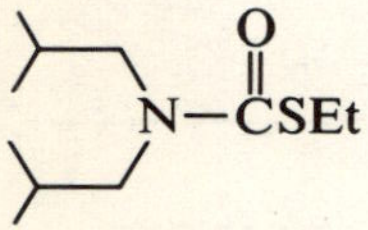	III. 20–60% MeCN in H_2O	UV 220	μBondapak C_{18}	225
Cycloate (Eurex™, Ro-Neet™)	IV. 0·4% isoPrOH in heptane	UV 220	Si-10, CN-10, NH_2-10	225
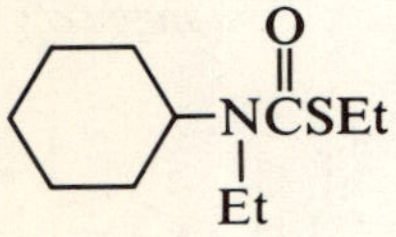	V. MeOH : H_2O (1 : 1, 1 : 2); MeCN; MeOH; isoPrOH; isoPrOH : hexane (1 : 1)	UV	Partisil-10 ODS	4
	(also I–III)			225
Di-allate (Avadex™)	VI. MeCN : H_2O (25–75 : 75–25 grad.)	UV 220	LiChrosorb RP-18	213
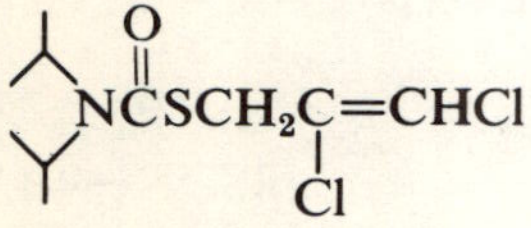	(also I–III)			225
EPTC (Eptam™) 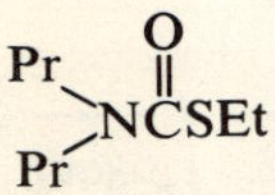	I–III, V			4, 225

Table 14 (*cont.*)

Compound	Mobile phase	Detector	Column	Reference
Pebulate Bu—NCSPr (C=O; N—Et) 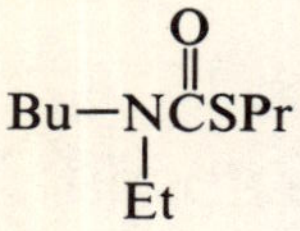	I–III			225
Tri-allate (Avadex™ BW) NCSCH$_2$C=CCl$_2$ (C=O; C—Cl) 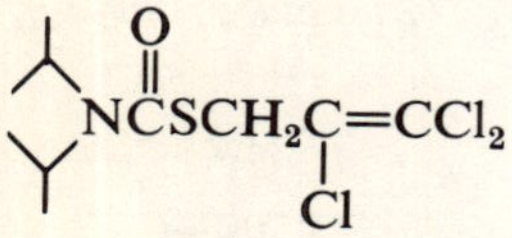	I–III			225
Vernolate Pr$_2$NCSPr (C=O) 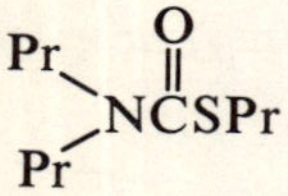	I–III			225

Table 15 LC conditions for acylanilines and N-phenylcarbamates

Compound	Mobile phase	Detector	Column	Reference
Alachlor	I. MeCN : H_2O (1 : 1)	UV 235	Partisil ODS	166
Barban	II. 4% isoPrOH : 96% hexane	UV	Permaphase ETH	155, 237
	III. 20–60% MeCN in H_2O	UV 220	μBondapak C_{18}	225
	IV. MeCN : H_2O (30–50 : 70–50 grad.)	UV	μBondapak C_{18}	155
	V. MeCN : H_2O (25–75 : 75–25 grad.)	UV 220	LiChrosorb RP-18	213
Benzoylpropethyl	VI. 2% isoPrOH in isooctane	UV	LiChrosorb SI 60 (5 μm)	132
Chlorpropham (CIPC)	VII. MeCN : H_2O (56 : 44)	UV	Bondapak C_{18}/Porasil B	229
	VIII. 0·4% isoPrOH in heptane	UV 220	Si-10, CN-10, NH_2-10	225
	IX. 5% MeOH in hexane	fluor.	0·5% ODPN on Zipax	60
	X. MeOH : H_2O (1 : 1, 1 : 2); MeCN; MeOH; isoPrOH; isoPrOH : hexane (1 : 1)	UV	Partisil-10 ODS	4
(also Isopropyl 4-hydroxycarbanilate)	XI. MeOH : H_2O (60 : 40)	UV	Zorbax ODS	71
	XII. hexane : EtOH : ether (93 : 5 : 2) (also III, IV)	UV	Zorbax SIL	100 155, 225

Table 15 (*cont.*)

Compound	Mobile phase	Detector	Column	Reference
4-Hydroxychlorpropham	VII			229
S-Cysteinyl hydroxychlorpropham; 4-O-Glucosylchlorpropham	XIII. MeOH : H$_2$O (26 : 74)	UV	Bondapak C$_{18}$/Porasil B	229
Methoxychlorprophram disulphide	XIV. 22% CHCl$_3$ in hexane	UV	Durapak Carbowax 400/Porasil C	229
Phenmedipham (Betanal™) 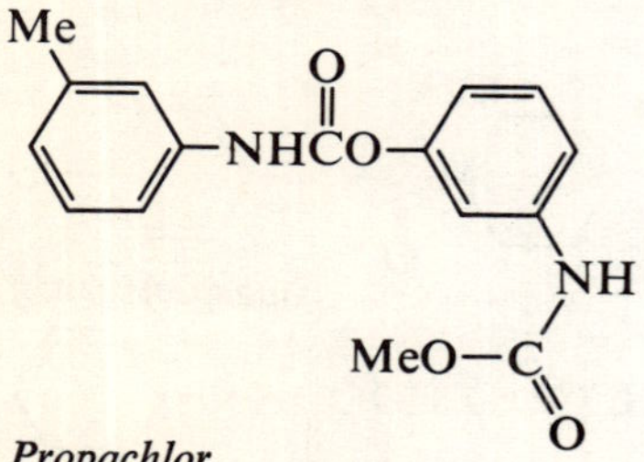	III			225
Propachlor 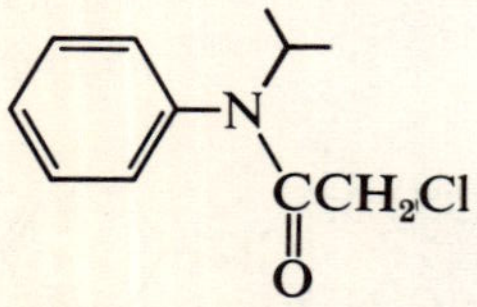	I (260 nm)			166
Propanil 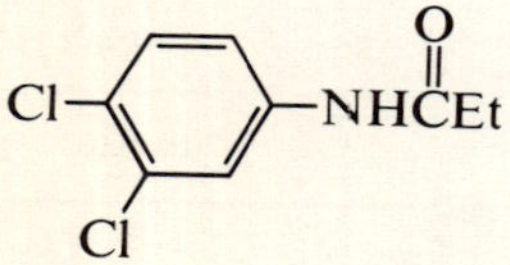	XV. 10% isoPrOH in isooctane	UV	LiChrosorb SI 60 (5 μm)	132

Propham (IPC)	XVI. MeCN : H$_2$O (1 : 1)	UV	μBondapak C$_{18}$, Bondapak C$_{18}$/Porasil B	228
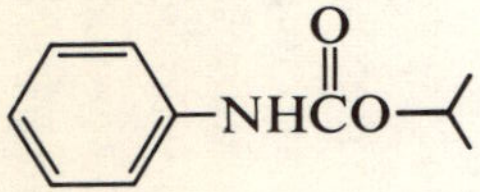	(also III, IV, VIII, IX)			60, 155, 225
2- and 4-Acetoxypropham	XVI			228
2-Hydroxyaniline sulphate ester; 4-Hydroxyaniline as unknown conjugate	XVII. EtOH : hexane (1 : 3)	UV	Permaphase ETH	167
Swep (Nia 2995)	XVIII. 5% isoPrOH in isooctane (also II)	UV	LiChrosorb SI 60 (5 μm)	133 155, 237

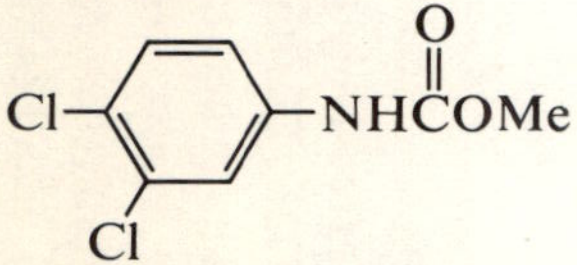

conventional infrared and g.l.c. methods for metribuzin assay. L.c. alone was dubbed as 'more time consuming than g.l.c.' because of longer l.c. retention times. Kawano *et al* (1975) used a Vydac cation-exchange resin for analysis of paraquat formulations.

Metabolism. Krzeminski *et al* (1972) determined the degradation of diphenamid and appearance of N-demethylated metabolites in soya beans by l.c. Lamoureux and Stafford (1977) studied the translocation and metabolism of perfluidone in peanuts. 3-Hydroxyperfluidone and its glucoside were purified by l.c. for subsequent structural verification by m.s.

Residue analysis. In order to improve sensitivity, Selim and Cook (1978) hydrolysed the acetal herbicide, FMC 25213, to propionaldehyde which was derivatized to its 2,4-dinitrophenylhydrazone. This derivative allowed detection of residues in soil and soya beans at 0·025 and 0·1 ppm, respectively. Pryde and Darby (1975) claimed the first silylation of alumina for the purposes of l.c. They assayed for paraquat and diquat in urine at 0·1 ppm.

Fungicides

A summary of the chromatographic analysis of fungicides, including l.c. methods, was given by Sherma (1975).

Imides

Carlstrom (1977) reported a collaborative study of folpet analysis in formulations. A baseline separation of folpet, captan, and captafol was obtained in 7 minutes using a silica gel column (10 μm). Carlstrom (1977) concluded that this l.c. method was more precise than a standard g.l.c. procedure.

Chlorobenzenes

Porcaro and Shubiak (1972) detected nanogram quantities (0·03 ppm) of hexachlorophene in blood samples using a Sil-X silica column and u.v. detection of the *p*-methoxybenzoate diester. Plimmer and Klingebiel (1976) followed the photolysis of hexachlorobenzene under various conditions. Reductive photoproducts such as penta- and tetrachlorobenzene, as well as chlorinated benzyl alcohols, were resolved on a Permaphase ODS column using methanol–water mixtures as the mobile phase.

Imidazoles and thiophanates

Kirkland and coworkers have used l.c. extensively to determine the metabolic fate of benomyl in animals (Kirkland, 1973b; Gardiner *et al*, 1974) and in soil or plant tissues (Kirkland *et al*, 1973). The general analytical procedure consisted of initial hydrolysis followed by l.c. analysis of methyl 2-benzimidazole-carbamate and its 4- or 5-hydroxy metabolites with a Zipax cation-exchange column. This procedure was suitable for residues in cow milk, faeces, urine, and tissues with 0·02, 0·1, 0·2, and 0·1 ppm limits of detection, respectively. These workers demonstrated conclusively (at an early stage of l.c. application development) the usefulness of l.c. for sensitive, selective analysis for pesticide residues and metabolites, particularly those compounds that are not suitable for g.l.c. techniques.

Benomyl and thiabendazole were analysed in plant samples by Maeda and Tsuji (1976) using fluorimetric detection with limits of 0·02 ppm for benomyl (as 2-aminobenzimidazole) and 0·001 ppm for thiabendazole. Austin *et al* (1976) reported comprehensive l.c. data for benomyl, carbendazim, and several related compounds using a variety of normal- and reversed-phase conditions. Farrow *et al* (1977) used both LiChrosorb SI 60 and Spherisorb ODS to determine post-harvest residues of carbendazim, thiabendazole, and thiophanate-methyl in citrus fruit.

Miscellaneous fungicides

Residues of biphenyl and *o*-hydroxybiphenyl in citrus are detectable by l.c. (Reeder, 1974, 1975, 1976; Farrow *et al*, 1977). Davis and Munroe (1977) used a µBondapak C_{18} column to monitor biphenyl residues in impregnated pads of shipping cartons. Cassidy *et al* (1974) derivatized hydroxybiphenyls with dansyl chloride for fluorimetric detection in urine samples.

The thermal decomposition of ethylenebisthiocarbamates to ethylenethiourea (ETU) was monitored with a silanized LiChrosorb SI 60 column by Marshall (1977). A Permaphase ETH column was used by Onley *et al* (1977) to compare l.c. with g.l.c. for the analysis of ETU in vegetable crops, fruits, milk, and cooked foods.

Wolkoff *et al* (1975) analysed carboxin and two of its photoproducts in natural waters. Lawrence (1976b) could detect dicloran at 0·2 ppm in corn. Cox (1976) determined 2-mercaptobenzothiazole in waste dumps.

Rodenticides, Pheromones, and Mycotoxins

Rodenticides

Vanhaelen-Fastre and Vanhaelen (1976) and Van den Berg *et al* (1977) have reported the resolution of several 4-hydroxycoumarin anticoagulants, including warfarin. Most of the l.c. methodology for warfarin relates to drug applications, in particular, analysis in plasma (Bjornsson *et al*, 1977) and in liver, blood, urine, and foodstuffs (Mundy *et al*, 1976). Several papers have detailed simultaneous determination of warfarin and its metabolites in blood (Vesell and Shively, 1974; O'Reilly and Motley, 1976; Fasco *et al*, 1977; Wong *et al*, 1977). Warfarin analysis in rodenticide formulations was reported by Billings *et al* (1976). Mundy and Machin (1977) detected difenacoum at 5–0·025 ppm in plasma. This compound was considered too non-volatile for reliable analysis by g.l.c. Bushway *et al* (1975a) assayed grain baits for strychnine using a µPorasil column with a 7-minute separation. Strychnine and 23 other alkaloids were

Table 16 LC conditions for miscellaneous herbicides

Compound	Mobile phase	Detector	Column	Reference
Chloramben	I. MeCN : H_2O (50 : 50)	UV 240	Partisil ODS	166
Chlorthal, dimethyl (Dacthal™)	II. cyclohexane	—	Bio-Beads S-X2	68
Dinoseb	III. MeCN : H_2O (25–75 : 75–25)	UV 220	LiChrosorb RP-18	213
Diphenamid	IV. MeOH : H_2O (1 : 4) (also mono- and didemethyldiphenamid)	UV	HCP (DuPont)	123, 155

Compound	Conditions	Detection	Column	Ref.
Diquat	V. 0·01 M $KH_2PO_4 + H_3PO_4$, pH 2·45 : MeOH (53 : 47, 3 : 2)	UV 258, 210	Spherisorb A2OY bonded to γ-aminopropyltriethoxy-silane	176
Ethofumesate	VI. MeOH : H_2O (25 : 75)	UV 225	C_{18} Sil-X-II	24
1-Methyl-3-phenyl-5-[3-(trifluoromethyl) phenyl]-4-(1H)-pyridinone	VII. MeCN : MeOH : H_2O (30 : 28 : 42)	UV	μBondapak C_{18}	104
Metribuzin (Sencor™)	VIII. cyclohexane : THF (92·5 : 7·5)	UV	Corasil II	7
Naphthylacetic acid (Planofix™)	IX. 0·1 M citrate buffer, pH 4·3	UV, fluor.	Permaphase ETH	155
	X. 0·1 M phosphate buffer, pH 7	UV, fluor.	μCN	155
Paraquat	V. (also 11 : 14, 23 : 27, 258 nm only)			176
	XI. 0·2 M dimethylamine HCl in MeOH	UV 264	Vydac cation exchange	101

Table 16 (*cont.*)

Compound	Mobile phase	Detector	Column	Reference
Perfluidone	XII. hexane : $CHCl_3$: HOAc (25 : 65 : 10), also 3-hydroxyperfluidone	radio. count	Biosil A	128
3-Hydroxyperfluidone glucoside	XIII. MeOH : H_2O (1 : 1)	UV	μBondapak C_{18}	128
Picloram	XIV. 0·01 M sodium tetraborate + + 0·002 M sodium perchlorate	UV 280	Zipax SAX	217
	XV. MeCN : H_2O (20 : 80, pH 3), also methyl and isooctyl esters	UV 280	Partisil ODS (10–25 μm)	218
Pyrazone	XVI. MeOH : H_2O (2·5 : 97·5)	UV 230	C_{18} Sil-X-II	24
Velpar™	XVII. MeOH : H_2O (20 : 80)	UV 245	C_{18} Sil-X-II	24

FMC-25213   Me   XVIII. MeCN : H$_2$O (47 : 53)   UV 336   μBondapak C$_{18}$ 209
converted to propionaldehyde, then
derivatized as 2,4-dinitrophenyl-
hydrazone

Table 17   LC conditions for imides

Compound	Mobile phase	Detector	Column	Reference
Captafol	I. 20–60% MeCN in H$_2$O	UV 220	μBondapak C$_{18}$	225
	II. CH$_2$Cl$_2$	UV	silica gel (10 μm)	30
Captan	III. MeOH : H$_2$O (80 : 20)	UV, CEC	Vydac 201 TP RP	42
	(also II)			30
Folpet	IV. CHCl$_3$: isooctane (25 : 75)	UV	Corasil II, μPorasil	21
	V. MeCN : H$_2$O (25–75 : 75–25)	UV 220	LiChrosorb RP-18	213
	(also II)			30

Table 18 LC conditions for chlorobenzenes

Compound	Mobile phase	Detector	Column	Reference
Hexachlorobenzene (HCB)	I. cyclohexane	—	Bio-Beads S-X2	68
	II. toluene : EtOAc (1 : 3)	glc fract.	Bio-Beads S-X3	98
	III. CH_2Cl_2; CH_2Cl_2 : cyclohexane mixtures	UV	Bio-Beads S-X2	124
	IV. hexane	EC	Partisil (5 and 10 μm)	43, 81
	V. hexane	UV	Merckosorb SI 60 (10 μm), Merck Alox-T (10 μm)	195
	VI. hexane	UV 254, 205	LiChrosorb SI 60 (5 μm)	15
	VII. hexane : CH_2Cl_2 (9 : 1)	UV, glc	Porasil A	262
(photoproducts)	VIII. MeOH : H_2O mixtures	UV	Permaphase ODS	170
	IX. MeOH : H_2O (80 : 20)	UV, CEC	Vydac 201 TP RP	42
Hexachlorophene	X. hexane : butyl chloride (55 : 45)	UV	Sil-X (36–40 μm)	173
Pentachloroaniline	I, III			68, 124

Pentachloroanisole 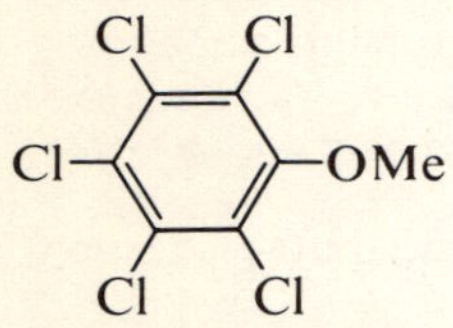	III, IX			42, 124
PCP (Pentachlorophenol) 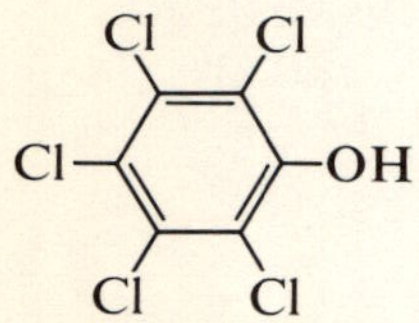	XI. 20% $CHCl_3$ in isooctane (also III, IX)	UV	Carbowax 400/Porasil	33 42, 124
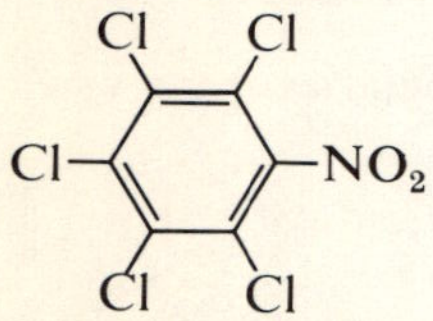 *Quintozene* (PCNB, Pentachloro- nitrobenzene)	XII. CH_2Cl_2 (also I, IX)	UV	silica gel (10 μm)	30 42, 68
Tecnazene (TCNB) 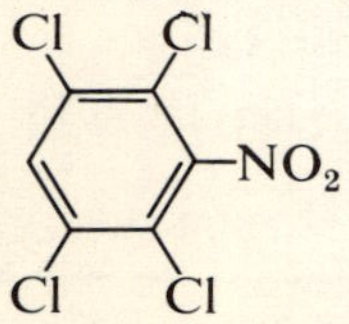	I			68

Table 19 LC conditions for imidazoles and thiophanates

Compound	Mobile phase	Detector	Column	Reference
Benomyl (Benlate™)	I. grad. 1–10% isoPrOH in heptane	UV 220	Si-10, CN-10, NH_2-10	225
	II. 5% isoPrOH in hexane	UV	Zorbax-SIL (10 μm)	5
	III. isoPrOH in hexane (2 : 98, 5 : 95, 10 : 90)	UV	Merckosorb SI 60	5
	IV. 25–60% MeCN in H_2O grad.	UV 220	μBondapak C_{18}	225
(also Me 2-benzimidazolecarbamate)	V. 0·025 M tetramethylammonium nitrate : 0·025 M HNO_3	UV	Zipax SCX	116, 155
(deriv. as Me 2-benzimidazole-carbamate; also 4- and 5-Hydroxy-2-benzimidazolecarbamates)	VI. 0·1 M HOAc : 0·1 M NaOAc, pH 5·15 (3 : 7)	UV	Zipax SCX	63, 114, 115, 155
	VII. MeOH : H_2O (25 : 75, 50 : 50, 75 : 25)	UV	Permaphase ODS	5
	VIII. MeOH : H_2O (20 : 80, 10 : 90, 5 : 95)	UV	Permaphase ETH	5
	IX. MeOH : H_2O (1 : 1, 1 : 2); MeCN; MeOH; isoPrOH; isoPrOH : hexane (1 : 1)	UV	Partisil-10 ODS	4
	X. MeCN : H_2O : NH_3 (30 : 70 : 0·6) to (50 : 50 : 0·6)	UV	Spherisorb ODS	213
(deriv. as 2-Aminobenzimidazole)	XI. 0·1% HOAc in MeOH	UV 277, fluor.	Hitachi Gel 3010 (20–23 μm)	143
(deriv. as Me 2-benzimidazole-carbamate)	XII. MeOH : H_2O (19 : 1)	fluor.	Hitachi Gel 3010	212
2-Aminobenzimidazole	XIII. butyl ether (also III, V, VII, VIII)	UV	1% ODPN on CSP support	109 5, 116, 155

Compound	Solvent system	Detection	Column	Ref.
Benzimidazole, 2-Methylbenzimidazole, Benzimidazol-2-yl urea, BUB	III, VII, VIII			5
Carbendazim 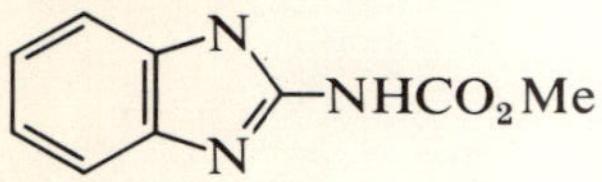	XIV. 1% EtOH, 0·2% morpholine in $CHCl_3$	UV 288	LiChrosorb SI 60	55, 213
	XV. $MeOH : H_2O : NH_3$ (60 : 40·0 : 0·6)	UV 288	Spherisorb ODS	55, 213
	XVI. $MeCN : H_2O : NH_3$ (30 : 70 : 0·6) to (50 : 50 : 0·6)	UV	Spherisorb ODS	213
	XVII. $MeOH : 0·3 \text{ M } KH_2PO_4$ (25 : 75)	UV 288	LiChrosorb CO_2H (weak cation exchange)	55
	(also II, III, VII, VIII)			5
Fuberidazole 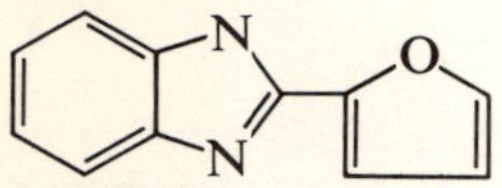	XVI			213
Thiabendazole 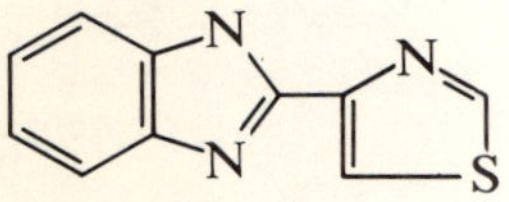	XVIII. 5% HOAc : 95% MeOH	UV 277, fluor.	Hitachi Gel 3010-CH_2OH (20–23 μm)	143
	XIX. 3 solvents (unreported) (also II, III, VII, VIII, XIV–XVII)	UV	silica gel (20 μm)	188 / 5, 55, 213
Thiophanate (R = Et) 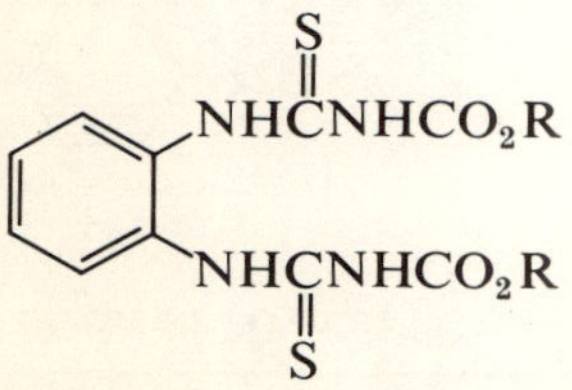	III, VII, VIII, XVI			5, 213
Thiophanate methyl (R = Me)	III, VII, VIII, XVI, XII (as Me 2-benzimidazolecarbamate) XIV, XV			5, 55, 212, 213

Table 20 LC conditions for miscellaneous fungicides

Compound	Mobile phase	Detector	Column	Reference
Anilazine (Dyrene™)	I. 29 and 50% aq. MeOH or EtOH	UV	Vydac RP	206
Biphenyl	II. MeOH : H_2O (45 : 55)	UV	Permaphase ODS	261
	III. hexane	UV	Merckosorb SI 60 (10 μm); Merck Alox-T (10 μm)	195
	IV. isooctane	UV	0·88% 1,2,3-tricyanoethoxy-propane on Corasil I	29
	V. 3 solvents (unreported)	UV	silica gel (20 μm)	188
	VI. EtOH	UV	μBondapak C_{18}	39
	VII. heptane	UV	LiChrosorb SI 60 (20 μm)	189
	VIII. hexane	UV 254, 205	LiChrosorb SI 60 (5 μm)	15
	IX. CH_2Cl_2; CH_2Cl_2 : cyclohexane mixtures	UV	Bio-Beads S-X2	124
	X. 90% MeCN or EtOH in H_2O, 70 °C	UV	pyrocarbon–silica	73
	XI. 80 or 100% MeCN, 55 °C	UV	graphitized carbon	73
	XII. MeCN : H_2O (90 : 10)	UV 205	LiChrosorb RP-18	213
	XIII. MeCN : H_2O : NH_3 (30 : 70 : 0·6) to (50 : 50 : 0·6)	UV	Spherisorb ODS	213
	XIV. isooctane	UV	LiChrosorb SI 60	55, 213
	XV. MeOH : H_2O : NH_3 (60 : 40 : 0·6)	UV 288	Spherisorb ODS	55
	XVI. 1% EtOH in isooctane	UV	Spherisorb CN	55

Carboxin (Vitavax™) 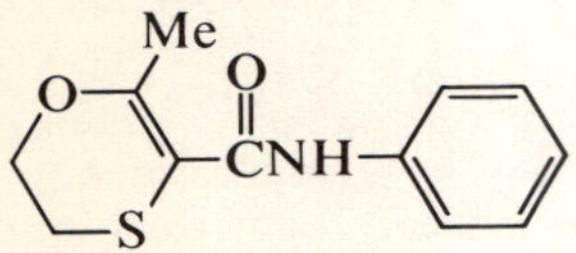	XVII. MeCN : H_2O (20 : 80) (also photoproducts: carboxin sulphoxide and sulphone)	UV, fluor.	Bondapak C_{18}/Corasil	257
Dazomet (Mylone™) 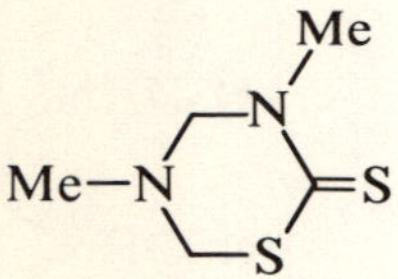	XVIII. 4% isoPrOH : 96% hexane	UV	Permaphase ETH	155, 237
Dicloran (Botran™, DCNA) 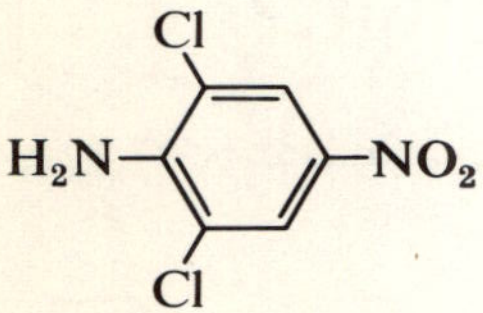	XIX. cyclohexane	—	Bio-Beads S-X2	68
	XX. 2% isoPrOH in isooctane	UV	LiChrosorb SI 60 (5 μm)	132
Dithianon 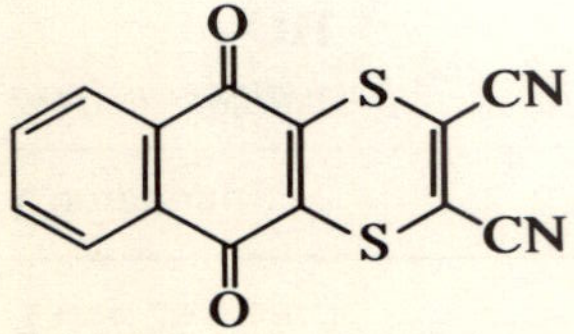	XXI. heptane : EtOAc (96·5 : 3·5)	UV	Perisorb A	49, 59

Table 20 (*cont.*)

Compound	Mobile phase	Detector	Column	Reference
o-Hydroxybiphenyl (structure: OH-substituted biphenyl)	XXII. MeOH : H_2O (1 : 1)	UV	Vydac RP	26
	XXIII. heptane : CH_2Cl_2 : HOAc (84·5 : 15 : 0·5, 90 : 10 : 0·5)	UV	Corasil II	190
	XXIV. hexane : $CHCl_3$ (9 : 1, 7 : 3) as dansyl der.	UV, fluor.	silica gel (7–18 μm)	29
	XXV. 1 % EtOH in isooctane (also V, XIII, XV, XVI)	UV	LiChrosorb SI 60	55, 213 55, 188, 213
MBT (2-Mercaptobenzothiazole) (structure: benzothiazole-SH)	XXVI. EtOH : isooctane (1 : 9)	UV 325	Merckosorb SI 60 (5 μm)	36
Nabam (structure: NHCSNa–CH₂CH₂–NHCSNa)	XXVII. MeOH : H_2O (15 : 85)	UV 240	LiChrosorb SI 60 (10 μm, silanized)	146
ETU (Ethylene thiourea)	XXVIII. EtOH : isooctane (7 : 93) (also XXVII)	UV	Permaphase ETH	161 146
Ethylenediamine (reacted with fluorescamine)	XXIX. 20 % MeOH in borate buffer, pH 8, 0·05 M	UV 410	LiChrosorb SI 60 (10 μm, silanized)	146
Thiram $(Me)_2NCSSCN(Me)_2$	XXX. CH_2Cl_2	UV	silica gel (10 μm)	30
	XXXI. MeCN : H_2O (25–75 : 75–25)	UV 220	LiChrosorb RP-18	213

investigated by Verpoorte and Svendsen (1974) using a Merckosorb SI 60 column. Formulations of Vacor™ rodenticide were analysed on Partisil-10 (Sims and Gard, 1977)

Pheromones

Synthetic insect pheromones are used mostly for monitoring insect populations, allowing more effective timing of insecticide sprays. Most pheromones are unsaturated alkanols or their acetates, although other functionality and cyclic structures are known. Response to these chemicals is usually species specific. Geometry of unsaturation is frequently of great importance for maximal activity.

It in fact appears that the key developments in silver nitrate loaded l.c. supports ('argentation' l.c.) have been made with the specific purpose of separating geometrical isomers of pheromones. Heath *et al* (1975) reported the use of three different silica gels coated with 20% silver nitrate (by evaporating an acetonitrile solution of $AgNO_3$ onto the silica in a rotary evaporator) for separation of mono- and diunsaturated pheromones. Extremely selective separations of *cis-* and *trans-*isomers were obtained, allowing preparative separation of 100 mg quantities on 50×0.93 cm columns. Heath *et al* (1977) reported improved techniques for packing columns of $AgNO_3$-laden 5 μm silica gels and studied the effect of the % loading of $AgNO_3$ on separation. All four isomers of 3,13-octadecadien-1-ol acetate were separated on a 5% loaded column, but not on 3, 7, or 10% loaded columns. This technique has been valuable for isolation and identification of pheromones (e.g. Tumlinson *et al*, 1974).

An alternate approach was described by Houx *et al* (1974; see also Houx and Voerman, 1976), who utilized a cation-exchange resin equilibrated with silver ion and eluted with methanol. Extremely selective separations of *cis-* and *trans-*isomers were achieved, with best selectivity at lower temperatures (10 °C). Unlike $AgNO_3$-coated silica, the effluent from the columns appeared to be free of silver ions.

Reversed-phase l.c. on a microparticulate C_{18} column has also been used for analytical and preparative separations of *cis-* and *trans-*isomers of synthetic pheromones (Warthen, 1975). Selectivity for *cis-* versus *trans-*isomers is substantially lower than with $AgNO_3$-laden columns, but considerable selectivity is observed between homologues, as would be expected for a r.p. system. Little separation of homologues is expected on $AgNO_3$ columns, so the techniques are complementary.

Isolation of pheromones is usually difficult because of their low titres in insects. Extracts of abdominal tips or whole bodies have been purified by sequential g.p.c. and l.c. on silica gel eluted with non-polar solvents (Ohta *et al*, 1976; Tumlinson and Heath, 1976).

Mycotoxins

While aflatoxins and other mycotoxins are certainly not pesticides, analysts working with pesticides may be called upon to analyse these natural products

Table 21   LC conditions for rodenticides

Compound	Mobile phase	Detector	Column	Reference
Warfarin	0.0025 M H_3PO_4 : MeOH ($1:2$)	UV 283	μBondapak C_{18}	8
(also 6- and 7-Hydroxywarfarin)	isooctane : CH_2Cl_2 : MeOH ($68:22:10$)	UV 308	Spherisorb	162
	CCl_4 : benzene : HOAc ($40:50:1$); CCl_4 : benzene : dioxane : HOAc ($40:50:5:1$ and $37:27:25:1$)	UV 313	μPorasil	244
	94% EtOH : H_2O containing 0.1% HOAc ($1:1$ and $3:2$)	UV 313	μBondapak C_{18}	244
	isoPrOH : isooctane ($2:98$)	UV 270	Corasil II	157, 158
(also 7-Hydroxywarfarin)	dioxane : H_2O ($10:90$), pH 4	UV	Permaphase ODS	247
(also 6- and 7-Hydroxywarfarin; Warfarin alcohol)	dioxane : H_2O ($40:60$), pH 4.2	UV 305	MicroPak CH-10	258
	MeOH : H_2O with 0.5% HOAc ($1:1$)	UV 308	MicroPak CH-10	9
(also Dicoumarol, Marcoumer, Sintrom)	CH_2Cl_2 : EtOH : H_2O ($98.8:1.0:0.2$)	UV 281	LiChrosorb SI 60 (5 μm)	243
Warfarin alcohols; 4-, 6-, 8-, 7-Hydroxywarfarin; Benzylic hydroxywarfarin	1.5% HOAc (pH 4.7 with conc. NH_4OH) : MeCN ($69:31$ or $9:1$)	UV 313	μBondapak C_{18}	56
	0.1 M ammonium acetate in MeCN : H_2O ($30:70$), pH 5	UV 305	LiChrosorb SI 60 (10 μm)	258
Difenacoum	isoPrOH : $CHCl_3$: isooctane ($1:2:397$)	UV	Corasil II	157
Strychnine	$CHCl_3$: MeOH ($9:1$, $8:2$, $7:3$); ether : MeOH ($8:2$, $7:3$, $6:4$)	UV	Merckosorb SI 60 (5 μm)	246
	MeOH : $CHCl_3$ ($10:90$)	UV	μPorasil (8–12 μm)	20
Vacor™	MeOH : CH_2Cl_2 ($10:90$)	UV	Partisil-10	215

as well. Existing t.l.c. methods for aflatoxin analysis are both selective and sensitive. With fluorodensitometric detection on t.l.c. plates, aflatoxins can be determined in foodstuffs at part per billion levels. A great deal of research has been conducted on l.c. analysis of aflatoxins. Most of the earlier reports have substantially poorer selectivity and sensitivity than t.l.c. methods, although precision and reproducibility may be better, and are not reviewed herein. A simple procedure has been described for clean-up of aflatoxin-containing samples prior to l.c. analysis (Lansden, 1977). Pons (1976) reported a highly reproducible system for separation of aflatoxins B_1, B_2, G_1, and G_2 on 10 μm silica l.c., but no applications were given. Engstrom et al (1977) have presented conditions for separation of seven mycotoxins by reversed-phase l.c. Aflatoxins B_1 and G_1 were selectively detected at 365 nm; the other mycotoxins examined (patulin, penicillic acid, rubratoxin B, ochratoxin A, zearalenone, roseotoxin B, and trichothecin) were not detectable at this wavelength but were at 254 nm. Detectability of aflatoxins is about 25 times better at the longer wavelength, and most coextractives do not interfere as much at the longer wavelength so detection at 365 nm is common. Fluorescence detection is even more sensitive and selective, but the most carcinogenic component, aflatoxin B_1, has much weaker fluorescence than aflatoxin B_2 or B_{2a}.

Recently, Takahashi (1977a, b) has developed methods for analysis of six aflatoxins (B_1, B_2, G_1, G_2, B_{2a}, G_{2a}) in wines and fruit juices using reversed-phase l.c. separation and fluorescence detection. Samples were treated with trifluoroacetic acid which catalyses hydration of the furanoid double bond of B_1 and G_1 to give the more strongly fluorescent hemiacetal aflatoxins B_{2a} and G_{2a} (aflatoxins B_2 and G_2 are unaffected by this treatment). Detection limits of 0·02 ppb were achieved; the method had greater resolution, sensitivity, precision, reproducibility, and rapidity than the t.l.c. method. Diebold and Zare (1977) subsequently reported detection of aflatoxins by laser-induced fluorescence with 0·75 pg reported as the minimum detectable quantity. Their procedure also utilized reversed-phase l.c. separation and acidic hydration of B_1 and G_1, but they found 1 M HCl to be superior to trifluoroacetic acid as catalyst. They reported a limit of detection of 2 ppb of aflatoxin B_1 in corn oil. Pons and Franz (1977) developed an analysis for aflatoxins B_1 and B_2 in cottonseed extracts using l.s.c. on 10 μm silica gel for separation and u.v. detection at 365 nm. Residues as low as 2–4 ppb of these aflatoxins could be determined, and the method was found to be much more precise than t.l.c. analysis. Stubblefield and Shotwell (1977) analysed for aflatoxins M_2, M_1, G_2, G_1, and B_1 in corn extracts by reversed-phase l.c. with u.v. detection at 350 nm. Values obtained by l.c. analysis averaged 25% less than t.l.c. values; numerous extraneous peaks and interferences in extracts made interpretation of data difficult. Seitz (1975) compared several methods for separation of aflatoxins B_1, B_2, G_1, and G_2, and obtained best results with l.c. on 10 μm silica gel with u.v. detection at 350 nm. However, no microparticulate reversed-phase packings were evaluated. A limit of detection was estimated as 10 ppb in yellow corn. Blanc et al (1976) reported a similar procedure for B_1, B_2, G_1, and G_2 using a 5 μm silica gel and detection at 362 nm. They reported detection limits of 5 ppb in oilseed cakes and feeds. L.c. has been utilized for separation of aflatoxin metabolites (Hsieh *et al*, 1976; Unger *et al*, 1977).

Holder *et al* (1977) described an analysis for the potent oestrogenic mycotoxins zearalenone and zearalanol in animal chow. Reversed-phase l.c. was used for separation with u.v. detection at 254 nm giving a sensitivity of 10 ppb. Methods have been developed for analysis of the carcinogenic mycotoxin patulin in apple juice (Ware *et al*, 1974) and apple butter (Ware, 1975). Both methods utilized 5–6 μm silica gel l.c. columns with detection at 254 nm; a detection limit of 11 ppb was obtained for apple juice. Stack *et al* (1976) described a modified procedure for analysis of the carcinogenic mycotoxin sterigmatocystin, using reversed-phase l.c. separation with u.v. detection at 254 nm. Detection limits in g.p.c. and column chromatography-purified extracts of oats and corn were apparently less than 25 ppb.

CONCLUSIONS

Utilization of l.c. methodology in pesticide chemistry has increased rapidly in the last few years. The nearly exponential increase in reports of new applications is evidenced by the references in this review—70% have publication dates between 1975 and January 1978, and half of those are dated 1977 to January 1978. It is quite evident that by the time this article appears, numerous new applications will be available. We hope therefore that this review will provide both a basis for understanding the principles and promise of l.c., and a means of rapid searching for many concrete examples of specific applications.

The rapid evolution of modern l.c. does not threaten totally to displace g.l.c. Each technique has its relative merits, and it is increasingly clear that l.c. and g.l.c. are complementary in utility. L.c. certainly has great advantages in analysis of thermally sensitive, extremely polar, or high molecular weight compounds. G.l.c. still offers a wider selection of both non-selective ('universal') and selective detectors with sensitivity frequently superior to l.c. detectors. Also, the coupling of the g.l.c. apparatus to a mass spectrometer is easier, and the extraordinary value of this technique is well appreciated. For preparative isolation work on either a micro- or macro-scale, l.c. has substantial advantages over g.l.c.; hence, it is not surprising that l.c. has become widely used in pesticide biochemistry for metabolite isolation. The most common method for metabolism studies appears to be reversed-phase l.c. using the newer packings consisting of silica with covalently bonded functionality. However, normal-phase l.c. with silica packing is also much used. It is anticipated that ion-pair chromatography, using reversed-phase packings, will prove valuable in isolating ionic, conjugated metabolites.

In analysis of formulations, l.c. appears to offer considerable advantages over g.l.c., since minimal pretreatment of formulations before l.c. analysis is required. Analysis of environmental samples for residues of pesticides has long been dominated by methods using g.l.c. with various detection devices for final qualitative and quantitative analysis. Usage of l.c. methodology for final detection in this area has been largely confined to those pesticides too unstable for g.l.c. analysis. Recent studies, especially from Lawrence and coworkers, have shown that l.c. can frequently be substituted for g.l.c. in many existing residue analyses with little change in clean-up procedures. In view of the ever-existing need for methodology for verification of residue data, l.c. appears to be a promising alternative approach, especially as experimenters gain a better understanding of the manipulation of selectivity in l.c. systems.

In summary, l.c. is useful in the analysis of compounds with diverse structures and polarities. The technique will continue to provide an expanding role in xenobiotic chemistry.

ACKNOWLEDGEMENTS

We thank our wives for their forbearance during the writing of the manuscript, M. A. Ratcliff and G. K. Kohn for critical reading of a draft, and the patient Ms. S. Dillow for typing several drafts and correcting inconsistencies.

APPENDIX

Abbreviations used in Tables

Certain standard abbreviations have been used for solvents such as: MeCN, MeOH, EtOH, EtOAc, etc.

aq. = aqueous
CEC = Coulson electrolytic conductivity
ChE inhib. = cholinesterase inhibition
CSP = controlled surface porosity
dansyl der = dansylated derivative
EC = electron capture
flame ioniz. = transport flame ionization
fluor. = fluorimetric
fluor. enz. inhib. = fluorimetric enzyme inhibition
grad. = gradient
glc fract. = gas–liquid chromatography of fractions
ms = mass spectral
nitro. spec. = nitrosamide specific
ODPN = β,β-oxydipropionitrile
polar = polarographic
radio. count. fract. = liquid scintillation counting of fractions
RI = refractive index
RP = reversed-phase
therm. energy = thermal energy analyser
UV = ultraviolet absorbance at 254 nm
UV 280, etc. = ultraviolet absorbance at indicated wavelength

Table Layout

Within a given table, analytical (solvent, column, and detection) conditions are indicated by Roman numerals. Thus, similar compounds analysed with the same conditions are listed together with the Roman numeral. Each table is independent, i.e. the Roman numerals are *not* comparable between two different tables.

REFERENCES

1. Aitzetmüller, K. (1975), *J. Chromatogr.*, **107**, 411.
2. Argauer, R. J. and Warthen, J. D. Jr (1975), *Anal. Chem.*, **47**, 2472.
3. Arpino, P. J., Dawkins, B. G. and McLafferty, F. W. (1974), *J. Chromatogr. Sci.*, **12**, 574.
4. Aten, C. F. and Bourke, J. B. (1977), *J. Agr. Food Chem.*, **25**, 1430.
5. Austin, D. J., Lord, K. A. and Williams, I. H. (1976), *Pestic. Sci.*, **7**, 211.
6. Bakalyar, S. R., McIlwrick, R. and Roggendorf, E. (1977), *J. Chromatogr.*, **142**, 353.
7. Betker, W. R., Smead, C. F. and Evans, R. T. (1976), *J. Ass. Offic. Anal. Chem.*, **59**, 278.
8. Billings, T. J., Hanks, A. R. and Colvin, B. M. (1976), *J. Ass. Offic. Anal. Chem.*, **59**, 1104.
9. Bjornsson, T. D., Blaschke, T. F. and Meffin, P. J. (1977), *J. Pharm. Sci.*, **66**, 142.
10. Blanc, M., Midler, O. and Karleskind, A. (1976), in Naudet, M., Ucciani, E. and Uzzan, A. (eds), *Actes Congr. Mond—Soc. Int. Etude Corps Gras, 13th*, Sect. D, p. 61, Paris, France.
11. Boehme, W. and Engelhardt, H. (1977), *J. Chromatogr.*, **133**, 67.
12. Borch, R. F. (1975), *Anal. Chem.*, **47**, 2437.
13. Bowman, M. C., Holder, C. L. and Rushing, L. G. (1978), *J. Agr. Food Chem.*, **26**, 35.
14. Brinkman, U. A. Th., de Kok, A., de Vries, G. and Reymer, H. G. M. (1976a), *J. Chromatogr.*, **128**, 101.
15. Brinkman, U. A. Th., Seetz, J. W. F. L. and Reymer, H. G. M. (1976b), *J. Chromatogr.*, **116**, 353.
16. Brown, N. D. and Sleeman, H. K. (1977), *J. Chromatogr.*, **138**, 449.
17. Brown, P. R. (1973), *High pressure liquid chromatography: biochemical and biomedical applications*, Academic, New York.
18. Burkhard, N. and Guth, J. A. (1976), *Pestic Sci.*, **7**, 65.
19. Bush, P. B., Tanner, M., Kiker, J. T., Page, R. K., Booth, N. H. and Fletcher, O. J. (1978), *J. Agr. Food Chem.*, **26**, 126.
20. Bushway, R. J., Cramer, C. W., Hanks, A. R. and Colvin, B. M. (1975a), *J. Ass. Offic. Anal. Chem.*, **58**, 957.
21. Bushway, R. J., Engdahl, B. S., Colvin, B. M. and Hanks, A. R. (1975b), *J. Ass. Offic. Anal. Chem.*, **58**, 965.
22. Bushway, R. and Hanks, A. (1977), *J. Chromatogr.*, **134**, 210.
23. Byast, T. H. (1975), *Analyst*, **100**, 325.
24. Byast, T. H. (1977), *J. Chromatogr.*, **134**, 216.
25. Byast, T. H. and Cotterill, E. G. (1975), *J. Chromatogr.*, **104**, 211.
26. Byrne, M. J. (1976), *J. Ass. Offic. Anal. Chem.*, **59**, 693.
27. Byrne, S. H. (1971), in Kirkland, J. J. (ed.), *Modern practice of liquid chromatography*, p. 108, Wiley, New York.
28. Byrne, S. H., Schmit, J. A. and Johnson, P. E. (1971), *J. Chromatogr. Sci.*, **9**, 592.

29. Callmer, K. and Nilsson, O. (1973), *Chromatographia*, **6**, 517.
30. Carlstrom, A. A. (1977), *J. Ass. Offic. Anal. Chem.*, **60**, 1157.
31. Cassidy, R. M., LeGay, D. S. and Frei, R. W. (1974), *J. Chromatogr. Sci.*, **12**, 85.
32. Colin, H. and Guiochon, G. (1977), *J. Chromatogr.*, **141**, 289.
33. Colvin, B. M., Engdahl, B. S. and Hanks, A. R. (1974), *J. Ass. Offic. Anal. Chem.*, **57**, 648.
34. Consden, R., Gordon, A. H. and Martin, A. J. P. (1944), *Biochem. J.*, **38**, 224.
35. Corley, C., Miller, R. W. and Hill, K. R. (1974), *J. Ass. Offic. Anal. Chem.*, **57**, 1269.
36. Cox, G. B. (1976), *J. Chromatogr.*, **116**, 244.
37. Cox, G. B. (1977), *J. Chromatogr. Sci.*, **15**, 385.
38. Crawford, M. J. and Hutson, D. H. (1977), *Pestic. Sci.*, **8**, 579.
39. Davis, P. L. and Munroe, K. A. (1977), *J. Agr. Food Chem.*, **25**, 426
40. Deelder, R. S. and Hendricks, P. J. H. (1973), *J. Chromatogr.*, **83**, 343.
41. Diebold, G. J. and Zare, R. N. (1977), *Science*, **196**, 1439.
42. Dolan, J. W. and Seiber, J. N. (1977), *Anal. Chem.*, **49**, 326.
43. Dolphin, R. J., Willmott, F. W., Mills, A. D. and Hoogeveen, L. P. J. (1976), *J. Chromatogr.*, **122**, 259.
44. Done, J. N., Kennedy, G. J. and Knox, J. H. (1972), *Nature*, **237**, 77.
45. Dorn, S., Oesterhelt, G., Suchy, M., Trautmann, K. H. and Wipf, H.-K. (1976), *J. Agr. Food Chem.*, **24**, 637.
46. Dorough, H. W. and Thorstenson, J. H. (1975), *J. Chromatogr. Sci.*, **13**, 212.
47. Dubsky, H. (1972), *J. Chromatogr.*, **71**, 395.
48. Durst, H. D., Milano, M., Kikta jr, E. J., Connelly, S. A. and Grushka, E. (1975), *Anal. Chem.*, **47**, 1797.
49. Eisenbeiss, F. and Sieper, H. (1973), *J. Chromatogr.*, **83**, 439.
50. Engelhardt, H. (1977), *J. Chromatogr. Sci.*, **15**, 380.
51. Engelhardt, H. and Wiedemann, H. (1973), *Anal. Chem.*, **45**, 1641.
52. Engstrom, G. W., Richard, J. L. and Cysewski, S. J. (1977), *J. Agr. Food Chem.*, **25**, 833.
53. Ettre, L. S. and Horvath, C. (1975), *Anal. Chem.*, **47**, 422A.
54. Farrington, D. S., Hopkins, R. G. and Ruzicka, J. H. A. (1977), *Analyst*, **102**, 377.
55. Farrow, J. E., Hoodless, R. A., Sargent, M. and Sidwell, J. A. (1977), *Analyst*, **102**, 752.
56. Fasco, M. J., Piper, L. J. and Kaminsky, L. S. (1977), *J. Chromatogr.*, **131**, 365.
57. Feil, V. J., Lamoureux, C. H. and Zaylskie, R. G. (1975), *J. Agr. Food Chem.*, **23**, 382.
58. Fine, D. H., Ross, R., Rounbehler, D. P., Silvergleid, A. and Song, L. (1976), *J. Agr. Food Chem.*, **24**, 1069.
59. Fishbein, L. (1974), *J. Chromatogr.*, **98**, 177.
60. Frei, R. W. and Lawrence, J. F. (1973), *J. Chromatogr.*, **83**, 321.
61. Frei, R. W., Lawrence, J. F., Hope, J. and Cassidy, R. M. (1974), *J. Chromatogr. Sci.*, **12**, 40.
62. Freudenthal, R. I., Emmerling, D. C. and Baron, R. L. (1977), *J. Chromatogr.*, **134**, 207.
63. Gardiner, J. A., Kirkland, J. J., Klopping, H. L. and Sherman, H. (1974), *J. Agr. Food Chem.*, **22**, 419.
64. Giddings, J. C. (1965), *Dynamics of chromatography, Part 1*, p. 294, Dekker, New York.
65. Gloor, R. and Johnson, E. L. (1977), *J. Chromatogr. Sci.*, **15**, 413.
66. Golab, T., Bishop, C. E., Donoho, A. L., Manthey, J. A. and Zornes, L. L. (1975), *Pestic. Biochem. Physiol.*, **5**, 196.
67. Gonnet, C. and Rocca, J. L. (1975), *J. Chromatogr.*, **109**, 297.

108

68. Griffitt, K. R. and Craun, J. C. (1974), *J. Ass. Offic. Anal. Chem.*, **57**, 168.
69. Grushka, E. (ed.) (1974), *Bonded stationary phases in chromatography*, Ann Arbor Science Publishers, Ann Arbor, Mich.
70. Grushka, E., Durst, H. D. and Kikta, E. J. (1975), *J. Chromatogr.*, **112**, 673.
71. Guzik, F. F. (1978), *J. Agr. Food Chem.*, **26**, 53.
72. Hammock, B. D., Mumby, S. M. and Lee, P. W. (1977), *Pestic. Biochem. Physiol.*, **7**, 261.
73. Hanai, T. and Walton, H. F. (1977), *Anal. Chem.*, **49**, 1954.
74. Hara, S. (1977), *J. Chromatogr.*, **137**, 41.
75. Hass, J. R., McConnell, E. E. and Harvan, D. J. (1978), *J. Agr. Food Chem.*, **26**, 94.
76. Heath, R. R., Tumlinson, J. H., Doolittle, R. E. and Proveaux, A. T. (1975), *J. Chromatogr. Sci.*, **13**, 380.
77. Heath, R. R., Tumlinson, J. H. and Doolittle, R. E. (1977), *J. Chromatogr. Sci.*, **15**, 10.
78. Heck, H. d'A., Dyer, R. L., Scott, A. C. and Anbar, M. (1977), *J. Agr. Food Chem.*, **25**, 901.
79. Henry, R. A., Schmit, J. A., Dieckman, J. F. and Murphey, F. J. (1971), *Anal. Chem.*, **43**, 1053.
80. Holder, C. L., Nony, C. R. and Bowman, M. C. (1977), *J. Ass. Offic. Anal. Chem.*, **60**, 272.
81. Hoogeveen, L. P. J., Willmott, F. W. and Dolphin, R. J. (1976), *Z. Anal. Chem.*, **282**, 401.
82. Horgan, jr, D. F. (1973), in Zweig, G. (ed.), *Analytical methods for pesticides and plant growth regulators*, vol. VII, p. 89, Academic, New York.
83. Horvath, C. and Melander, W. (1977), *J. Chromatogr. Sci.*, **15**, 393.
84. Hosler jr, C. F. (1974), *Bull. Environ. Contam. Toxicol.*, **12**, 599.
85. Houx, N. W. H. and Voerman, S. (1976), *J. Chromatogr.*, **129**, 456.
86. Houx, N. W. H., Voerman, S. and Jongen, W. M. F. (1974), *J. Chromatogr.*, **96**, 25.
87. Howard, G. A. and Martin, A. J. P. (1950), *Biochem. J.*, **46**, 532.
88. Hsieh, D. P. H., Fitzell, D. L., Miller, J. L. and Seiber, J. N. (1976), *J. Chromatogr.*, **117**, 474.
89. Hunt, J. A. (1968), *Anal. Biochem.*, **23**, 289.
90. Hunt, L. M. and Gilbert, B. N. (1976), *J. Agr. Food Chem.*, **24**, 669.
91. Ishii, Y. (1976), *Kagaku No Ryoiki, Zokan (J. of Japan. Chem. Supplement)*, **109**, 241.
92. Ishii, Y. and Otake, T. (1973), *Noyaku Kensasho Hokoku (Bull. Agric. Chem. Inspect. Sta.)*, **13**, 32.
93. Isshiki, K., Tsumura, K. and Watanabe, T. (1976), *Proc. Annu. Meet. Food Hyg. Soc. Japan*, **32**, 29.
94. Isshiki, K., Tsumura, S. and Watanabe, T. (1977), *Shokuhin Eiseigaku Zasshi (J. Food Hyg. Soc. Japan)*, **18**, 159.
95. Jackson, E. R. (1976), *J. Ass. Offic. Anal. Chem.*, **59**, 740.
96. Jackson, E. R. (1977), *J. Ass. Offic. Anal. Chem.*, **60**, 724.
97. James, A. T. and Martin, A. J. P. (1951), *Biochem. J. Proc.*, **48**, vii.
98. Johnson, L. D., Waltz, R. H., Ussary, J. P. and Kaiser, F. E. (1976), *J. Ass. Offic. Anal. Chem.*, **59**, 174.
99. Jork, H. and Roth, B. (1977), *J. Chromatogr.*, **144**, 39.
100. Katayama, J. (1976), *Osaku-fu Norin Gijutsu Senta Kenkyu Hokoku*, **13**, 63.
101. Kawano, Y., Audino, J. and Edlund, M. (1975), *J. Chromatogr.*, **115**, 289.
102. Kearney, P. C., Plimmer, J. R., Williams, V. P., Klingebiel, U. I., Isenee, A. R., Laanio, T. L., Stolzenberg, G. E. and Zaylskie, R. G. (1974), *J. Agr. Food Chem.*, **22**, 856.

103. Kearney, P. C., Plimmer, J. R., Wheeler, W. B. and Konston, A. (1976), *Pestic. Biochem. Physiol.*, **6**, 229.
104. Kennedy, J. H. (1977), *J. Chromatogr. Sci.*, **15**, 79.
105. Kikta jr, E. J. and Stange, A. E. (1977), *J. Chromatogr.*, **138**, 41.
106. Kikta jr, E. J., Stange, A. E. and Lam, S. (1977), *J. Chromatogr.*, **138**, 321.
107. Kirkland, J. J. (1968), *Anal. Chem.*, **40**, 391.
108. Kirkland, J. J. (1969a), *J. Chromatogr. Sci.*, **7**, 7.
109. Kirkland, J. J. (1969b), *J. Chromatogr. Sci.*, **7**, 361.
110. Kirkland, J. J. (1969c), *Anal. Chem.*, **41**, 218.
111. Kirkland, J. J. (ed.), (1971a), *Modern practice of liquid chromatography*, Wiley, New York.
112. Kirkland, J. J. (1971b), *Anal. Chem.*, **43**, 36A.
113. Kirkland, J. J. (1973a), *J. Chromatogr.*, **83**, 149.
114. Kirkland, J. J. (1973b), *J. Agr. Food Chem.*, **21**, 171.
115. Kirkland, J. J. (1974), *Analyst*, **99**, 859.
116. Kirkland, J. J., Holt, R. F. and Pease, H. L. (1973), *J. Agr. Food Chem.*, **21**, 368.
117. Kissinger, P. T., Refshauge, C., Dreiling, R. and Adams, R. N. (1973), *Anal. Lett.*, **6**, 465.
118. Koen, J. G. and Huber, J. F. K. (1970), *Anal. Chem. Acta*, **51**, 303.
119. Koen, J. G., Huber, J. F. K., Poppe, H. and den Boef, G. (1970), *J. Chromatogr. Sci.*, **8**, 192.
120. Kojima, M., Shiga, N., Matano, O. and Goto, S. (1977), *Nippon Noyaku Gakkaishi*, **2**, 311.
120a. Kok, J. J. de, Kok, A. de, Brinkman, U. A. Th. and Kok, R. M. (1977), *J. Chromatogr.*, **142**, 367.
121. Krull, I. S. (1977), *Residue Rev.*, **66**, 185.
122. Krupcik, J., Kriz, J., Prusova, D., Suchanek, P. and Cervenka, Z. (1977), *J. Chromatogr.*, **142**, 797.
123. Krzeminski, L. F., Cox, B. L. and Neff, A. W. (1972), *Anal. Chem.*, **44**, 126.
124. Kuehl, D. W. and Leonard, E. N. (1978), *Anal. Chem.*, **50**, 182.
125. Kvalvag, J., Elliot, D. L., Iwata, Y. and Gunther, F. A. (1977a), *Bull. Environ. Contam. Toxicol.*, **17**, 253.
126. Kvalvag, J., Ott, D. E. and Gunther, F. A. (1977b), *J. Ass. Offic. Anal. Chem.*, **60**, 911.
127. Lam, S. and Grushka, E. (1977), *J. Chromatogr. Sci.*, **15**, 234.
128. Lamoureux, G. L. and Stafford, L. E. (1977), *J. Agr. Food Chem.*, **25**, 512.
129. Lansden, J. A. (1977), *J. Agr. Food Chem.*, **25**, 969.
130. Larose, R. H. (1974), *J. Ass. Offic. Anal. Chem.*, **57**, 1046.
131. Lawrence, J. F. (1976a), *J. Ass. Offic. Anal. Chem.*, **59**, 1066.
132. Lawrence, J. F. (1976b), *J. Chromatogr. Sci.*, **14**, 557.
133. Lawrence, J. F. (1977), *J. Agr. Food Chem.*, **25**, 211.
134. Lawrence, J. F. and Frei, R. W. (1974), *J. Chromatogr.*, **98**, 253.
135. Lawrence, J. F. and Frei, R. W. (1976), *Chemical derivatization in liquid chromatography*, Elsevier, Amsterdam.
136. Lawrence, J. F. and Leduc, R. (1977), *J. Agr. Food Chem.*, **25**, 1362.
137. Lawrence, J. F., Lewis, D. A. and McLeod, H. A. (1977), *J. Chromatogr.*, **138**, 143.
138. Lawrence, J. F., Renault, C. and Frei, R. W. (1976), *J. Chromatogr.*, **121**, 343.
139. Leitch, R. E. (1971), *J. Chromatogr. Sci.*, **9**, 531.
140. Little, J. N., Horgan, D. F. and Bombaugh, K. J. (1970), *J. Chromatogr. Sci.*, **8**, 625.
141. Lovins, R. E., Ellis, S. R., Tolbert, G. D. and McKinney, C. R. (1973), *Anal. Chem.*, **45**, 1553.
142. Lubkowitz, J. A. and Petit, L. R. (1976), *J. Chromatogr.*, **121**, 161.

110

143. Maeda, M. and Tsuji, A. (1976), *J. Chromatogr.*, **120**, 449.
144. Majors, R. E. (1973), in Zlatkis, A. (ed.), *Advances in chromatography 1973*, p. 376, Chromatography Symposium, Houston, Texas.
145. Majors, R. E. (1977), *J. Chromatogr. Sci.*, **15**, 334.
146. Marshall, W. D. (1977), *J. Agr. Food Chem.*, **25**, 357.
147. Marshall, W. D., Greenhalgh, R. and Batora, V. (1974), *Pestic. Sci.*, **5**, 781.
148. Martin, A. J. P. and Synge, R. L. M. (1941), *Biochem. J.*, **35**, 1358.
149. McFadden, W. H., Bradford, D. C., Games, D. E. and Gower, J. L. (1977), *Amer. Lab.*, October 1977, p. 55.
150. McFadden, W. H., Schwartz, H. L. and Evans, S. (1976), *J. Chromatogr.*, **122**, 389.
151. McNair, H. M. and Chandler, C. D. (1976), *J. Chromatogr. Sci.*, **14**, 477.
152. Miller, L. L., Nordblom, G. D. and Yost, G. A. (1974), *J. Agr. Food Chem.*, **22**, 853.
153. Mittelstaedt, W., Still, G. G., Dürbeck, H. and Führ, F. (1977), *J. Agr. Food Chem.*, **25**, 908.
154. Moring, S. E. (1977), M.A. thesis, University of Kansas.
155. Moye, H. A. (1975), *J. Chromatogr. Sci.*, **13**, 268.
156. Moye, H. A. and Wade, T. E. (1976), *Anal. Lett.*, **9**, 891.
157. Mundy, D. E. and Machin, A. F. (1977), *J. Chromatogr.*, **139**, 321.
158. Mundy, D. E., Quick, M. P. and Machin, A. F. (1976), *J. Chromatogr.*, **121**, 335.
159. Oehler, D. D. and Holman, G. M. (1975), *J. Agr. Food Chem.*, **23**, 590.
160. Ohta, K., Tatsuki, S., Uchiumi, K., Kurihara, M. and Fukami, J. (1976), *Agr. Biol. Chem.*, **40**, 1897.
161. Onley, J. H., Giuffrida, L., Ives, N. F. and Watts, R. R. (1977), *J. Ass. Offic. Anal. Chem.*, **60**, 1105.
162. O'Reilly, R. A. and Motley, C. H. (1976), *Fed. Proc.*, **35**, 756.
163. Ott, D. E. (1977), *Bull. Environ. Contam. Toxicol.*, **17**, 269.
164. Pacco, J. M. and Mukherji, A. K. (1977), *J. Chromatogr.*, **144**, 113.
165. Papa, L. J. and Turner, L. P. (1972), *J. Chromatogr. Sci.*, **10**, 747.
166. Paschal, D. C., Bicknell, R. and Dresbach, D. (1977), *Anal. Chem.*, **49**, 1551.
167. Paulson, G. D., Jacobsen, A. M., Zaylskie, R. G. and Feil, V. J. (1973), *J. Agr. Food. Chem.*, **21**, 804.
168. Perry, S. G., Amos, R. and Brewer, P. I. (1972), *Practical liquid chromatography*, Plenum, New York.
169. Pflugmacher, J. and Ebing, W. (1975), *J. Chromatogr.*, **109**, 199.
170. Plimmer, J. R. and Klingebiel, U. I. (1976), *J. Agr. Food Chem.*, **24**, 721.
171. Pons jr, W. A. (1976), *J. Ass. Offic. Anal. Chem.*, **59**, 101.
172. Pons jr, W. A. and Franz jr, A. O. (1977), *J. Ass. Offic. Anal. Chem.*, **60**, 89.
173. Porcaro, P. J. and Shubiak, P. (1972), *Anal. Chem.*, **44**, 1865.
174. Pribyl, J. and Herzel, F. (1976), *J. Chromatogr.*, **125**, 487.
175. Pryde, A. (1974), *J. Chromatogr. Sci.*, **12**, 486.
176. Pryde, A. and Darby, F. J. (1975), *J. Chromatogr.*, **115**, 107.
177. Quistad, G. B., Staiger, L. E. and Schooley, D. A. (1974), *J. Agr. Food Chem.*, **22**, 582.
178. Quistad, G. B., Staiger, L. E. and Schooley, D. A. (1975a), *J. Agr. Food Chem.*, **23**, 743.
179. Quistad, G. B., Staiger, L. E. and Schooley, D. A. (1975b), *J. Agr. Food Chem.*, **23**, 750.
180. Quistad, G. B., Staiger, L. E. and Schooley, D. A. (1975c), *Pestic. Biochem. Physiol.*, **5**, 233.
181. Quistad, G. B., Staiger, L. E. and Schooley, D. A. (1976a), *J. Agr. Food Chem.*, **24**, 644.

182. Quistad, G. B., Schooley, D. A., Staiger, L. E., Bergot, B. J., Sleight, B. H. and Macek, K. J. (1976b), *Pestic. Biochem. Physiol.*, **6**, 523.
183. Quistad, G. B., Staiger, L. E. and Schooley, D. A. (1978a), *J. Agr. Food Chem.*, **26**, 60.
184. Quistad, G. B., Staiger, L. E. and Schooley, D. A. (1978b), *J. Agr. Food Chem.*, **26**, 66.
185. Quistad, G. B., Staiger, L. E. and Schooley, D. A. (1978c), *J. Agr. Food Chem.*, **26**, 71.
186. Quistad, G. B., Staiger, L. E. and Schooley, D. A. (1978d), *J. Agr. Food Chem.*, **26**, 76.
187. Ramsteiner, K. A. and Hörmann, W. D. (1975), *J. Chromatogr.*, **104**, 438.
188. Reeder, S. K., *ACS Abstracts LA Meeting*, Spring 1974, PEST 85.
189. Reeder, S. K. (1975), *J. Ass. Offic. Anal. Chem.*, **58**, 1013.
190. Reeder, S. K. (1976), *J. Ass. Offic. Anal. Chem.*, **59**, 162.
191. Reeve, D. R. and Crozier, A. (1977), *J. Chromatogr.*, **137**, 271.
192. Reichstein, T. and Van Euw, J. (1938), *Helv. Chim. Acta*, **21**, 1197.
193. Roberts, T. R. and Standen, M. E. (1977a), *Pestic. Sci.*, **8**, 305.
194. Roberts, T. R. and Standen, M. E. (1977b), *Pestic. Sci.*, **8**, 600.
195. Rohleder, H., Staudacher, H. and Soemmermann, W. (1976), *Z. Anal. Chem.*, **279**, 152.
196. Ross, M. S. F. (1977), *J. Chromatogr.*, **141**, 107.
197. Ross, R. D., Morrison, J., Rounbehler, D. P., Fan, S. and Fine, D. H. (1977), *J. Agr. Food Chem.*, **25**, 1416.
198. Schaefer, C. H. and Dupras jr, E. F. (1976), *J. Agr. Food Chem.*, **24**, 733.
199. Schaefer, C. H. and Dupras, jr, E. F. (1977), *J. Agr. Food Chem.*, **25**, 1026.
200. Schill, G., Borg, K. O., Modin, R. and Persson, B. A. (1977), in Bridges, J. W. and Chasseaud, L. F. (eds), *Progress in drug metabolism*, vol. 1, p. 219, Wiley, London.
201. Schmit, J. A. (1971), in Kirkland, J. J. (ed.), *Modern practice of liquid chromatography*, p. 398, Wiley, New York.
202. Schooley, D. A., Bergot, B. J., Dunham, L. L. and Siddall, J. B. (1975a), *J. Agr. Food Chem.*, **23**, 293.
203. Schooley, D. A., Creswell, K. M., Staiger, L. E. and Quistad, G. B. (1975b), *J. Agr. Food Chem.*, **23**, 369.
204. Schooley, D. A. and Nakanishi, K. (1973), in Heftmann, E. (ed.), *Modern methods of steroid analysis*, p. 37, Academic, New York.
205. Scott, R. P. W. and Kucera, P. (1977), *J. Chromatogr.*, **142**, 213.
206. Seiber, J. N. (1974), *J. Chromatogr.*, **94**, 151.
207. Seitz, L. M. (1975), *J. Chromatogr.*, **104**, 81.
208. Self, C., McKerrell, E. H. and Webber, T. J. N. (1975), *Proc. Anal. Div. Chem. Soc.*, **12**, 288.
209. Selim, S. and Cook, R. F. (1978), *J. Agr. Food Chem.*, **26**, 106.
210. Selim, S., Cook, R. F. and Leppert, B. C. (1977), *J. Agr. Food Chem.*, **25**, 567.
211. Sherma, J. (1975), *J. Chromatogr.*, **113**, 97.
212. Shiga, N., Matano, O. and Goto, S. (1977), *Nippon Noyaku Gakkaishi*, **2**, 27.
213. Sidwell, J. A. (1977), *Med. Fac. Landbouww. Rijksuniv. Gent.*, **42**, 1803.
214. Sidwell, J. A. and Ruzicka, J. H. A. (1976), *Analyst*, **101**, 111.
215. Sims, C. W. and Gard, R. K. (1977), *J. Ass. Offic. Anal. Chem.*, **60**, 1375.
216. Singer, G. M., Singer, S. S. and Schmidt, D. G. (1977), *J. Chromatogr.*, **133**, 59.
217. Skelly, N. E., Russell, R. J. and Porter, D. F. (1976), *J. Ass. Offic. Anal. Chem.*, **59**, 748.
218. Skelly, N. E., Stevens, T. S. and Mapes, D. A. (1977), *J. Ass. Offic. Anal. Chem.*, **60**, 868.

219. Slais, K. and Krejci, M. (1974), *J. Chromatogr.*, **91**, 181.
220. Smith, A. E. and Lord, K. A. (1975), *J. Chromatogr.*, **107**, 407.
221. Snyder, L. R. (1968), *Principles of adsorption chromatography*, p. 18, Dekker, New York.
222. Snyder, L. R. (1971), in Kirkland, J. J. (ed.), *Modern practice of liquid chromatography*, p. 130, Wiley, New York.
223. Snyder, L. R. and Kirkland, J. J. (1974), *Introduction to modern liquid chromatography*, Wiley, New York.
224. Spackman, D. H., Stein, W. H. and Moore, S. (1958), *Anal. Chem.*, **30**, 1190.
225. Sparacino, C. M. and Hines, J. W. (1976), *J. Chromatogr. Sci.*, **14**, 549.
226. Stack, M. E., Nesheim, S., Brown, N. L. and Pohland, A. E. (1976), *J. Ass. Offic. Anal. Chem.*, **59**, 966.
227. Stalling, D. L., Tindle, R. C. and Johnson, J. L. (1972), *J. Ass. Offic. Anal. Chem.*, **55**, 32.
228. Still, G. G. and Mansager, E. R. (1975), *Pestic. Biochem. Physiol.*, **5**, 515.
229. Still, G. G. and Rusness, D. G. (1977), *Pestic. Biochem. Physiol.*, **7**, 210.
230. Stubblefield, R. D. and Shotwell, O. L. (1977), *J. Ass. Offic. Anal. Chem.*, **60**, 784.
231. Subach, D. J., Barnes, D. and Wyche, C. (1976), *J. Chromatogr.*, **125**, 435.
232. Szalontai, G. (1976), *J. Chromatogr.*, **124**, 9.
233. Takahashi, D. M. (1977a), *J. Chromatogr.*, **131**, 147.
234. Takahashi, D. M. (1977b), *J. Ass. Offic. Anal. Chem.*, **60**, 799.
235. Thean, J. E., Fong, W. G., Lorenz, D. R. and Stephens, T. L. (1978), *J. Ass. Offic. Anal. Chem.*, **61**, 15.
236. Thomas, J.-P., Brun, A. and Brounine, J.-P. (1977). *J. Chromatogr.*, **139**, 21.
237. Thruston jr, A. D. (1972), EPA–R2–72–079, N.E.R.C., U.S., EPA, Corvallis, OR 97330.
238. Tindle, R. C. and Stalling, D. L. (1972), *Anal. Chem.*, **44**, 1768.
239. Tumlinson, J. H. and Heath, R. R. (1976), *J. Chem. Ecol.*, **2**, 87.
240. Tumlinson, J. H., Yonce, C. E., Doolittle, R. E., Heath, R. R., Gentry, C. R. and Mitchell, E. R. (1974), *Science*, **184**, 614.
241. Unger, P. D., Mehendale, H. M. and Hayes, A. W. (1977), *Toxicol. Appl. Pharmacol.*, **41**, 523.
242. Van Deemter, J. J., Zuiderweg, F. J. and Klinkenberg, A. (1956), *Chem. Eng. Sci.*, **5**, 271.
243. Van den Berg, J. H. M., Wielders, J. P. M. and Scheeren, P. J. H. (1977), *J. Chromatogr.*, **144**, 266.
244. Vanhaelen-Fastre, R. and Vanhaelen, M. (1976), *J. Chromatogr.*, **129**, 397.
245. Vermont, J., Deleuil, M., de Vries, A. J. and Guillemin, C. L. (1975), *Anal. Chem.*, **47**, 1329.
246. Verpoorte, R. and Svendsen, A. B. (1974), *J. Chromatogr.*, **100**, 227.
247. Vesell, E. S. and Shively, C. A. (1974), *Science*, **184**, 466.
248. Viricel, M. and Lemar, M. (1976), *J. Chromatogr.*, **116**, 343.
249. Vivilecchia, R. V., Lightbody, B. G., Thimot, N. Z. and Quinn, H. M. (1977), *J. Chromatogr. Sci.*, **15**, 424.
250. Ware, G. M. (1975), *J. Ass. Offic. Anal. Chem.*, **58**, 754.
251. Ware, G. M., Thorpe, C. W. and Pohland, A. E. (1974), *J. Ass. Offic. Anal. Chem.*, **57**, 1111.
252. Warthen, J. D. (1975), *J. Amer. Oil Chem. Soc.*, **52**, 151.
253. Waters, J. L., Little, J. N. and Horgan, D. F. (1969), *J. Chromatogr. Sci.*, **7**, 293.
254. Wheals, B. B. and Jane, I. (1977), *Analyst*, **102**, 625.
255. Willmott, F. W. and Dolphin, R. J. (1974), *J. Chromatogr. Sci.*, **12**, 695.
256. Wise, S. A. and May, W. E. (1977), *Research and Development*, October 1977, p. 54.

257. Wolkoff, A. W., Onuska, F. I., Comba, M. E. and Larose, R. H. (1975), *Anal. Chem.*, **47**, 754.
258. Wong, L. T., Solomonraj, G. and Thomas, B. H. (1977), *J. Chromatogr.*, **135**, 149.
259. Yost, G. A. and Miller, L. L. (1976), *J. Agr. Food Chem.*, **24**, 724.
260. Zehner, J. M. and Simonaitis, R. A. (1976), *J. Ass. Offic. Anal. Chem.*, **59**, 1101.
261. Zehner, J. M. and Simonaitis, R. A. (1977), *J. Ass. Offic. Anal. Chem.*, **60**, 14.
262. Zimmerli, B. and Marek, B. (1975), *Mitt. Gebiete Lebens Hyg.*, **66**, 362.
263. Zulalian, J. and Blinn, R. C. (1977), *J. Agr. Food Chem.*, **25**, 1033.

Note Added in Proof

Subsequent to submission of this chapter, a brief tabular review of l.c. data for 166 pesticides has been published: Lawrence, J. F. and Turton, D. (1978), *J. Chromatogr.*, **159**, 207 [42 references].

CHAPTER 2

Rational analysis of drugs in biological fluids with particular reference to the tricyclic antidepressants

W. Riess, S. Brechbühler and J. P. Dubois

INTRODUCTION

The search for correlations between pharmacological or toxicological effects and drug concentrations in biological systems is the most prominent reason for the employment of quantitative analytical chemistry in the interdisciplinary profession of industrial development and clinical use of drugs. The recent progress in analytical technology and the supply of advanced instrumentation have caused a massive increase in the number of published papers. Currently the great potential of analytical techniques contrasts with a limited capability of quantitative pharmacological procedures to assess drug effects or side-effects. Frequently, the difficulties encountered in quantifying pharmacological effects lead to an abundance of pharmacokinetic data-interpretation which is then reported independently and without a clinical correlate that would have made the studies really worthwhile. The deficiencies in quantitative pharmacological data-acquisition may also have an adverse effect on the quality of analytical work. It is therefore justified to recall some aspects of the rational analysis of drugs in biological fluids which may help to guide the analyst.

AN ALARMING STATE OF THE ART OF DRUG ASSAY

The number of published analytical methods to determine xenobiotics, particularly drugs in biological material, is steadily increasing. This trend has been favoured by the requirements of regulatory authorities for documentation of drug properties, by the efforts to correlate drug concentrations in body fluids with their pharmacological effects, and by modern developments in instrumental analysis. For drugs of general interest, a multitude of different analytical techniques are available and still more methods are bound to appear. For instance up to 1974, thirty-two papers on the quantitative determination of carbamazepine in body fluids had been published (Gérardin and Hirtz, 1976). Since then an additional twenty-seven methods have been reported, of which ten resort to high pressure liquid chromatography. Many authors claim to have improved the analytical techniques published previously. In practice, the same method in the hands of different experimenters or, worse, different methods exercised in different laboratories may produce vastly discrepant results when analysing the same biological sample. Richens (1975) compared the performance of forty-four laboratories given the same specimen of pooled serum containing phenytoin, phenobarbitone, and primidone. Two samples, one labelled 'low level specimen', the other 'high level specimen', were distributed. All the laboratories had been informed that they were participating in an analytical test and that they should choose their own analytical technique for the analyses of the samples. The thirty-four laboratories which did the phenytoin determinations reported results ranging from 17·5 to 82·5 μM for the 'low level specimen' and from 25·8 to 130·8 μM for the 'high level specimen'. The twenty-four laboratories involved in the phenobarbitone determinations reported concentrations ranging from 82·8 to 189 μM for the 'low level specimen' and from 94·5 to 224 μM for the 'high level specimen'. The sixteen laboratories carrying out the primidone determinations reported values ranging from 5·0 to 29 μM for the 'low level specimen' and from 4·0 to 18·4 μM for the 'high level specimen'.

In a more stringent test (Pippenger *et al*, 1976), three pooled plasma samples containing phenytoin, phenobarbitone, primidone, and ethosuximide were sent to one hundred and twelve different laboratories, none of which was aware of being involved in a test. As might be expected, the results were even more devastating than those reported by Richens (1975) and have been described as 'completely unacceptable'. Eighty-eight different methods of modifications of commonly accepted methods were used. Most of the modifications were attempts to simplify the analysis. These simplifications very often rendered the methods completely non-specific and/or unreliable. The situation as described by Richens (1975) and Pippenger *et al* (1976) appears alarming enough to warrant discussion of a few basic rules in drug assay.

SOME POINTS TO BE CONSIDERED IN DRUG ASSAY WORK

Before starting the experimental work on any technique, a literature survey should be conducted. Information on the chemical and physical properties and on existing analytical methods for the drug or for chemically related compounds is essential.

Aside from systematic surveys of the older literature by computer or manually, recent developments can be followed in title abstracts, such as *Current Contents* or abstract papers like *Ringdoc*. At present the most popular journals for publishing new methods for drug assay in biological materials are *Journal of Chromatography, Analytical Chemistry, Journal of Pharmaceutical Sciences, Clinical Chemistry, and Analytica Chimica Acta.*

Methods used for different drugs are surveyed biennially in *Analytical Chemistry* (see review by Huettemann *et al*, 1975). Current aspects of pharmaceutical analysis are discussed in quarterly reviews by Fairbrother (1976).

The isolation of a drug from biological material requires special care, and so its extraction and purification rely on a careful choice of the optimal pH and solvent. Drugs which cannot be extracted may be isolated by adsorption to charcoal or resins like Amberlite XAD-2 and eluted with suitable solvents. A useful guide to sample preparation in the micro-determination of organic compounds has been compiled by Reid (1976).

The precision and sensitivity of a method depend largely on the quality of the internal standard chosen. Its properties should be closely related to those of the drug to be assayed especially with respect to yields of isolation, derivatization, and detector response. Ideally the internal standard should have the same structure as the drug to be assayed but incorporates either stable (Hawkins, 1977) or radioactive (Whitehead and Dean, 1968) isotopes so that it can be discriminated from the original drug by mass- or β-spectrometry respectively.

Once the different individual conditions are optimized, all the analytical steps of isolation, of derivative formation, of separation and detection have to be performed in sequences, beginning with the analysis of aqueous standard solutions of the drug. This is followed by the analysis of all specified biological fluids, with the drug added in concentrations that are expected to be present *in vivo*. Special attention has to be paid to equilibration of the added drug standard with the biological medium prior to addition of the extracting organic solvent. In no case should the drug standard be added after the extracting solvent. Precision, accuracy, and the limit of detection of the method can be estimated by repeatedly measuring spiked samples of various biological fluids containing concentrations of the drug unknown to the analyst but known only

118

to a referee. The interference of known metabolites can easily be tested by adding these to spiked samples. Ideally, biological samples from a suitable animal species following administration of the drug should be analysed by two methods including basically different separation steps to detect interferences by unknown metabolites.

DRUG ASSAY, A CHEMICAL OR AN INSTRUMENTAL PROBLEM?

The rapid development in instrumental equipment especially in gas chromatography has improved the specific and sensitive analysis of drugs in biological fluids. Yet even with more specific and more sensitive detector systems and the refinement in the choice of column material (Moffat, 1974), the development of quantitative analytical methods will essentially remain a chemical challenge. The selective isolation and formation of suitable derivatives will in the majority of all cases lead to a better analytical result than the use of highly sophisticated equipment only. This concept will be demonstrated by the following four examples. They do not represent a special selection but have been part of the normal analytical work of the authors during 1975–6.

Determination of Hydralazine in Plasma by Gas Chromatography

Problem: Hydralazine is practically non-extractable from biological fluids and is chemically unstable. The existing colorimetric method was not sufficiently sensitive to measure plasma levels of hydralazine after therapeutic doses.

Solution of problem: Hydralazine (**1**, R = H) is converted in the plasma to tetrazolo(1,5-*a*)phthalazine (**2**) by treatment with nitrite at low pH. The derivative is stable, can be extracted from biological material, and is sensitive to electron capture detection in the gas chromatograph. The 4-methyl analogue (**1**, R = CH$_3$) served as an internal standard for derivatization, extraction, and gas chromatography (Jack *et al* 1975). During the preparation of this manuscript, Zak *et al* (1977) and Reece *et al* (1978) have reported that this method determines the sum total of free hydralazine and acid labile hydrazones of hydralazine.

HN—NH$_2$ $\xrightarrow[\text{NaNO}_2,\ \text{HCl}]{\text{in Plasma,}}$

(1)   (2)

Determination of Clioquinol in Biological Material by Extractive Alkylation and Gas Chromatography

Problem: The published method used the O-acetyl derivative for gas chromatography. This derivative was unstable and the determination of small quantities was hampered by impurities from biological material.

Solution of problem: Clioquinol (**3**, R = I) and the internal standard, 5,7-dichloro-8-hydroxyquinoline (**3**, R = Cl), are extracted from the biological material in the form of their tetrahexyl ammonium salts into dichloromethane, where in the presence of methyl iodide, both clioquinol and the standard are spontaneously transformed to their O-methyl derivatives (**4**). These derivatives are stable and can be purified by a base-specific extraction. Detection limits for the determination can be improved to measure 10 ng clioquinol in the biological sample (Degen *et al*, 1976a).

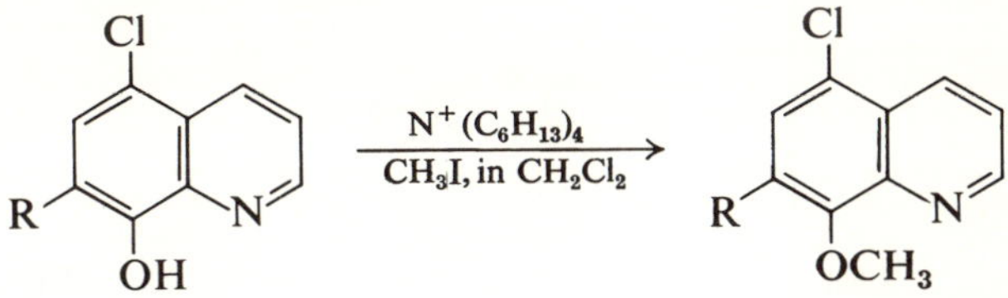

$$\text{(3)} \xrightarrow[\text{CH}_3\text{I, in CH}_2\text{Cl}_2]{\text{N}^+(\text{C}_6\text{H}_{13})_4} \text{(4)}$$

Determination of Baclofen in Biological Material by Gas Chromatography

Problem: Baclofen cannot be extracted from biological material by organic solvents.

Solution of problem: Baclofen (**5**, R = H) and its internal standard, γ-amino-β-(2,4-dichlorophenyl)butyric acid (**5**, R = Cl), are isolated from the biological sample by adsorption onto charcoal. After elution, both compounds are converted to their butyl esters (**6**). The esters are stable and can be extracted by base-specific solvent extraction. They are then N-acylated with heptafluorobutyryl imidazole. The neutral end-products (**7**) are isolated by solvent extraction and detected by gas chromatography (Degen and Riess, 1976).

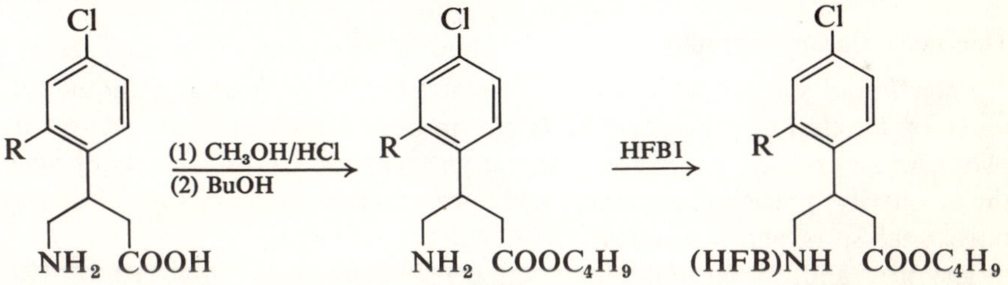

$$\text{(5)} \xrightarrow[\text{(2) BuOH}]{\text{(1) CH}_3\text{OH/HCl}} \text{(6)} \xrightarrow{\text{HFBI}} \text{(7)}$$

Determination of Phanquone in Biological Material by Gas Chromatography

Problem: In the body, phanquone, 4,7-phenanthroline-5,6-dione (**8**, R = H), is partially reduced to 4,7-phenanthroline-5,6-diol (**9**). Neither of these two compounds can be extracted from biological material by the usual organic solvents. Suitable derivatives have been lacking.

Solution of problem: Both phanquone (**8**, R = H) and its diol derivative (**9**) as well as the internal standard, 10-methyl-4,7-phenanthroline-5,6-dione (**8**, R = CH$_3$), can be reacted in the aqueous biological sample with methyl hydroxylamine to yield the dimethoxime derivatives (**10**). These bases can be extracted specifically, gas chromatographed, and measured by electron capture detection (Degen *et al*, 1976b).

(8)

(9)

$$\xrightarrow{\text{CH}_3\text{ONH}_2}$$
in Plasma, pH 3, 70°C, 2 h

(10)

MAIN ANALYTICAL METHODOLOGIES

References to introductory reading about each technique as well as information on equipment and applications are provided in this section. A more detailed treatment concerning the tricyclic antidepressants is given in the final section of this chapter.

Thin-layer Chromatography

Detection of substances on thin-layer plates can be performed semiquantitatively by an elution process or by *in situ* measurement of compounds on the plates. In general, only the direct evaluation (densitometry) of the plates offers the sensitivity, precision, accuracy, and speed that is necessary for the quantitative analysis of pharmaceuticals in biological specimens.

The first and so far only book on densitometry was published in 1973 (Touchstone, 1973). Advances, theory, apparatus, techniques, and applications have been reviewed biennially in *Analytical Chemistry* (see review by Zweig and Sherma, 1976). An updating on instrumentation has been published by Lott *et al* (1976).

The great advantage of thin-layer chromatography lies in its simplicity and speed. Additionally metabolites can be recognized and measured, very often by the same procedure as the unchanged drug. Success in the separation of different metabolites depends on the proper choice of solvents (Moffat, 1974) and coating materials of the thin-layer plates. Sensitivity is excellent, reaching nanogram levels with ultraviolet-detection (e.g. Breyer and Villumsen, 1976) and sub-nanogram levels with fluorimetric detection (e.g. Tripp *et al*, 1975). Yet reproducibility is sometimes difficult to achieve. Reproducibility is greatly influenced by the quality of the plates used, by the mode of application of the samples onto the plate, standardization of the separation procedures, and detection of the compounds on the plate. Application of samples may be improved by using plates with 'concentrating zones' (Halpaap and Krebs, 1977). The use of internal standards may correct for losses during working-up procedures and for differences in the application of samples and the uniformity of the plate layer. With the standardization of the separation and derivatization procedures, the distribution of a compound within the layer can be controlled. Considerable progress will probably be achieved in separation and reproducibility with the rapidly developing high performance thin-layer chromatography (HPTLC; Zlatkis and Kaiser, 1977; *Advances in Chromatography*, 1977).

Quantitative measurement of fluorescence, fluorescence quenching, or light absorption of the compounds on the thin-layer plates is performed on single- or double-beam instruments, in a reflectance or transmission mode or by a combination of the two modes. A comparison of transmission and reflectance measurements has recently been published by Pollak (1975). With instruments using the 'flying spot' technique or zigzag scan, the influence of varying spot sizes on the detector signal can be diminished (Ebel and Herold, 1976).

Thin-layer densitometry is a useful tool for the analysis of drugs in biological samples. Useful qualitative and quantitative information on drugs and their metabolites can be gained in a very short time with the minimum of equipment. For a larger series of samples and if higher precision is required, i.e. in pharmacokinetic studies, high performance liquid chromatography might be a more suitable tool than thin-layer chromatography.

High Performance Liquid Chromatography

High performance liquid chromatography (HPLC) has been developed in recent years to be a useful and versatile tool in pharmaceutical chemistry and biochemistry. With the increasing availability of commercial instruments, with improved column technologies, detectors, and automation, the number of papers dealing with HPLC has increased from less than one hundred papers in the six years before 1973 to about three hundred per annum today. The historical events that led to this explosive expansion in the past few years were described by Ettre and Horvath (1975).

Several textbooks published recently contain information on the theory, instrumentation, and application of HPLC (Done *et al*, 1974; Snyder and Kirkland, 1974; Engelhardt, 1975; Simpson, 1976). Reviews on HPLC are regularly published in *Analytical Chemistry* (see review by Walton, 1976). Equipment is regularly discussed in the *Journal of Chromatographic Science* (see paper by McNair and Chandler, 1976). Practical aspects in design, preparation, and operation of the HPLC-columns of today have been discussed by Majors (1977). Application of HPLC in the pharmaceutical industry was described by Bailey (1976) and Knox *et al* (1976). A review on the analysis of drugs and their metabolites has recently been published by Wheals and Jane (1977) and on pesticides by Schooley and Quistad in this volume (see Chapter 1).

High performance liquid chromatography today offers speed and specificity comparable to gas chromatography (GC). Detection limits have often been better in GC than in HPLC. The development of suitable chromophoric and fluorogenic derivatives (Frei and Santi, 1975) and the development of new types of detectors have improved sensitivity to the same level as GC. The great advantage of HPLC compared to GC lies in the fact that non-volatile and unstable compounds and especially conjugates can also be measured. Compounds are rarely degraded by HPLC and usually there is no need to prepare stable or volatile derivatives.

Compared to thin-layer chromatography, HPLC offers much better reproducibility and resolution. HPLC is easier to automate and therefore more efficient in handling large numbers of samples. The technical advances in detector (Simpson, 1976; Kissinger, 1977) and gradient elution systems (Saunders, 1977) allow the separation and quantitation of still more complex mixtures. The availability of a wide variety of packing materials (Majors, 1977) for normal and reversed-phase techniques (Karch *et al*, 1976; Scott and Kucera, 1977) will facilitate improvements in the sensitivity and resolution. Yet the cost of HPLC equipment is still relatively greater than that of GC equipment.

Gas Chromatography

An introduction to the technique of gas chromatography (GC) is given in the practical manual edited by Tranchant (1969) and recent developments in gas chromatography are reviewed by Cram and Juvet (1976). GC methods are frequently used to identify and to quantify drugs in biological fluids. Moffat (1974) describes the evaluation of different stationary phases used for GC identifications of unknown drugs. For accurate quantitation of a known drug in biological fluids, an internal standard with similar chemical structure is required. Identification or quantitation procedures need to be rapid, specific, sensitive, and reproducible.

In a first step, the drug and the internal standard have to be separated from the biological fluid (Reid, 1976) and their reactive groups may have to be chemically derivatized prior to GC separation (Drozd, 1975; Ahuja, 1976) to make the compounds sufficiently volatile for GC.

Gas chromatographic separation is usually achieved on packed glass columns. The packed column in GC has been described by Supina (1974). Recently, Bailey *et al* (1977) described an automated method for the determination of nomifensine in human plasma using a 50 m open tubular glass capillary column with a frequency of one chromatogram every 37 minutes. Shorter open tubular glass capillary columns with a length of 10 or 15 m also show a much better resolution than packed columns but a comparable retention time (Johansen, 1977). Isothermal GC is most frequently used for the quantitation of a known drug but linear temperature programming may be helpful for the simultaneous determination of a drug and one of its more polar metabolites or for the elution of impurities with long retention times.

The different types of detectors used to identify the eluted compounds have been described by Ševčík (1976) and the routine use of specific detectors by Pigliucci *et al* (1975). Unfortunately, the characterization of GC detectors by the smallest detectable sample that can be read above the noise level is of little interest for the analyst working with biological samples. In this case, not only the drug to be determined together with the internal standard, but also a multitude of other compounds extracted from the biological samples or introduced as a result of extraction or derivatization, are detected with comparable sensitivity. The noise level is therefore considerably increased and the smallest detectable amount of a drug in a biological fluid is about 10^3 times higher than for the pure compound. In favourable cases about 5–10 ng of a drug can be detected in 1 ml of plasma with a ^{63}Ni-electron capture detector (ECD) and about 20–40 ng per ml with a flame ionization detector (FID). The limit of detection for nitrogen-containing compounds in biological fluids detected with an alkali flame ionization or nitrogen/phosphorus detector lies between those for the ECD and the FID.

Gas Chromatography/Mass Spectrometry

Introduced as a detector to monitor the components of an unresolved gas chromatographic peak separately, the mass spectrometer has become a powerful tool in the quantitative analysis of drugs in the low nanogram range. Quantitation of the effluent of a gas chromatograph is performed by electron impact or chemical ionization and monitoring of two or more ions through their mass-to-charge ratios. The best application of this method is obtained through using stable isotope-labelled internal standards which are added to the biological fluid prior to extraction. When added in excess, such an almost ideal internal standard also serves as a carrier for the small amounts of drug during extraction and chromatography thereby minimizing drug losses. Due to the increased specificity of the detector, the smallest detectable amount of a drug in 1 ml of a biological fluid ranges in favourable cases between 0·5–1 ng per ml, being about 10 times lower than for the ^{63}Ni-ECD. The advantages of this technique have to be compared to the high costs of the instrument, the technical skill required of the operator, and the laboratory work necessary to synthesize stable isotope-labelled internal standards (for a recent review, see Hawkins, 1977).

The book edited by Waller (1972) gives an introduction to the biochemical applications of mass spectrometry. The first chapter of the first volume of *Progress in drug metabolism* describes the newer developments in the mass spectrometry of drugs and metabolites (Millard, 1976). The following reviews are also of interest: gas chromatography/mass spectrometry by Fenselau (1974) and by Junk (1972), the scope of mass spectrometry in clinical chemistry by Lawson (1975), and the application of mass fragmentography in high-accuracy analysis (Björkhem *et al*, 1976). A more detailed survey of the mass spectrometry literature is given in the biennial reviews of *Analytical Chemistry* (see review by Burlingame *et al*, 1976), in a list of 319 references on mass fragmentography literature up to the beginning of 1975 by Palmér and Holmstedt (1975) and in a review on gas chromatography and mass spectrometry by Politzer *et al* (1976).

124

Double Radioisotope Derivative Technique

The double radioisotope derivative (DRID) methodology, in which one isotope (for example ^{14}C) is used to label an internal standard and another (for example ^3H) is used to label the reagent, has originally been elaborated and applied to biochemical analytical problems. A survey of the literature up to 1968 has been published by Whitehead and Dean (1968). The usefulness of the DRID technique for the assay of drugs in biological samples has been underrated for a long time. Only a simplified version of this technique (Hammer and Brodie, 1967; Harris *et al*, 1970) has been applied. Without an internal standard and without a separation process the method, however, was poorly reproducible and non-specific.

Modern β-spectrometer equipment, ideal for automatic data processing, recently helped to revive the DRID method. Thus a method has been reported for the quantitative determination of maprotiline in biological material (Riess, 1974b) which gave results as satisfactory as those from a sensitive gas chromatographic technique (Geiger *et al*, 1975). Similarly, methods have been published to measure benzoctamine (Riess, 1974a), clomipramine and desmethylclomipramine (Carnis *et al*, 1976), nortriptyline (Maguire *et al*, 1976), and acenocoumarol (Le Roux and Richard, 1977).

A special attraction of the DRID technique is the simultaneous determination of a drug and its metabolites. This has been demonstrated by the simultaneous determination of opipramol and its deshydroxyethyl metabolite (Riess, 1977) and of maprotiline, its N-desmethyl metabolite, and an aromatic hydroxylated metabolite (Riess, 1974a).

Despite the obvious advantages of the DRID technique, a few disadvantages must not be overlooked. It requires the radioactively-labelled drug and metabolites as internal standards. In one case, a ^{14}C-labelled metabolite necessary for the determination has been isolated from animal urine (Riess, 1974a) since synthesis proved difficult. Special laboratory facilities are necessary to prevent radioactive contamination of samples and to protect the operator. Without adequate safety facilities the DRID method should not be considered.

Radioimmunoassay

In the past few years, radioimmunoassay (RIA) has become a useful tool, especially for the determination of steroids. Very recently the state of the art of the radioimmunoassay of steroid hormones was reviewed in a textbook by Gupta (1975) and for drugs in general by Landon and Moffat (1976).

The great advantage of RIA lies in its sensitivity which allows the use of small amounts of biological samples, and in the large number of assays that can be handled per day. Its ease in performance lends itself to automation (Brooker *et al*, 1976). The great disadvantage is the risk of cross-reactions which has to be compensated by specific purification of the biological sample. This difficulty can be overcome by the preparation of more specific antisera.

Establishing a new radioimmunoassay needs appropriate laboratory and animal facilities. Radioactive reagents of high purity and high specific activity are necessary. A number of commercial kits for the assay of several drugs are now available, thus enabling laboratories without extensive facilities to obtain good results. Initially results should, however, always be checked by comparison with a good chemical method.

PRACTICAL VALUE OF QUANTITATIVE DRUG ASSAY

There is increasing demand for the determination of plasma drug concentrations following the administration of drugs. One reason for this is the improvement in quality control *in vivo*. Different galenic forms of a drug have to be tested for their performance (bioavailability) in the body. Another reason is the control of patient compliance during the treatment and the follow-up period (Kragh-Sørensen *et al*, 1976c). For the evaluation of quality control and for patients compliance, even methods that do not differentiate between parent drug and metabolites may be used if the ratio between the drug and its metabolites is fairly constant in each individual. In both cases the volunteers or patients in a study serve as their own control.

The determination of pharmacokinetic parameters and the establishment of correlations between plasma levels and therapeutic effects or side-effects are the more demanding aims of plasma drug concentration measurements. For these studies, not only the precision but also the specificity of the analytical method need to be known. Pharmacokinetic parameters are usually estimated for a single compound. Very often, not only the unchanged drug but also the metabolites exert a pharmacological effect, and yet the extent and duration of this effect may be different. Thus the parent drug and active metabolites should be measured separately.

Therapeutic response is assumed to be dependent on the amount of drug present at the receptor site(s) which in turn is in equilibrium with the amount of drug in the body. Comparing different individuals, the amount of the drug in the body may be poorly related to the administered dose due to differences in absorption, elimination, extent of first-pass effect, and metabolism. The amount of the drug in the body may even be influenced by environmental factors as well as co-medications and diseases. Therefore, the determination of concentrations of a drug in the circulating blood, which are in equilibrium with those in the tissues, should give a much better correlation with the pharmacological effect exerted by that drug than does the administered dose. Furthermore, even under steady-state conditions, the plasma concentrations of a drug are not constant but fluctuate during each dosing interval (Levy, 1974). The pharmacological parameters to be correlated with drug concentrations on the other hand have to be quantitated accurately and precisely also.

The current state of the art to correlate plasma concentrations of drugs with therapeutic efficacy will be examined in an example chosen from psychiatry, tricyclic antidepressant therapy, where admittedly the clinical response to drug treatment is difficult to measure, and yet a multitude of data on steady-state blood levels have been published with varying claims for correlations.

AMBITIOUS AIM TO CORRELATE TRICYCLIC ANTIDEPRESSANT PLASMA LEVELS WITH CLINICAL EFFECTS OF DRUG TREATMENT

General Aspects

Review of the many papers dealing with blood level determinations of antidepressants reveals a striking variability in experimental findings. It is therefore almost impossible to combine data from different laboratories in order to reach statistically relevant conclusions. In the literature shortcomings of different kinds and degrees are apparent, namely:

1. The determination of the blood or plasma concentrations must be performed with a specific and sensitive method. Without the use of an internal standard and an appropriate chromatographic separation step, the quality of the chemical analytical data required cannot be achieved. Inappropriate blood collection methods may cause redistribution of the drug between plasma and red cells as shown for meperidine, quinidine, and some β-receptor antagonists (Piafsky and Borgå, 1976), and for tricyclic antidepressants (Brunswick and Mendels, 1977).

2. It is assumed that the pharmacological effect of tricyclic antidepressants correlates with the mean steady-state plasma drug concentration. The steady-state drug concentrations are fluctuating during each dosing interval, the amplitude of the fluctuations being dependent on the dose and dosage regimen. The mean steady-state concentration is defined (Levy, 1974) as the area under the steady-state concentration–time curve during a regular dosing interval divided by the length of this interval. In most studies only one single blood sample is assayed to determine the steady-state concentration.

3. A study which is aimed at achieving correlations between plasma concentrations and pharmacological effect should provide for equal frequency distribution of the individual concentrations in the whole concentration range under study. To reach equal distributions, patients have to be treated with different dosages. Figures 1 and 2 illustrate the plasma concentration distribution in patients receiving two standard doses of nortriptyline. With 150 mg nortriptyline per day, a homogeneous distribution of the plasma concentrations is obtained only for 65% of the patients, ranging between 50 and 150 ng/ml. The probability of finding patients with plasma concentrations below 50 ng/ml or above 150 ng/ml is much lower.

4. The selection of patients poses a paramount problem. Only 50–60% of depressed patients respond to tricyclic antidepressant treatment. Burrows *et al* (1974c) found that 21% of the patients with a primary depressive illness, who were admitted to the hospital for the first time, improved without drug treatment. Luchins and Ananth (1976) reported that about 20–30% of depressive disorders are resistant to drug treatment. A critical review on the prediction of tricyclic antidepressant response has been published by Bielski and Friedel (1976).

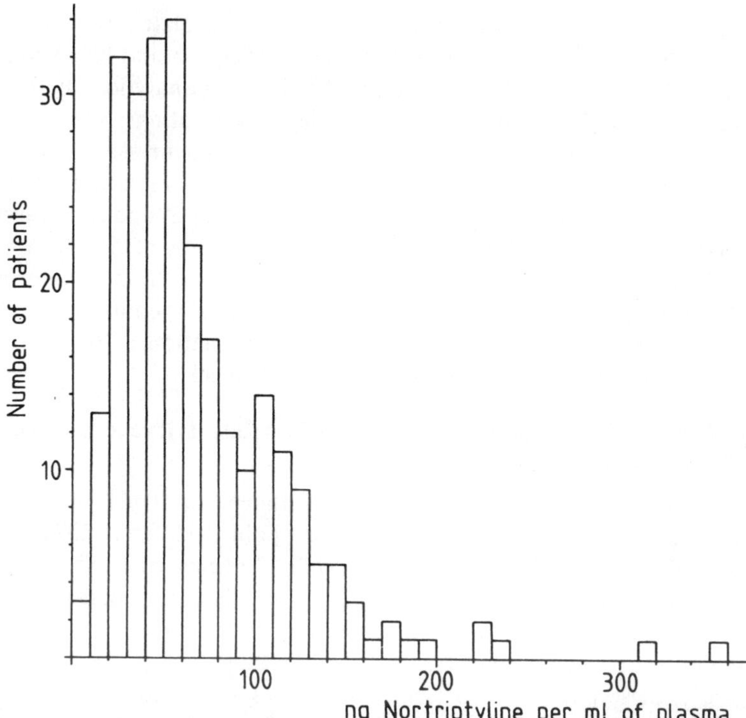

Figure 1 Plasma levels of nortriptyline obtained during therapy in 263 patients on a daily dose of 75 mg of the drug. From Åsberg, 1976, reproduced with permission of Georg Thieme Verlag

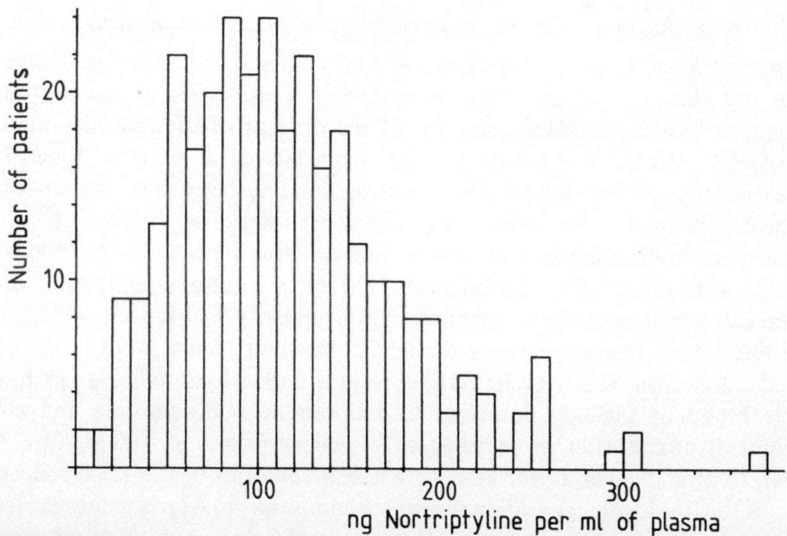

Figure 2 Plasma levels of nortriptyline obtained during therapy in 311 patients on a daily dose of 150 mg of the drug. From Åsberg, 1976, reproduced with permission of Georg Thieme Verlag

5. Accuracy and precision of both parameters to be correlated, that is the mean steady-state concentration and the therapeutic effect, should be documented. Whereas this is generally accessible for the chemical analytical methods, no relevant information is available for the depression ratings.

6. Based on the initial depression score S_i and the final depression score S_f, five different improvement indices have been defined: estimation of $S_i - S_f$, $(S_i - S_f)/S_i$, of S_f only, of S_f/S_i, and of the analysis of S_i and S_f using partial correlation (Shah and Kline, 1974). Partial correlation of S_i and S_f would seem the best approach yet it is not easily accessible. S_f/S_i lacks information on the level of improvement. S_f is not independent of the initial score S_i and by using S_f, the final score only, part of the information is lost. The differences $S_i - S_f$ or $(S_i - S_f)/S_i$ have too large a variance.

Survey of the Various Published Attempts to Correlate Tricyclic Antidepressant Concentrations and Therapeutic Effect

Several reviews of correlations of tricyclic antidepressant plasma concentrations with pharmacological effect have been published from 1974 to 1976 (Åsberg, 1974; Kragh-Sørensen *et al*, 1976b; Luchins and Ananth, 1976; Modestin and Petrin, 1976; Simpson *et al*, 1976) discussing papers published before the end of 1974. In the meantime another ten papers have appeared. With the exception of two papers, published by Haydu *et al* (1962) and Yates *et al* (1963), these papers are presented in Tables 1–6. The tables summarize on the one hand the analytical methodologies, the steady-state concentrations, and the daily doses of the tricyclic antidepressant drugs, and on the other hand the patient selection, the depression rating, and the results of the study.

Analytical methodology for the assay of tricyclic antidepressant drugs

Sample work-up. Common problems for all assays of tricyclic antidepressant drugs are the physical or chemical instability (e.g. losses by adsorption or decomposition) of standard solutions of the drug or of the internal standard, the specific extraction of the compounds from biological material, losses from the extracting solvent due to adsorption on glass surfaces, and the separation of the compounds to be determined from other interfering compounds.

Losses of imipramine hydrochloride and clomipramine hydrochloride of up to 20% were observed by Dubois *et al* (1976) in solutions containing 200 µg of the salt per litre of water, ethanol, or *n*-heptane. For solutions in 10 mmol/litre HCl, these losses were less than 5%. The best results were obtained by directly dissolving the tricyclic antidepressant amine hydrochloride in human whole blood or plasma. Solutions of imipramine hydrochloride and clomipramine hydrochloride in pyridine at a concentration of 100 mg/litre were shown to be stable for a year at 4 °C, whereas solutions of the same concentrations of the free bases in pyridine showed decomposition. At pH values exceeding 10, the tricyclic antidepressant amines are extracted in high yield with *n*-heptane/isopentyl alcohol (99 : 1 by volume) and there is no need for a multiple first extraction step. Using *n*-hexane instead of *n*-heptane, a lower extraction yield is obtained. To eliminate the large amount of neutral compounds in the solvent extract of the first extraction step, the amines can be re-extracted from the solvent at pH values below 2. Such a purification procedure shortens the duration of the gas chromatographic analysis by elimination of neutral compounds with long retention times, e.g. cholesterol, and increases the lifetime of the columns.

Losses from the extracting solvent by adsorption to glass surfaces can be reduced by adding 1% of isopentyl alcohol to the extracting solvent. However, the addition of 1% of isopentyl alcohol increases the amount of endogenous material extracted from the biological sample (Hammer and Brodie, 1967) and therefore may reduce the specificity of the assay or may complicate the gas chromatographic analysis of a large number of samples because of the presence of interfering compounds with long retention times.

Different analytical assays used in correlation studies

The analytical assays of the twenty studies reviewed in Tables 1 to 5 include six fluorimetric, six radioisotope derivative, two thin-layer chromatographic, four gas chromatographic, and two gas chromatographic/mass spectrometric methods.

Fluorimetric methods. Those used allowed separate determination of tertiary and secondary amines but they included neither an internal standard nor a chromatographic separation step. Purification was only achieved by repeated extraction steps. Dingell *et al* (1964) used a method with 4 single extraction steps separating imipramine and desipramine at pH 5·9. By acetylation of desipramine, Moody *et al* (1967) obtained a better separation from imipramine. Perel *et al* (1974) reported a modified version including only two single extraction steps and Moody *et al* (1973) published a method for the secondary amine protriptyline.

Radioisotope derivative methods. The assay described by Hammer and Brodie (1967) for the secondary amine desipramine includes only one single extraction step. Much effort therefore has to be spent to avoid increased blank values which may occur upon too vigorous and prolonged shaking during the extraction or upon addition of 1·5% of isopentyl alcohol to the extracting solvent to prevent adsorption. Sjöqvist *et al* (1969) extended this method to nortriptyline and stressed, in addition to the points outlined above, the need for high radiochemical purity of the ^{3}H-acetic anhydride and the use of fresh plasma. These authors noted further the interference by other tricyclic antidepressant drugs. Kline and Cooper (1974) combined the ^{3}H-acetylation of the secondary amine desmethyldoxepin with the ^{14}C-methylation of the tertiary amine doxepin following the procedure described by Harris *et al* (1970). To correct for the variable yields of the ^{3}H-acetyl derivative of maprotiline ranging between 38 and 77%, Riess (1974b) used ^{14}C-labelled maprotiline as an internal standard and to eliminate interfering background he added the non-radioactive N-acetyl derivative of maprotiline as a carrier after the ^{3}H-acetylation of the biological extract prior to two-dimensional thin-layer chromatography.

Thin-layer chromatographic methods. Modestin (1973) described a method for dibenzepin and its side-chain N-demethylated metabolite with colorimetric determination of the compounds eluted from the scraped thin-layer chromatographic spots. Nagy and Treiber (1973) determined imipramine and desipramine with direct densitometry of the thin-layer chromatograms after colour reaction on the plates with nitrous gases. To show the actual possibilities of this method, two recent techniques not included in this survey should be mentioned. Breyer and Villumsen (1976) reported the scan of unstained plates at the ultraviolet maximum in a reflectance mode and Fenimore *et al* (1977) described a high performance thin-layer chromatographic method for the quantitative determination of different tricyclic antidepressant drugs.

Gas chromatographic methods. The quantitative determination of unchanged amitriptyline and the trifluoroacetyl derivative of nortriptyline by gas chromatography with flame ionization detection was reported by Braithwaite and Widdop (1971). The internal standard triptycene was not added to the biological sample prior to extraction but only after trifluoroacetylation. Borgå and Garle (1972) described a method for the quantitative determination of nortriptyline and some of its metabolites after preparation of the heptafluorobutyryl derivative and separation on a gas chromatograph equipped with an electron capture detector. They added maprotiline as an internal standard to the biological fluid prior to extraction. Two recent gas chromatographic techniques are not included in this correlation survey: the electron capture gas chromatography of tertiary amines in the form of their pentafluorobenzyl or trichloroethyl carbamates (Hartvig *et al*, 1976) and gas chromatography with a nitrogen-specific detector (Bailey and Jatlow, 1976; Witts and Turner, 1977).

Gas chromatographic/mass spectrometric methods. Biggs *et al* (1976) described a method for the determination of several tricyclic antidepressant drugs, which has been used for correlation studies with amitriptyline and nortriptyline. N,N-Di-C^{2}H$_3$-amitriptyline and desmethyldoxepin were used as internal standards for the determination of amitriptyline and nortriptyline respectively. But in both assays the full advantages offered by the gas chromatographic/mass spectrometric method could not be realized, namely the use of a stable isotope-labelled internal standard combined with the detection of the molecular ions of the drug to be determined and of the internal standard. The electron-impact mass spectrum of amitriptyline shows only a single abundant ion at *m/e* 58 and it would need chemical ionization mass spectrometry to be able to measure the quasi-molecular ion (MH$^+$) at *m/e* 278 for amitriptyline and at *m/e* 284 for hexadeuteroamitriptyline (Garland, 1977; Wilson *et al*, 1977). Other gas chromatographic/mass spectrometric methods not included in the correlation survey using stable isotope-labelled internal standards and monitoring of the molecular ions were reported by Claeys *et al* (1976) for imipramine and desipramine, by Dubois *et al* (1976) for imipramine, clomipramine, and desmethylclomipramine and by Alfredsson *et al* (1977) for clomipramine and desmethylclomipramine.

Two analytical methods of importance not included at all in the reviewed correlation studies were *high performance liquid chromatography and radioimmunoassay*. Some recent papers on high performance liquid chromatography of tricyclic antidepressant drugs were published by Brodie *et al* (1977), Mellström and Tybring (1977), Van den Berg *et al* (1977), Watson and Stewart (1977), and Westenberg *et al* (1977). These assays were used to determine amitriptyline, nortriptyline, imipramine, desipramine, clomipramine, and desmethylclomipramine. The assay of Watson and Stewart (1977) also includes the determination of the metabolites of amitriptyline and imipramine. Radioimmunoassays have been reported by Spector *et al* (1975) for desipramine, by Aherne *et al* (1976) for nortriptyline, and by Aherne *et al* (1977) for amitriptyline and nortriptyline.

Other parameters used in the survey correlation studies

Aside from a specific, sensitive, and reproducible assay method, other parameters of importance in correlation studies are the dosage of the tricyclic antidepressant drug and the dosage regimen, the appropriate determination of the steady-state concentration of the drug and its active metabolites, the selection of patients who respond to the drug, and an appropriate index of improvement based on a reliable rating scale. The parameters chosen for the different correlation studies are listed in Tables 1 to 6. Unfortunately, the variety of each of the parameters chosen makes it impossible to pool the results of different studies. Though eight studies with nortriptyline comprising 298 patients were performed, each study has to be judged separately, thus giving much less information than if the data could be pooled.

Outcome of the surveyed correlation studies

Classifying the twenty studies surveyed in Tables 1 to 6, four studies show no correlation, five a curvilinear, and eleven a linear positive correlation between plasma concentration and therapeutic effect. The linear positive relationship was, with one exception, observed for tertiary amines only: six studies with imipramine, two studies with amitriptyline, and one with dibenzepin and doxepin each. Maprotiline is the only secondary amine where in a single study a positive linear relationship has been reported. All the other secondary amines show either no correlation (four studies with nortriptyline) or a curvilinear correlation (four studies with nortriptyline and one study with protriptyline). Although correlations have been established, the multitude of parameters used allow no general, acceptable guidelines on therapeutic ranges.

Table 1 No relationship between tricyclic antidepressant plasma concentration and pharmacological effect

| Study | Analysis | | | Tricyclic antidepressant | Dose in mg per day | Regimen | Blood collection (time after last dose) | Range of plasma concentrations | Other drugs |
	Method	Separation steps	Internal standard						
(1) Burrows *et al* (1972)	RID*	—	—	nortriptyline	150	TID 6/14/22	6–7 h	37–592 ng/ml after 4 weeks (*N* = 32) 24–468 ng/ml after 6 weeks (*N* = 19)	not men-tioned
(2) Burrows *et al* (1974a)	RID*	—	—	nortriptyline	variable	TID 6/14/22	not mentioned	intended plas-ma concentra-tions: below 49 ng/ml above 140 ng/ml	no other drugs than nitra-zepam
(3) Burrows *et al* (1974b, 1974c) Davies *et al* (1975)	RID*	—	—	nortriptyline	75–250	TID 6/14/22	6–7 h	20–590 ng/ml (*N* = 80)	no other drugs than nitra-zepam
(4) Collaborative study (1974)	GC/FID†	GC	added after ex-traction	nortriptyline	55–200	not men-tioned	not mentioned	20–355 ng/ml (*N* = 45)	in one case barbi-turate detected

RID: radioisotope derivative, GC: gas chromatography, FID: flame-ionization detector, TID: three times daily.
* Hammer and Brodie (1967); Burrows *et al* (1972).   † Braithwaite and Widdop (1971).

Table 2 Curvilinear relationship between tricyclic antidepressant plasma concentration and pharmacological effect

		Analysis							
Study	Method	Separation steps	Internal standard	Tricyclic antidepressant	Dose in mg per day	Regimen	Blood collection (time after last dose)	Range of plasma concentrations	Other drugs
(1) Åsberg et al (1971)	RID*	—	—	nortriptyline	75–225	TID 6/14/22	7 h	32–164 ng/ml ($N = 24$)	pentobarbitone, glutethimide, diazepam
(2) Kragh-Sørensen et al (1973a, b)	GC/ECD† GC	added before extraction		nortriptyline	150	TID 6/14/22	not mentioned	48–238 ng/ml ($N = 30$)	meprobamate, aspirin, oestrogens (1 case)
(3) Kragh-Sørensen et al (1976a)	GC/ECD† GC	added before extraction		nortriptyline	50–300	TID 6/14/22	7 h	intended plasma concentrations: below 150 ng/ml above 180 ng/ml	not mentioned
(4) Ziegler et al (1976b)	GC/MS‡ GC	added before extraction		nortriptyline	75–150	single bedtime dose	12–16 h	individual mean values: 53–252 ng/ml ($N = 18$)	no other drugs

Table 2 (*cont.*)

| Study | Analysis | | | Tricyclic antidepressant | Dose in mg per day | Regimen | Blood collection (time after last dose) | Range of plasma concentrations | Other drugs |
	Method	Separation steps	Internal standard						
(5) Whyte *et al* (1976)	FLUOR§	—	—	protriptyline	40	QID 10/14/ 18/22	11·5 h	106–378 ng/ml ($N = 28$)	nitraze-pam, sodium amylo-barbitone, laxatives, antibiotics (2 cases), chlorpro-mazine (1 case)

RID: radioisotope derivative, GC: gas chromatography, ECD: electron capture detector, MS: mass spectrometry, FLUOR: fluorimetry, TID, QID: three, four times daily.

* Hammer and Brodie (1967); Sjöqvist *et al* (1969).　† Borgå and Garle (1972); Kragh-Sørensen *et al* (1973b).　‡ Biggs *et al* (1976). § Moody *et al* (1973).

Table 3 Positive relationship between tricyclic antidepressant plasma concentration and pharmacological effect

| Study | Method | Analysis | | Tricyclic antidepressant | Dose in mg per day | Regimen | Blood collection (time after last dose) | Range of plasma concentrations | Other drugs |
		Separation steps	Internal standard						
(1) Wharton *et al* (1971)	FLUOR*	separation of IMI and DES	—	imipramine	150–225	TID no schedule	not mentioned	not mentioned	20 mg methyl-phenidate per day, chloral hydrate
(2) Zeidenberg *et al* (1971)	FLUOR*	separation of IMI and DES?	—	imipramine	max. 450	TID no schedule	2 h	IMI + DES: 170–750 ng/ml $(N = 7)$	sodium amobarbi-tone, chloral hydrate, 20 mg methylphe-nidate/day $(N = 4)$, 10 mg dex-troamphet-amine/day $(N = 1)$
(3) Walter (1971)	FLUOR*	separation of IMI and DES	—	imipramine	0·7 mg/kg $(N = 8)$ 150–225 $(N = 8)$	TID no schedule	14–15 h	IMI: 2·5–71·0 ng/ml $(N = 16)$	no other drugs than nitrazepam

Table 3 (*cont.*)

Study	Method	Separation steps	Internal standard	Tricyclic antidepressant	Dose in mg per day	Regimen	Blood collection (time after last dose)	Range of plasma concentrations	Other drugs
		Analysis							
(4) Braithwaite *et al* (1972)	GC/FID†	GC	added after ex-traction	amitriptyline	150	TID no schedule	average of 19 h (SD = 4·3)	AMI ($N = 15$): 20–162 ng/ml after 6 weeks NOR ($N = 15$): 20–206 ng/ml after 6 weeks	nitrazepam 1 case: phenobar-bitone + phenytoin
(5) Modestin (1973)	TLC/ COLOR‡	TLC	—	dibenzepin	8 mg/kg correspon-ding to 400–600	TID no schedule	4 h after the morning dose	individual mean values of dibenzepin ($N = 12$) 80–280 ng/ml	chloral hydrate

FLUOR: fluorimetry, GC: gas chromatography, FID: flame ionization detector, TLC: thin-layer chromatography, COLOR: colorimetry, IMI: imipramine, DES: desipramine, AMI: amitriptyline, NOR: nortriptyline, TID: three times daily.
* Moody *et al* (1967).   † Braithwaite and Widdop (1971).   ‡ Modestin (1973).

Table 3 (*cont.*)

| Study | | Analysis | | Tricyclic antidepressant | Dose in mg per day | Regimen | Blood collection (time after last dose) | Range of plasma concentrations | Other drugs |
	Method	Separation steps	Internal standard						
(6) Angst and Rothweiler (1974)	DRID*	TLC	^{14}C-labelled, added before extraction	maprotiline	150 ($N = 10$) 225 ($N = 10$)	150: evening dose 225: 150 evening + 75 morning dose	before morning dose	maprotiline: 107–1277 ng/ml blood levels ($N = 20$)	not mentioned
(7) Olivier-Martin *et al* (1975)	FLUOR†	separation of IMI and DES	—	imipramine	150	2 daily doses 7/12	19 h	IMI ($N = 18$): 50–220 ng/ml IMI + LEVO ($N = 6$): 170–240 ng/ml DES ($N = 18$): 50–300 ng/ml DES + LEVO ($N = 6$): 100–380 ng/ml	levomepromazine ($N = 6$) diazepam, methaqualone
(8) Gram *et al* (1976)	TLC/ DENSIT‡	TLC	—	imipramine	150–225	TID 8/13/17	15 h	IMI ($N = 24$): 22–232 ng/ml DES ($N = 24$): 22–585 ng/ml	no other drugs than nitrazepam
(9) Kline *et al* (1976)	RID§	separation of DOX and DESDOX	—	doxepin	30 ($N = 5$) 150 ($N = 5$)	TID no schedule	not mentioned	not mentioned	not mentioned

DRID: double radioisotope derivative, FLUOR: fluorimetry, TLC: thin-layer chromatography, DENSIT: densitometry, RID: radioisotope derivative, IMI: imipramine, DES: desipramine, DOX: doxepin, DESDOX: desmethyldoxepin, LEVO: levomepromazine, TID: three times daily.
* Riess (1974b). † Dingell *et al* (1964). ‡ Nagy and Treiber (1973). § Kline and Cooper (1974).

Table 3 (*cont.*)

| Study | Method | Analysis | | Tricyclic antidepressant | Dose in mg per day | Regimen | Blood collection (time after last dose) | Range of plasma concentrations | Other drugs |
		Separation steps	Internal standard						
(10) Perel *et al* (1976) Glassman *et al* (1973, 1975)	FLUOR*	separation of IMI and DES	—	imipramine	3·5 mg/kg	TID no schedule	before morning dose	IMI+DES: 95–1020 ng/ml ($N = 29$)	flurazepam
(11) Ziegler *et al* (1976a)	GC/MS†	GC	D_6-label-led, added before extrac-tion	amitriptyline	max. 150	single bedtime	12–16 h	individual mean values AMI+NOR: 55–315 ng/ml ($N = 18$)	no other drugs

FLUOR: fluorimetry, GC: gas chromatography, MS: mass spectrometry, IMI: imipramine, DES: desipramine, AMI: amitriptyline, NOR: nortriptyline, TID: three times daily.
* Moody *et al* (1967); Perel *et al* (1974).   † Biggs *et al* (1976).

Table 4 No relationship between tricyclic antidepressant plasma concentration and pharmacological effect

Study	Patient selection			Depression rating			Results of the study
	Number of in/outpatients	Selection criteria	Initial observation period	Rating scale	Index of improve-ment	Duration of active medication	
(1) Burrows *et al* (1972)	32 inpatients	primary depressive illness, E.C.T. not necessary	1 week	Hamilton DRS Beck self-RS	change score	4 week ($N = 32$) 6 weeks ($N = 19$)	no significant correlation between plasma concentration and pharmacological effect
(2) Burrows *et al* (1974a)	40 inpatients	primary depressive illness, E.C.T. not necessary	1 week	Hamilton DRS	change score $\geqslant 8$	4 weeks	matched pairs of patients, one below 49 ng/ml, the other above 140 ng/ml 8 cases in favour of high, 4 cases in favour of low plasma concentrations, 8 cases with no preference
(3) Burrows *et al* (1974b, 1974c) Davies *et al* (1975)	80 inpatients	primary depressive illness, E.C.T. not necessary	1 week	Hamilton DRS	percent change score	4 weeks ($N = 80$) 6 weeks ($N = 12$)	no significant correlation between plasma concentration and pharmacological effect ($N = 80$) out of these patients, 12 responders showed a positive linear relationship on an individual evaluation
(4) Collaborative study (1974)	45 inpatients	depressed patients admitted to hospital	—	—	progress satisfactory, unsatisfactory	min. 2 weeks	no significant correlation between plasma concentration and pharmacological effect satisfactory responders ($N = 26$) unsatisfactory responders ($N = 15$)

E.C.T.: electroconvulsive therapy, DRS: depression rating scale.

Table 5 Curvilinear relationship between tricyclic antidepressant plasma concentration and pharmacological effect

Study	Patient selection			Depression rating			Results of the study
	Number of in/outpatients	Selection criteria	Initial observation period	Rating scale	Index of improvement	Duration of active medication	
(1) Åsberg *et al* (1971)	29 inpatients	endogenous depression	4–7 days placebo period	Cronholm–Ottosson RS	change score	2 weeks	curved relationship between plasma concentration and pharmacological effect optimum range: 50–139 ng/ml
(2) Kragh-Sørensen *et al* (1973a, b)	30 inpatients	endogenous depression (diagnostic inventory of Gurney)	4–7 days placebo period COR score > 8	Cronholm–Ottosson RS	final score	4 weeks	only 1 patient with a plasma concentration below 50 ng/ml, best therapeutic effect with plasma concentrations below 175 ng/ml
(3) Kragh-Sørensen *et al* (1976a)	24 inpatients	endogenous depression (diagnostic inventory of Gurney)	1 week placebo period COR score > 8	Cronholm–Ottosson RS	final score	6 weeks	all 16 patients with plasma concentrations below 150 ng/ml recovered; from 7 patients with plasma concentrations above 180 ng/ml only 1 recovered recommended range: 50–150 ng/ml
(4) Ziegler *et al* (1976b)	18 outpatients	primary or secondary depression (criteria of Feighner *et al*) Hamilton DR score ≥ 22	—	Hamilton DRS Zung self-RS depression scale	final score	6 weeks	no patient with a plasma concentration below 50 ng/ml all 9 patients with plasma concentrations below 130 ng/ml recovered, from 9 patients with plasma concentrations above 140 ng/ml 3 recovered
(5) Whyte *et al* (1976)	28 inpatients	depressive illness	1 week	global assessment	improvement score	3½ weeks	patients within a range of 166–238 ng/ml showed better responses

DRS: depression rating scale, RS: rating scale, COR: Cronholm–Ottosson rating

Table 6 Positive relationship between tricyclic antidepressant plasma concentration and pharmacological effect

Study	Patient selection			Depression rating			Results of the study
	Number of in|outpatients	Selection criteria	Initial observation period	Rating scale	Index of improvement	Duration of active medication	
(1) Wharton *et al* (1971)	7 inpatients	recurrent refractory psychotic depression with delusion formation	—	—	clinical remission	3 weeks IMI + 2–3 weeks IMI and methyl-phenidate	5 of 7 patients treated with the combination therapy had complete clinical remission
(2) Zeidenberg *et al* (1971)	7 inpatients	severe depression of psychotic or near psychotic intensity	—	clinical RS brief psychiatric RS	final score	6 weeks 2 weeks in between with IMI + methyl-phenidate	6 out of 7 patients improved rapidly on very high doses of IMI, IMI + DES > 170 ng/ml
(3) Walter (1971)	16 inpatients	endogenous depression (diagnostic scale of Carney), admission to hospital	—	Hamilton DRS Self-RS	final score	4 weeks	all the responders showed IMI plasma concentrations above 20 ng/ml ($N = 10$) and all non-responders below 20 ng/ml ($N = 6$)

Table 6 (*cont.*)

Study	Patient selection			Depression rating			Results of the study
	Number of in/ outpatients	Selection criteria	Initial observation period	Rating scale	Index of improvement	Duration of active medication	
(4) Braithwaite *et al* (1972)	9 outpatients 6 inpatients	depressive illness	—	Hamilton DRS Wakefield self-assessment depression inventory	final score in % of the baseline	6 weeks	2 weeks: no significant correlation 4 weeks: some degree of correlation 6 weeks: highly significant correlation between plasma concentration and pharmacological effect, good clinical response for AMI + NOR above 120 ng/ml
(5) Modestin (1973)	12 inpatients	endogenous depression	—	Hamilton DRS	% change score	3 weeks	tendency toward a positive linear correlation age and baseline rating included as covariables

DRS: depression rating scale, RS: rating scale, IMI: imipramine, DES: desipramine, AMI: amitrityline, NOR: nortriptyline.

Table 6 (*cont.*)

Study	Patient selection			Depression rating			Results of the Study
	Number of in/ outpatients	Selection criteria	Initial observation period	Rating scale	Index of improve-ment	Duration of active medication	
(6) Angst and Rothweiler (1974)	20 inpatients	depressive psychoses (diagnosis ICD 296)	— —	Hamilton DRS 12 dimensions of the AMP-system	change score	30 days	significant positive correlation after exclusion of 2 patients with maprotiline concentra-tions above 800 ng/ml no significant difference be-tween 150 mg or 225 mg daily
(7) Olivier-Martin *et al* (1975)	24 inpatients	endogenous or psychotic depression	—	modified Hamilton DRS	% change score	3 weeks	positive correlation of clinical response and plasma concen-trations of DES or IMI+ DES, but not with IMI alone
(8) Gram *et al* (1976)	24 inpatients	endogenous depression, selection based on Hamilton DRS	7 days pla-cebo period	Hamilton DRS	final score	4 weeks	11 of the 12 recovered patients had plasma concentrations of IMI $\geqslant$ 45 ng/ml and DES > 75 ng/ml, whereas the others had plasma concentrations of one or both compounds below these limits
(9) Kline *et al* (1976)	10 outpatients	psycho-neurotic with mild to moderate anxiety Hopkins symptom checklist	—	Hamilton DRS Hamilton ARS	global assessment	4 weeks	Clinical response appears related to desmethyldoxepin concentrations in serum, but not to doxepin concentrations higher doses of doxepin appeared useful

DRS: depression rating scale, ARS: anxiety rating scale, IMI: imipramine, DES: desipramine.

Table 6 (*cont.*)

| Study | Patient selection | | | Depression rating | | Duration of active medication | Results of the Study |
	Number of in/ outpatients	Selection criteria	Initial observation period	Rating scale	Index of improve-ment		
(10) Perel *et al* (1976) Glassman *et al* (1973, 1975)	29 inpatients	primary affective disorder	1 week + 1 week placebo period (Hamilton DR score ≥ 18)	modified Hamilton DRS, mood scale, global RS	—	4 weeks	delusional depressive patients are unresponsive to IMI smokers have markedly lower plasma concentrations than non-smokers clinical outcome was related to the plasma concentrations of IMI + DES high probability of recovery for IMI + DES above 180 ng/ml
(11) Ziegler *et al* (1976a)	18 outpatients	primary or secondary depression (criteria of Feighner *et al*) Hamilton DR score ≥ 22	—	Hamilton DRS	final score, % change score	6 weeks	positive correlation between the plasma concentrations of AMI + NOR and therapeutic response patients with concentrations of AMI + NOR above 95 ng/ml had a better response ($N = 10$)

DRS: depression rating scale, IMI: imipramine, DES: desipramine, AMI: amitriptyline, NOR: nortriptyline.

CONCLUSIONS

The statistically conclusive analysis of beneficial therapeutic effects or unwanted side-effects of drugs in relation to their concentrations in body compartments requires large sample sizes. To reach that critical mass of information, it is a paramount requisite that analytical data from different research institutes can be pooled. Because of the current state of the variable quality of drug and therapeutic effect monitoring, the pooling of data is rarely warranted. In this review, the difficulty in correlating plasma levels with therapeutic effects has been analysed for the tricyclic antidepressants. It is shown that, if ever useful correlations are to be established, the most accurate, precise analytical methods must be used and that the measurements of clinical parameters have to be of similar quality. The experimental design should additionally define the plasma concentrations to be correlated, i.e. mean steady state, or if possible the actual concentration and assure a homogeneous frequency distribution of the concentrations to be correlated. The clinical parameters should be adequately chosen and strictly defined. Only if the same clinical parameters are used and the same standard in assessing them is guaranteed can the results from different clinics be compared and pooled.

To improve the situation on the chemical analytical side, Richens (1977) gave practical proposals of how analytical standards could be developed and made available 'to alert the analyst to an erroneous result'. The U.S. FDA regulations on 'Good Laboratory Practices', imposed upon institutes which submit data for drug registration purposes, will exert some pressure towards improvements. A similar effect will result for academic institutes from the more stringent criteria under which research grants can be obtained in the future.

The most natural and attractive approach, however, would be to accept that quantitative analytical chemistry is a co-discipline of pharmacology and to teach appropriate courses in the curriculum of pharmacologists.

REFERENCES

Advances in Chromatography, Amsterdam (1977), *J. Chromatogr.*, **142**, chapter on HPTLC.

Aherne, G. W., Piall, E. M. and Marks, V. (1976), *Brit. J. Clin. Pharmacol.*, **3**, 561.

Aherne, G. W., Marks, V., Mould, G. and Stout, G. (1977), *Lancet*, **1**, 1214.

Ahuja, S. (1976), *J. Pharm. Sci.*, **65**, 163.

Alfredsson, G., Wiesel, F. A., Fyrö, B. and Sedvall, G. (1977), *Psychopharmacology (Berlin)*, **52**, 25.

Angst, J. and Rothweiler, R. (1974), in Symposia Medica Hoechst 8, *Classification and prediction of outcome of depression*, p. 237, Schattauer, Stuttgart.

Åsberg, M. (1974), *Clin. Pharmacol. Ther.*, **16**, 215.

Åsberg, M. (1976), *Pharmakopsychiat. Neuro-Psych.*, **9**, 18.

Åsberg, M., Crönholm, B., Sjöqvist, F. and Tuck, D. (1971), *Brit. Med. J.*, **3**, 331.

Bailey, D. N. and Jatlow, P. I. (1976), *Clin. Chem. (Winston-Salem)*, **22**, 1697.

Bailey, E., Fenoughty, M. and Richardson, L. (1977), *J. Chromatogr.*, **131**, 347.

Bailey, F. (1976), *J. Chromatogr.*, **122**, 73.

Bielski, R. J. and Friedel, R. O. (1976), *Arch. Gen. Psychiat.*, **33**, 1479.

Biggs, J. T., Holland, W. H., Chang, S., Hipps, P. P. and Sherman, W. R. (1976), *J. Pharm. Sci.*, **65**, 261.

Björkhem, I., Blomstrand, R., Lantto, O., Svensson, L. and Oehman, G. (1976), *Clin. Chem.* (Winston-Salem), **22**, 1789.

Borgå, O. and Garle, M. (1972), *J. Chromatogr.*, **68**, 77.

Braithwaite, R. A. and Widdop, B. (1971), *Clin. Chim. Acta*, **35**, 461.

Braithwaite, R. A., Goulding, R., Theano, G., Bailey, J. and Coppen, A. (1972), *Lancet*, **1**, 1297.

Breyer, U. and Villumsen, K. (1976), *Eur. J. Clin. Pharmacol.*, **9**, 457.

Brodie, R. R., Chasseaud, L. F. and Hawkins, D. R. (1977), *J. Chromatogr.*, **143**, 535.

Brooker, G., Terasiki, W. L. and Price, M. G. (1976), *Science*, **194**, 270.

Brunswick, D. J. and Mendels, J. (1977), *Commun. Psychopharmacol.*, **1**, 131.

Burlingame, A. L., Kimble, B. J. and Derrick, P. J. (1976), *Anal. Chem.*, **48**, 368R.

Burrows, G. D., Davies, B. and Scoggins, B. A. (1972), *Lancet*, **2**, 619.

Burrows, G., Turecek, L. R., Davies, B., Mowbray, R. and Scoggins, B. A. (1974a), *Aust. N.Z. J. Psychiat.*, **8**, 21.

Burrows, G., Scoggins, B. A. and Davies, B. (1974b), in Symposia Medica Hoechst 8, *Classification and prediction of outcome of depression*, p. 173, Schattauer, Stuttgart.

Burrows, G., Scoggins, B. A., Turecek, L. R. and Davies, B. (1974c), *Clin. Pharmacol. Ther.*, **16**, 639.

Carnis, G., Godbillon, J. and Metayer, J. P. (1976), *Clin. Chem.* (*Winston-Salem*), **22**, 817.

Claeys, M., Muscettola, G. and Markey, S. P. (1976), *Biomed. Mass Spectrom.*, **3**, 110.

Collaborative Study (1974), *Postgrad. Med. J.*, **50**, 282.

Cram, S. P. and Juvet, R. S. (1976), *Anal. Chem.*, **48**, 411R.

Davies, B., Burrows, G. and Scoggins, B. (1975), *Aust. N.Z. J. Psychiat.*, **9**, 249.

Degen, P. H. and Riess, W. (1976), *J. Chromatogr.*, **117**, 399.

Degen, P. H., Schneider, W., Vuillard, P., Geiger, U. P. and Riess, W. (1976a), *J. Chromatogr.*, **117**, 407.

Degen, P. H., Brechbühler, S., Schäublin, J. and Riess, W. (1976b), *J. Chromatogr.*, **118**, 363.

Dingell, J. V., Sulser, F. and Gillette, J. R. (1964), *J. Pharmacol. Exp. Ther.*, **143**, 14.

Done, J. N., Knox, J. H. and Loheac, J. (1974). *Applications of high-speed liquid chromatography*, Wiley, London.

Drozd, J. (1975), *J. Chromatogr.*, **113**, 303.

Dubois, J. P., Küng, W., Theobald, W. and Wirz, B. (1976), *Clin. Chem.* (*Winston-Salem*), **22**, 892.

Ebel, S. and Herold, G. (1976), *Arch. Pharm.* (*Weinheim*), **309**, 660.

Engelhardt, H. (1975), *Hochdruck-Flüssigkeits-Chromatographie*, Springer, Berlin.

Ettre, L. S. and Horvath, C. (1975), *Anal. Chem.*, **47**, 422A.

Fairbrother, J. E. (1976), *Pharm. J.*, **216**, 537; **217**, 210, 623.

Fenimore, D. C., Meyer, C. J., Davies, C. M., Hsu, F. and Zlatkis, A. (1977), *J. Chromatogr.*, **142**, 399.

Fenselau, C. (1974), *Appl. Spectrosc.*, **28**, 305.

Frei, R. W. and Santi, W. (1975), *Fresenius' Z. Anal. Chem.*, **277**, 303.

Garland, W. A. (1977), *J. Pharm. Sci.*, **66**, 77.

Geiger, U. P., Rajagopalan, T. G. and Riess, W. (1975), *J. Chromatogr.*, **114**, 167.

Gérardin, A. and Hirtz, J. (1976), in Birkmeyer, W. (ed.), *Epileptic seizures—behaviour —pain*, p. 151, Huber, Bern.

Glassman, A. H., Hurwic, M. J. and Perel, J. M. (1973), *Amer. J. Psychiat.*, **130**, 1367.

Glassman, A. H., Kantor, S. J. and Shostak, M. (1975), *Amer. J. Psychiat.*, **132**, 716.

Gram, L. F., Reisby, N., Ibsen, I., Nagy, A., Dencker, S. J., Bech, P., Petersen, G. O. and Christiansen, J. (1976), *Clin. Pharmacol. Ther.*, **19**, 318.

Gupta, D. (1975), *Radioimmunoassay of steroid hormones*, Verlag Chemie, Weinheim.

Halpaap, H. and Krebs, K. F. (1977), *J. Chromatogr.*, **142**, 823.

Hammer, W. M., Brodie, B. B. (1967), *J. Pharmacol. Exp. Ther.*, **157**, 503.

Harris, S. R., Gaudette, L. E., Efron, D. H. and Manian, A. A. (1970), *Life Sci.*, **9**, Part 1, 781.

Hartmann, C. H. (1971), *Anal. Chem.*, **43**, 113A.

Hartvig, P., Ahnfelt, N. O. and Karlsson, K. E. (1976), *Acta Pharm. Suec.*, **13**, 181.

Hawkins, D. R. (1977), in Bridges, J. W. and Chasseaud, L. F. (eds), *Progress in drug metabolism*, vol. 2, p. 163, Wiley, London.

Haydu, G. G., Dhrymiotis, A. and Quinn, G. P. (1962), *Amer. J. Psychiat.*, **119**, 574.

Huettemann, R. E., Cotter, M. L., Shaw, C. J., Janicki, C. A., Almond, H. R., Moyer, E. S., Shroff, A. P. and Vestano, F. (1975), *Anal. Chem.*, **47**, 233R.

Jack, D. B., Brechbühler, S., Degen, P. H., Zbinden, P. and Riess, W. (1975), *J. Chromatogr.*, **115**, 87.

Johansen, N. (1977), *Chromatogr. Newsl.*, **5**, 14.

Junk, G. A. (1972), *Int. J. Mass Spectrom. Ion Phys.*, **8**, 1.

Karch, K., Sebestian, I., Halász, I. and Engelhardt, H. (1976), *J. Chromatogr.*, **122**, 171.

Kissinger, P. T. (1977), *Anal. Chem.*, **49**, 447A.

Kline, N. S. and Cooper, T. B. (1974), in Symposia Medica Hoechst 8, *Classification and prediction of outcome of depression*, p. 207, Schattauer, Stuttgart.

Kline, N. S., Cooper, T. and Johnston, B. (1976), in Gottschalk, L. A. and Merlis, S. (eds), *Pharmacokinetics of psychoactive drugs*, p. 221, Spectrum, New York.

Knox, J. H., Jurand, J. and Pryde, A. (1976), *Proc. Anal. Div. Chem. Soc.*, **1976**, 14.

Kragh-Sørensen, P., Åsberg, M. and Hansen, C. E. (1973a), *Lancet*, **1**, 113.

Kragh-Sørensen, P., Hansen, C. E. and Åsberg, M. (1973b), *Acta Psychiat. Scand.*, **49**, 444.

Kragh-Sørensen, P., Hansen, C. E., Baastrup, P. C. and Hvidberg, E. F. (1976a), *Psychopharmacologia (Berlin)*, **45**, 305.

Kragh-Sørensen, P., Hansen, C. E., Baastrup, P. C. and Hvidberg, E. F. (1976b), *Pharmakopsychiat. Neuro-Psych.*, **9**, 27.

Kragh-Sørensen, P., Hvidberg, E. F., Hansen, C. E. and Baastrup, P. C. (1976c), *Pharmakopsychiat. Neuro-Psych.*, **9**, 178.

Landon, J. and Moffat, A. C. (1976), *Analyst (London)*, **101**, 225.

Lawson, A. M. (1975), *Clin. Chem. (Winston-Salem)*, **21**, 803.

Le Roux, Y. and Richard, J. (1977), *J. Pharm. Sci.*, **66**, 997.

Levy, G. (1974), *Clin. Pharmacol. Ther.*, **16**, 130.

Lott, F. G., Dias, J. R. and Hurtubise, R. J. (1976), *J. Chromatogr. Sci.*, **14**, 488.

Luchins, D. and Ananth, J. (1976), *J. Nerv. Ment. Dis.*, **162**, 430.

Maguire, K. P., Burrows, G. D., Coghlan, J. P. and Scoggins, B. A. (1976), *Clin. Chem. (Winston-Salem)*, **22**, 761.

Majors, R. E. (1977), *J. Ass. Offic. Anal. Chem.*, **60**, 186.

McNair, H. M. and Chandler, C. D. (1976), *J. Chromatogr. Sci.*, **14**, 477.

Mellström, B. and Tybring, G. (1977), *J. Chromatogr.*, **143**, 597.

Millard, B. J. (1976), in Bridges, J. W. and Chasseaud, L. F. (eds), *Progress in drug metabolism*, vol. 1, p. 1, Wiley, London.

Modestin, J. (1973), *Pharmakopsychiat. Neuro-Psych.*, **6**, 29.

Modestin, J. and Petrin, A. (1976), *Int. J. Clin. Pharmacol. Ther. Toxicol.*, **13**, 11.

Moffat, A. C. (1974), in CIBA Foundation Symposium 26 (New Series), *The poisoned patient: the role of the laboratory*, p. 83, Elsevier, Amsterdam.

Moody, J. P., Tait, A. C. and Todrick, A. (1967), *Brit. J. Psychiat.*, **113**, 183.

Moody, J. P., Whyte, S. F. and Naylor, G. J. (1973), *Clin. Chim. Acta*, **43**, 355.

Nagy, A. and Treiber, L. (1973), *J. Pharm. Pharmacol.*, **25**, 599.

Olivier-Martin, R., Marzin, D., Buschsenschutz, E., Pichot, P. and Boissier, J. (1975), *Psychopharmacologia* (*Berlin*), **41**, 187

Palmér, L. and Holmstedt, B. (1975), *Sci. Tools* (the LKB Instrument Journal), **22**, 25, 38.

Perel, J. M., O'Brien, L., Black, N. B., Bellward, G. D. and Dayton, P. G. (1974), in Forrest, I. S., Carr, C. J. and Usdin, E. (eds), *The phenothiazines and structurally related drugs*, p. 201, Raven, New York.

Perel, J. M., Shostak, M., Gann, E., Kantor, S. J. and Glassman, A. H. (1976), in Gottschalk, L. A. and Merlis, S. (eds), *Pharmacokinetics of psychoactive drugs*, p. 229, Spectrum, New York.

Piafsky, K. M. and Borgå, O. (1976), *Lancet*, **2**, 963.

Pigliucci, R., Averill, W., Purcell, J. E. and Ettre, L. S. (1975), *Chromatographia*, **8**, 165.

Pippenger, C. E., Penry, J. K., White, B. G., Daly, D. D. and Buddington, R. (1976), *Arch. Neurol.* (*Chicago*), **33**, 351.

Politzer, I. R., Dowty, B. J. and Laseter, J. L. (1976), *Clin. Chem.* (*Winston-Salem*), **22**, 1775.

Pollak, V. (1975), *J. Chromatogr.*, **105**, 279.

Reece, P. A., Stanley, P. E. and Zacest, R. (1978), *J. Pharm. Sci.*, **67**, 1150.

Reid, E. (1976), *Analyst* (*London*), **101**, 1.

Richens, A. (1975), in Schneider, H., Janz, D., Gardner-Thorpe, C., Meinardi, H. and Sherwin, A. L. (eds), *Clinical pharmacology of anti-epileptic drugs*, p. 293, Springer, Berlin.

Richens, A. (1977), *Brit. Med. J.*, **1**, 1411.

Riess, W. (1974a), in CIBA Foundation Symposium 26 (New Series), *The poisoned patient: the role of the laboratory*, p. 139, Elsevier, Amsterdam.

Riess, W. (1974b), *Anal. Chim. Acta*, **68**, 363.

Riess, W. (1977), *Anal. Chim. Acta*, **88**, 109.

Saunders, D. L. (1977), *J. Chromatogr. Sci.*, **15**, 129.

Scott, R. P. W. and Kucera, P. (1977), *J. Chromatogr.*, **142**, 213.

Ševčík, J. (1976), *Detectors in gas chromatography*, *J. Chromatogr.* Library, vol. 4, Elsevier, Amsterdam.

Shah, B. K. and Kline, N. S. (1974), in Symposia Medica Hoechst 8, *Classification and prediction of outcome of depression*, p. 219, Schattauer, Stuttgart.

Simpson, C. F. (1976), *Practical high performance liquid chromatography*, Heyden, London.

Simpson, G. M., Cooper, T. B. and Lee, J. H. (1976), in Gallant, D. M. (ed.), *Depression*, p. 109, Spectrum, New York.

Sjöqvist, F., Hammer, W., Borgå, O. and Azarnoff, D. L. (1969), in Cerletti, A. and Boré, F. J. (eds), *The present status of psychotropic drugs* (*ICS 180*), p. 128, Excerpta Medica, Amsterdam.

Snyder, L. R. and Kirkland, J. J. (1974), *Introduction to modern liquid chromatography*, Wiley, New York.

Spector, S., Spector, N. L. and Almeida, M. P. (1975), *Psychopharmacol. Commun.*, **1**, 421.

Supina, W. R. (1974), *The packed column in gas chromatography*, Supelco, Bellefonte, Pa.

Touchstone, J. C. (1973), *Quantitative thin layer chromatography*, Wiley, New York.

Tranchant, J. (ed.) (1969), *Practical manual for gas chromatography*, Elsevier, Amsterdam.

Tripp, S. L., Williams, E., Wagner, W. E. and Lukas, G. (1975), *Life Sci.*, **16**, 1167.

Van den Berg, J. H. M., De Ruwe, H. J. J. M., Deelder, R. S. and Plomp, T. A. (1977), *J. Chromatogr.*, **138**, 431.

Waller, G. R. (ed.) (1972), *Biochemical applications of mass spectrometry*, Wiley–Interscience, New York.

Walter, C. J. S. (1971), *Proc. Roy. Soc. Med.*, **64**, 282.

Walton, H. F. (1976), *Anal. Chem.*, **48**, 52R.

Watson, I. D. and Stewart, M. J. (1977), *J. Chromatogr.*, **134**, 182.

Westenberg, H. G. M., Drenth, B. F. H., De Zeeuw, R. A., De Cuyper, H., Van Praag, H. M. and Korf, J. (1977), *J. Chromatogr.*, **142**, 725.

Wharton, R. N., Perel, J. M., Dayton, P. G. and Malitz, S. (1971), *Amer. J. Psychiat.*, **127**, 1619.

Wheals, B. B. and Jane, I. (1977), *Analyst (London)*, **102**, 625.

Whitehead, J. K. and Dean, H. G. (1968), in Glick, D. (ed.), *Methods of biochemical analysis*, vol. 16, p. 1, Interscience, New York.

Whyte, S. F., Macdonald, A. J., Naylor, G. J. and Moody, J. P. (1976), *Brit. J. Psychiat.*, **128**, 384.

Wilson, J. M., Williamson, L. J. and Raisys, V. A. (1977), *Clin. Chem. (Winston-Salem)*, **23**, 1012.

Witts, D. J. and Turner, P. (1977), *Brit. J. Clin. Pharmacol.*, **4**, 249.

Yates, C. M., Todrick, A. and Tait, A. C. (1963), *J. Pharm. Pharmacol.*, **15**, 432.

Zak, S. B., Lukas, G. and Gilleran, T. G. (1977), *Drug Metab. Disp.*, **5**, 116.

Zeidenberg, P., Perel, J. M., Kanzler, M. Wharton, R. N. and Malitz, S. (1971), *Amer. J. Psychiat.*, **127**, 1321.

Ziegler, V. E., Bun Tee Co, Taylor, J. R., Clayton, P. J. and Biggs, J. T. (1976a), *Clin. Pharmacol. Ther.*, **19**, 795.

Ziegler, V. E., Clayton, P. J., Taylor, J. R., Bun Tee Co and Biggs, J. T. (1976b), *Clin. Pharmacol. Ther.*, **20**, 458.

Zlatkis, A. and Kaiser, R. E. (1977), *HPTLC—high performance thin-layer chromatography*, J. Chromatogr. Library, vol. 9, Elsevier, Amsterdam.

Zweig, G. and Sherma, J. (1976), *Anal. Chem.*, **48**, 66R.

CHAPTER 3

The metabolism of xenobiotics in insects

G. T. Brooks

INTRODUCTION

The last decade has witnessed an ever-increasing emphasis on the need to control the amounts of synthetic chemicals of all kinds that are added to the environment. It is now widely appreciated that although such foreign compounds (drugs, pesticides, other toxicants; xenobiotics) are often greatly modified by chemical hydrolysis, atmospheric oxidation, or photochemical changes in sunlight, the major burden of environmental transformations nevertheless falls on those enzymic processes of the biosphere that occur in animals, plants, and microorganisms. These biotransformations, which may not necessarily be beneficial to the biosphere as a whole, can profoundly affect the environmental levels of the parent chemicals, and studies of the biodegradation of xenobiotics have therefore attained a greater significance than ever before.

Investigations of drug metabolism in man and other mammals form a well-established branch of the study of xenobiotic biodegradation and a great deal of information about the principles of mammalian metabolism is already available. Thus, it is well known that for mammals interspecific differences in sensitivity to the effects of drugs frequently depend on qualitative and/or quantitative differences in ability to effect biotransformations. The wider study of the enzymic degradation of environmental xenobiotics (such as pesticides, plasticizers, detergents, flame retardants, and other compounds that may occur in industrial wastes) by any contacting target or non-target organism comprises a second branch for which much less information is available, although the principles appear to be similar. Most information is available for plants and for pest arthropods, because of their economic importance. However, concern for the environment has produced a new emphasis on comparative metabolism and a consequent increase in studies on vertebrate and invertebrate aquatic organisms, birds, and non-pest arthropods.

The study of drug metabolism in insects is mainly that of insecticide metabolism, although drugs as understood by the pharmacologist are sometimes used as model compounds or for other purposes. Since the phylum Arthropoda is the largest in the animal kingdom (75% of all known animal species) and the class Insecta (about 26 major orders) constitutes some 90% of known arthropod species (up to 10 million species estimated), the scope for investigations is obviously unlimited.

The first serious studies of xenobiotic metabolism in insects were initiated by the dramatic appearance of resistance to DDT in houseflies in Sweden in 1946, only two years after it was first used there with excellent results. Two decades later, the combined total of public health and agricultural insect pest species that were resistant to one or more of the major classes of insecticides was well over 200. This situation has produced a considerable body of knowledge about insecticide metabolism in a number of common pests, extending even to the location of genes controlling different metabolic (and non-metabolic) mechanisms in insects such as houseflies, mosquitoes, and cockroaches. The consequences of inhibiting toxicant detoxication *in vivo* in insects are often spectacularly evident and sometimes commercially valuable for extending the use of insecticides. Synergists derived from 1,3-benzodioxole ('methylenedioxyphenyl' synergists) have long been known to increase the insecticidal potency of natural pyrethrins, and it was soon discovered that certain non-toxic DDT analogues and other compounds could potentiate DDT against insects resistant to it. Therefore, the study of insecticide synergists developed alongside investigations of insecticide metabolism, and synergists have proved to be highly valuable aids in metabolic studies.

Resistance studies have provided much information about insecticide metabolism but few practical solutions to the problem except to suggest structural modifications which might enable new toxicants to evade specific detoxication mechanisms, or to indicate the order in which different classes of insecticides should be used in order to delay the onset of resistance. Nevertheless, the information accumulated, together with that from comparative studies between insect species and between insects and mammals, provides a basis for the research needed to meet the increasing demand for insecticides that have both improved species selectivity and environmental degradability.

Relevant reviews are available for insecticides in general (O'Brien, 1967; Brooks, 1972; Corbett, 1974; Matsumura, 1975; Metcalf and McKelvey, 1976; Wilkinson, 1976b), pyrethrins (Casida, 1973), chlorinated insecticides (Brooks, 1974b), organophosphorus insecticides (Eto, 1974), and carbamate insecticides (Kuhr and Dorough, 1976). Other texts contain relevant information on naturally occurring insecticides (Jacobson and Crosby, 1971) and insect juvenile hormone analogues (Menn and Beroza, 1971).

The following account considers:

1. The development of insect metabolism studies in a historical context;
2. The present state of knowledge of basic metabolic processes in insects;
3. The application of metabolism studies to the improvement of selectivity and biodegradability of the major classes of insecticides.

DEVELOPMENT OF METABOLISM STUDIES

Table 1, which is not intended to be exhaustive, summarizes some of the major developments in metabolic studies in insects between 1950 and 1970.

With the introduction for insect control of DDT (1) in 1942, γ-HCH (2) in 1942–3, TEPP (3) in 1943, parathion (4) in 1944, chlordane (5) in 1945 and

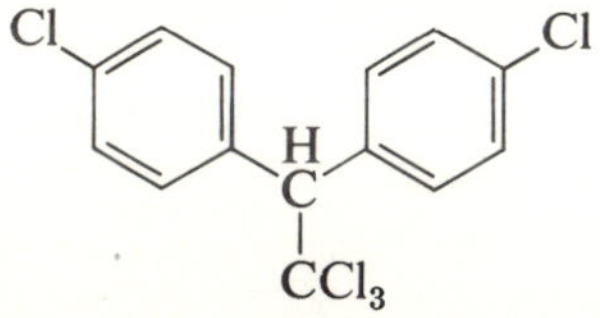

DDT
(1)

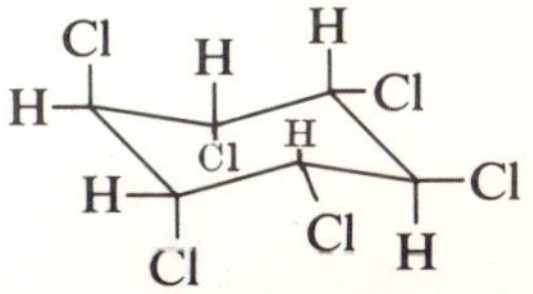

HCH (γ-isomer; lindane)
(2)

$$(C_2H_5O)_2P(O)-O-P(O)(OC_2H_5)_2$$
TEPP
(3)

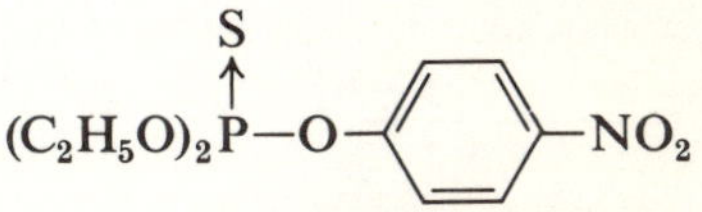

parathion
(4)

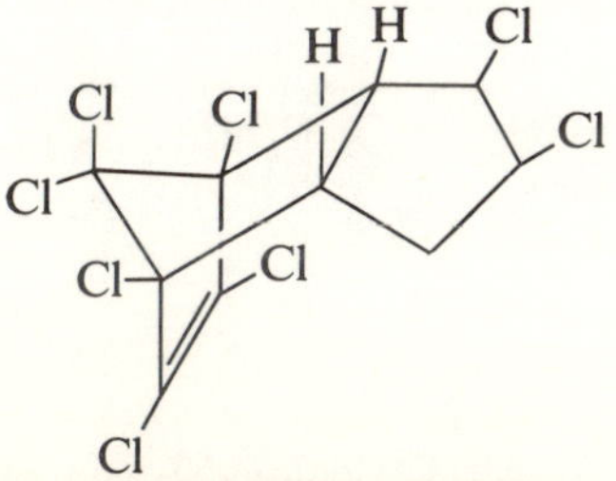

chlordane (isomeric mixture)
(5)

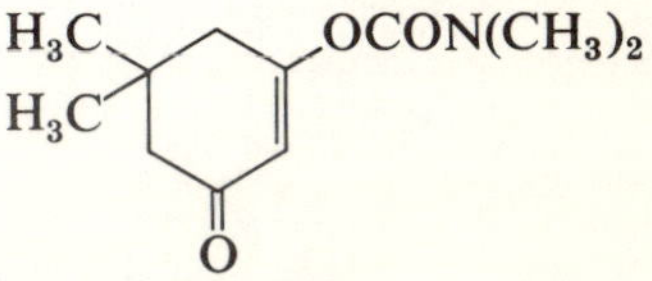

dimetan
(6)

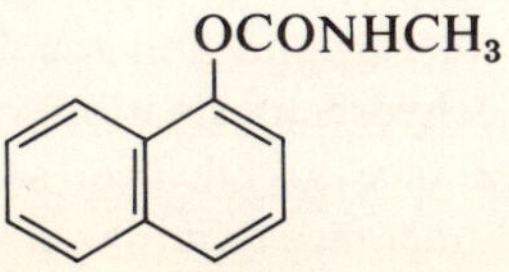

carbaryl
(7)

camphechlor (toxaphene) in 1948 (camphechlor is a complex mixture of chlorinated camphenes containing 67–69% chlorine), and the development of the carbamate anticholinesterases (e.g. **6** and **7**) for this purpose in the early 1950s, it is seen that four classes of chlorinated insecticides and two classes of anticholinesterase insecticides suddenly became available about 25 years ago— a somewhat unique situation.

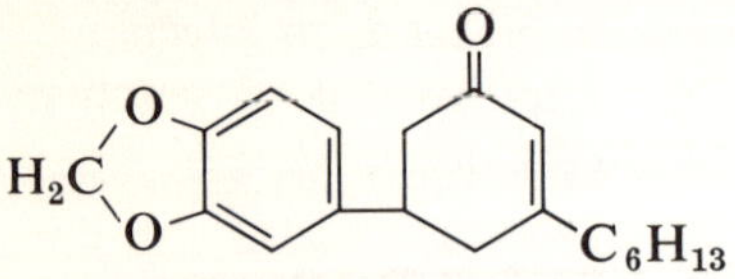

major component of
piperonyl cyclonene
(8)

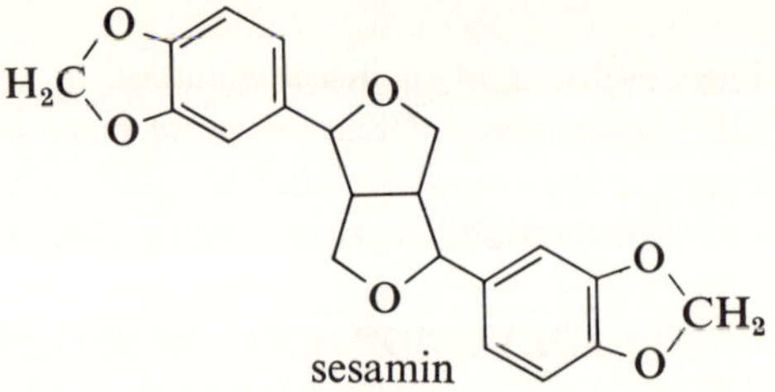

sesamin
(9)

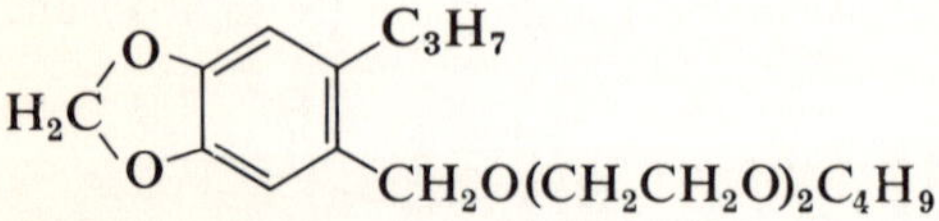

piperonyl butoxide
(10)

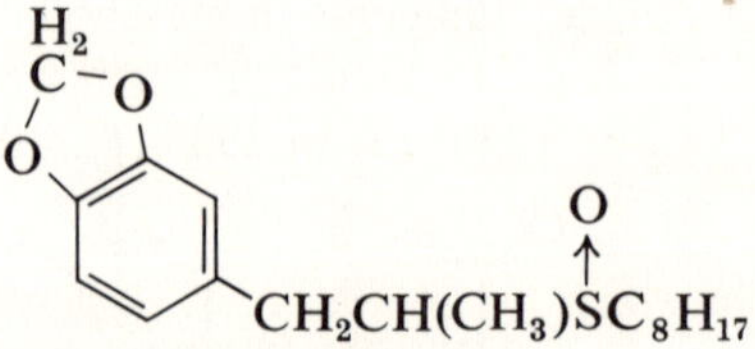

sulfoxide
(11)

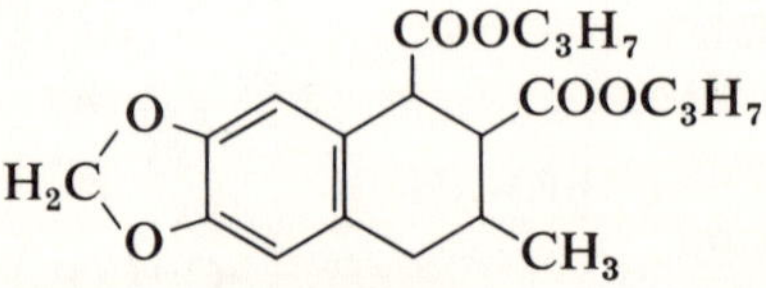

propyl isome
(12)

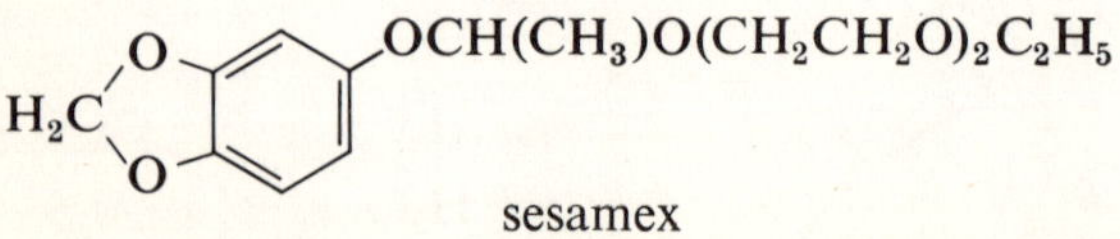

sesamex
(13)

The study of what has become known as 'Insect Toxicology' began, at least as far as organic insecticides are concerned, with the appearance of DDT-resistance in 1946. Research in England and the United States soon showed that the enzymic conversion (dehydrochlorination) of DDT to DDE was largely responsible for acquired resistance to DDT in some insects (e.g. houseflies, *Musca domestica*) and natural tolerance to it in others (e.g. Mexican bean beetle, *Epilachna varivestis*). A substantial purification of the DDT-dehydrochlorinase (DDT-ase) from resistant houseflies in 1954 was followed by an extensive examination of its properties and substrate specificity (Lipke and Kearns, 1960). A low titre of a similar enzyme occurs in normal houseflies; its natural function is unknown and DDT-ase is still under investigation.

The role of DDT-ase in detoxication was proven by the fact that non-toxic DDT analogues which inhibited it *in vitro* and *in vivo* synergized DDT in resistant houseflies (Moorefield and Kearns, 1955). This observation generated a new interest in insecticide synergists, especially since piperonyl cyclonene (**8**), a pyrethrins synergist of the 1,3-benzodioxole (methylenedioxyphenyl) type, appeared to block DDT metabolism by this route. Interest in such compounds actually dates from 1942, when sesamin (**9**) was identified (Haller *et al*, 1942) as one of the active constituents of sesame oil, which was already used to enhance the toxicity of natural pyrethrins. Several other compounds of this type (**10, 11, 12**) later reached commercial development, while sesamex (**13**) has been widely used as a research tool in studies of insecticide metabolism.

In addition to the effect of synergists on DDT metabolism, structural modifications such as the introduction of an *ortho*-chlorine into one benzene ring of DDT (Hennessy *et al*, 1961) or replacement of the benzylic hydrogen by deuterium (Barker, 1960; Dachauer *et al*, 1963) suppressed enzymic dehydrochlorination.

However, these investigations revealed interesting interspecific differences in the substrate specificity of the enzyme, since benzylic deuteration suppressed dehydrochlorination in certain mosquitoes but not in houseflies, whereas *o*-chloro-DDT was effective against both houseflies and some other species of mosquitoes that resisted deutero-DDT.

Reports on the metabolism of insecticides such as the natural pyrethrins and nicotine appeared in the early 1950s (Table 1) and some of them (as well as some of the DDT researches) provide early examples of the use of radiotracer techniques in this field. The belief that the pyrethrins would be detoxified mainly by hydrolysis of their central ester groups persisted until 1960 and considerably hindered an understanding of the behaviour of these compounds in insects.

Resistance to lindane (γ-HCH), chlordane, toxaphene, and dieldrin (**15**) soon followed their use against DDT-resistant houseflies in the late 1940s, and resistance to lindane was found to extend to chlordane, dieldrin (cyclodiene insecticides), and toxaphene but not to DDT. The spread of resistance to these chlorinated insecticides (OC) and, from 1949 onwards, to the organophosphorus anticholinesterases (OP) has been well documented by Brown (1969) for agricultural pests and by Brown and Pal (1971) for public health pests. These alarming developments led to the metabolism studies on lindane and the cyclodiene insecticides mentioned in Table 1. From the work on lindane came early evidence for the involvement of reduced glutathione (GSH) in insect detoxication mechanisms, and from the investigations on aldrin (**14**), isodrin, and heptachlor (**16**) the first examples of an oxidative process (epoxidation) converting the unsaturated precursors (themselves undoubtedly toxic) into stable and equally toxic or more toxic products (depending on the insects examined). At the time, these cyclodienes appeared to be otherwise metabolically inert, in

Table 1 Developments in metabolic studies on insecticides and other xenobiotics in insects, 1950–1970

Observation or event	References
Discovery the DDT is converted into DDE (dehydrochlorination) by DDT-resistant houseflies	Perry and Hoskins, 1950; Sternburg *et al*, 1950; Winteringham *et al*, 1951; Winteringham, 1952
Early studies on the metabolism of botanical insecticides (pyrethrins, nicotine)	Chamberlain, 1950; Zeid *et al*, 1953; Winteringham *et al*, 1955; Hopkins and Robbins, 1957; Guthrie *et al*, 1957
Resistance to lindane, cyclodienes, and toxaphene from 1949	Brown, 1969; Brown and Pal, 1971
First investigations of lindane metabolism in insects	Bradbury and Standen, 1956, 1959; Bradbury, 1957; Oppenoorth, 1954, 1955, 1956; Sternburg and Kearns, 1956
Early metabolic studies on hexachlorocyclopentadiene derivatives (cyclodiene insecticides; aldrin, heptachlor, chlordane, etc.)	Giannotti *et al*, 1956; Perry *et al*, 1958; Winteringham and Harrison, 1959; Brooks, 1960; Perry, 1960; Cohen and Smith, 1961; Korte *et al*, 1962; Brooks *et al*, 1963
First observation of epoxide formation from aldrin, isodrin, and heptachlor in insects	
Resistance to organophosphorus insecticides from 1949 onwards	Brown, 1969; Brown and Pal, 1971
Discovery of the oxidative activation of certain organophosphorus insecticides by insect tissues	Metcalf and March, 1953; O'Brien and Spencer, 1953, 1955; Kok and Walop, 1954; Fenwick *et al*, 1957; Fenwick, 1958; Arthur and Casida, 1959
Degradation (detoxication) of organophosphorus insecticides	Fernando *et al*, 1951; Metcalf *et al*, 1956; Plapp and Casida, 1958; van Asperen and Oppenoorth, 1959; Krueger and O'Brien, 1959; Krueger *et al*, 1960; Mengle and Casida, 1960; Fukami and Shishido, 1963, 1966; Lewis (1969)
Studies on metabolism and conjugation of non-insecticidal and insecticidal aromatic compounds, including carbamate insecticides	Myers and Smith, 1954; Smith, 1955; Terriere and Schonbrod, 1955; Kikal and Smith, 1959; Gessner and Smith, 1960; Eldefrawi and Hoskins, 1961; Terriere *et al*, 1961; Cohen *et al*, 1964; Dorough and Casida, 1964; Dutton and Ko, 1964; Smith, 1968
Investigations on the effect of 'drug extenders' such as SKF 525A and Lilly 18947 on the metabolism and/or toxicity of pyrethrins, organophosphate, and carbamate insecticides *in vivo*	Moorefield, 1958; Moorefield and Tefft, 1959; Metcalf *et al*, 1960; Hewlett *et al*, 1961; O'Brien, 1961; Hadaway *et al*, 1963

Discovery of powerful synergistic interactions between 1,3-benzodioxole 'pyrethrins' synergists' and carbamate insecticides	
Development of insect resistance to carbamates in the laboratory and its suppression by 1,3-benzodioxole synergists	Moorefield, 1960; Georghiou and Metcalf, 1961; Georghiou *et al*, 1961
Proposal that the synergism or antagonism of organophosphorus insecticide toxicity by pyrethrin synergists (1,3-benzodioxole type) is related to their inhibitory effects on oxidative activating or detoxifying reactions *in vivo*. Suggestion that synergism of pyrethrins is also due to inhibition of oxidation	Sun and Johnson, 1960
Discovery that the hydroxylation (benzylic) of DDT and of naphthalene is effected by insect microsomal enzymes having similar characteristics to those of mammalian liver	Agosin *et al*, 1961; Arias and Terriere, 1962
Discovery of enzyme induction in insects	Morello, 1964; Ilevicky *et al*, 1964; Ishaaya and Chefurka, 1968; Agosin *et al*, 1969; Perry and Buckner, 1970; Matthews and Casida, 1970; Walker and Terriere, 1970
Demonstration that the synergism of various analogues of cyclodiene insecticides by 1,3-benzodioxole synergists is related to inhibition of their oxidative detoxication	Brooks and Harrison, 1963, 1964a, b, 1966, 1967a, b; Brooks, 1968
Discovery of cyclodiene epoxide hydrase in microsomes from mammalian liver and insects	Brooks, 1966; Brooks *et al*, 1968, 1970
Oxidation of alkyl benzenes and their derivatives by insect fat body, etc.	Chakraborty and Smith, 1964, 1967; Hook and Smith, 1967; Hook *et al*, 1968
Demonstration that insect homogenates or microsomes plus NADPH can oxidatively metabolize phosphorothioates, carbamates, pyrethrins, aldrin, 1,3-benzodioxole synergists	Nakatsugawa and Dahm, 1962, 1965; Fukami and Shishido, 1963; Nakatsugawa *et al*, 1965; Schonbrod *et al*, 1965; Leeling and Casida, 1966; Yamamoto and Casida, 1966; Casida *et al*, 1966a, b; Lewis *et al*, 1967; Ray, 1967; Oonnithan and Casida, 1968; Casida, 1970

Table 1 (*cont.*)

Observation or event	References
Demonstration of a P-450 type cytochrome in microsomes from houseflies, German cockroaches, American cockroaches, and several other insects and its involvement in insecticide metabolism	Ray, 1965, 1967; Lewis, 1967; Brooks, 1968
Studies on mode of action and structure–activity relations of insecticide synergists	Haller *et al*, 1942; Beroza and Barthel, 1957; Moore and Hewlett, 1958; Moorefield, 1958; Moorefield and Tefft, 1959; Moorefield and Weiden, 1964; Fahmy and Gordon 1965; Hennessy, 1965; Wilkinson *et al*, 1966; Hewlett and Wilkinson, 1967; Wilkinson, 1967; Wilkinson and Hicks, 1969; Casida, 1970

159

contrast to the situation with lindane, which was evidently detoxified to aromatic compounds and their conjugation products.

The intense interest in the mode of action of OP in mammals soon led to the recognition that phosphorothioates such as parathion (4) are toxic by virtue of their oxidation *in vivo* to the corresponding phosphates, which are active anticholinesterases. In the case of schradan (19), hydroxylation of a single methyl group attached to nitrogen was required for activation. Together with the development of insect resistance to OP, these findings aroused interest in

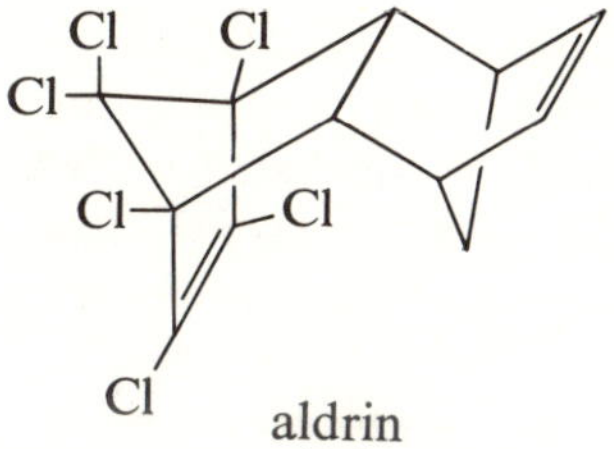

aldrin
(14)

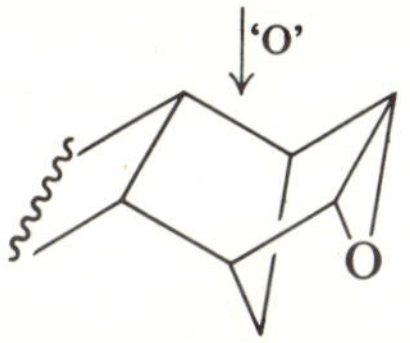

'O'

dieldrin
(15)

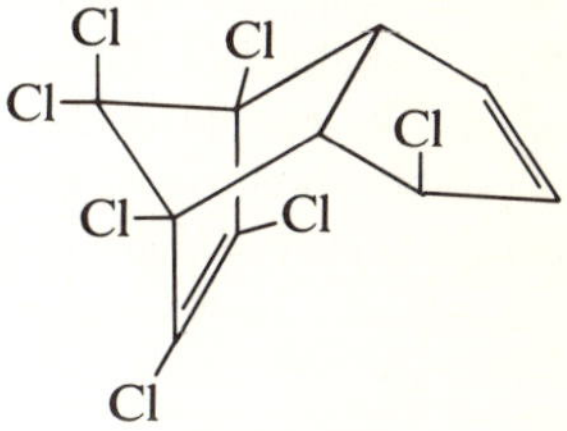

heptachlor
(16)

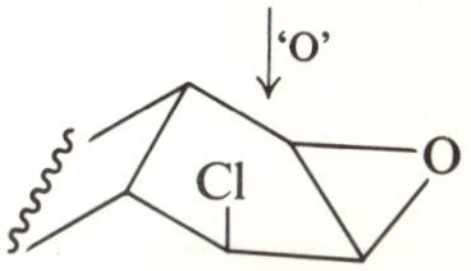

'O'

heptachlor
epoxide
(17)

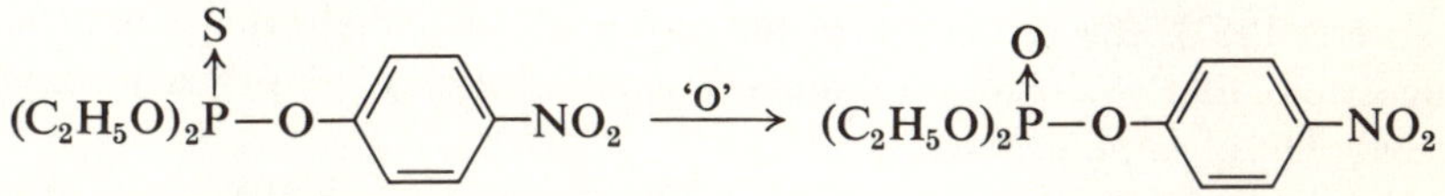

$(C_2H_5O)_2P—O$⟨⟩$—NO_2$ $\xrightarrow{\text{'O'}}$ $(C_2H_5O)_2P—O$⟨⟩$—NO_2$

parathion
(4)

paraoxon
(18)

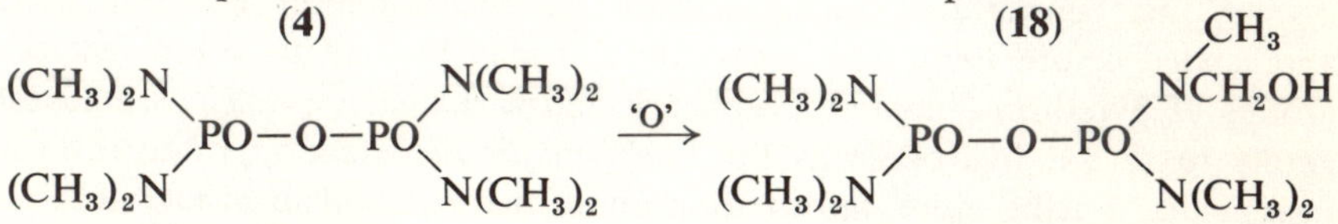

schradan
(19)

schradan activation
product

their metabolism in insects and intact insect tissues were found to effect similar activations. However, tissue homogenates, e.g. from cockroach gut, supplemented with NADH were ineffective (Fenwick *et al*, 1957; O'Brien, 1957) in contrast to NADH-supplemented homogenates of mammalian liver (Davison, 1954). Fenwick's (1958) later report represents a considerable advance, since it showed that schradan was activated by locust (*Schistocerca gregaria*) fat body homogenates in sucrose, or particles (plus NADH) from the corresponding 18,000 **g** supernatants. Commenting on 'this strange need for a reducing agent in an oxidative process', Fenwick (1958) surmised that the reaction was of the

160

type discussed by Mason *et al* (1955), catalysed by the enzymes now called mixed function oxidases.

Since organic esters of phosphorus, especially phosphates, are susceptible to hydrolysis, the early work on their metabolism in insects is much concerned with the role of this mechanism in the intoxication process. It was thought at first that the O-dealkylation of such esters was effected entirely hydrolytically by phosphatases, but two new mechanisms were discovered subsequently; namely, transfer of a single alkyl group (especially methyl) to GSH, mediated by soluble enzymes of insect gut and fat body that are probably GSH S-transferases (Fukami and Shishido, 1963, 1966) and oxidative O-dealkylation (Lewis, 1969) or O-dearylation (Nakatsugawa and Dahm, 1967; Nakatsugawa *et al*, 1968; El Bashir and Oppenoorth, 1969; Lewis, 1969) mediated by NADPH-dependent microsomal oxidases. Thus, it was soon discovered that, as in mammals, the insect toxicity of a phosphorothioate is the result of a balance between its activation to the toxic phosphate and the metabolic destruction of both the phosphate and its inactive precursor by one or more of the above mechanisms.

The studies of comparative metabolism in intact insects and insect tissues initiated by Smith (Table 1) showed that locusts produce phenols from benzene derivatives and further conjugate them with glucose and sulphate; the evidence for conjugations involving GSH appeared later (Gessner and Smith, 1960; Cohen and Smith, 1964). Houseflies converted naphthalene into 1-naphthol and 1,2-dihydro-1,2-dihydroxynaphthalene and 1-naphthol was conjugated with glucose, sulphate, N-acetylcysteine, and phosphate (Terriere *et al*, 1961; Dutton and Ko, 1964; Smith and Turbert, 1964; Binning *et al*, 1967; Boose and Terriere, 1967); the formation of the diol and 1-naphthyl-premercapturic acid suggested that 1,2-epoxy-1,2-dihydronaphthalene is a primary oxidative metabolite of naphthalene.

Despite a variety of evidence from *in vivo* studies for oxidative mechanisms in insects, their importance for insecticide biotransformation was not widely appreciated before 1960. One reason for this may be that the prominent ester groups of pyrethrins, organophosphates, and carbamates predisposed investigators to regard hydrolysis as the likely major detoxication route for such insecticides. Furthermore, information about the metabolism of OC in insects was at that time virtually limited to the DDT→DDE conversion and the formation of chlorinated benzene derivatives from lindane. The heavily chlorinated cyclodiene insecticides were thought to be metabolically rather inert, apart from the epoxidation reaction.

This situation was changed by several important discoveries between 1958 and 1960. Moorefied and others (Table 1) found that 1,3-benzodioxole derivatives were powerful synergists for carbamate insecticides as well as pyrethrins. Almost simultaneously, Sun and Johnson (1960) showed that sesamex (**13**) and other 1,3-benzodioxoles synergized the toxicity of certain OP and antagonized the action of others. They concluded that the pyrethrin synergists inhibit mainly biological oxidations which either activate or detoxify OP depending on their structure, and on this basis suggested that the pyrethrins were also probably detoxified by oxidation rather than hydrolysis. DDT was then found to be hydroxylated at the benzylic carbon by an enzyme system from cockroaches and houseflies that had the properties of a microsomal mixed function oxidase (Agosin *et al*, 1961). Shortly afterwards Arias and Terriere (1962) reported the conversion of naphthalene into 1-naphthol and 1,2-dihydroxy-1,2-dihydro-naphthalene by a microsomal preparation from whole houseflies. The preparation of microsomes from whole insects presented difficulties due to instability of the enzymes and the presence of endogenous inhibitors (see below) and the efforts of numerous laboratories were directed to these problems.

The value of an enzyme preparation that permits investigation of the primary metabolism of insecticides without the problems of distribution, conjugation, and excretion met with in intact insects is self-evident. Besides most classes of insecticides, various model compounds (e.g. alkyl benzenes) were exposed to insect microsomal preparations during the next few years (Table 1). By this time there was great concern about the selectivity of insecticides (mammal versus insect and insect versus insect) and the new ability to compare the microsomal metabolism of different species greatly stimulated research in this direction. The links between insect and vertebrate biochemical pharmacology were completely established in 1965 when Ray (1965, 1967) demonstrated that microsomal preparations from several insects contain a P-450 type cytochrome.

INSECT MICROSOMES AND CYTOCHROME P-450

Biochemical Aspects

Microsomes were at first made from whole insects by methods similar to those established for mammalian liver and were often spontaneously inactivated by endogenous inhibitors such as the ommochrome eye pigment, xanthommatin (Jordan and Smith, 1970; Schonbrod and Terrier, 1971; Wilson and Hodgson, 1972), and digestive proteases of the insect gut (Krieger and Wilkinson, 1970; Brattsten and Wilkinson, 1973a). Xanthommatin accepts electrons at the flavoprotein level, and thereby prevents cytochrome P-450 reduction by NADPH, whereas the proteases appear to attack the microsomal protein; both inhibitions are somewhat alleviated by bovine serum albumin (BSA). The removal of insect heads and careful washing of isolated insect gut often results in remarkably active microsomal preparations (Hook *et al*, 1968; Krieger and Wilkinson, 1970).

Smith and colleagues (references in Table 1) studied the oxidation of *p*-nitrotoluene in intact locust organs, in whole homogenates of organs, and in various fractions from locust fat body and found the fat body to be most active in producing *p*-nitrobenzoic acid. Midgut tissue was most active in the southern armyworm (*Prodenia eridania*) (Krieger and Wilkinson, 1969) and Malpighian tubules in the house cricket (*Acheta domesticus*) (Benke and Wilkinson, 1971), using aldrin epoxidation as the measure of activity. Casida avoided some of the problems found with microsomes from whole houseflies by making the preparations from abdomens and showed that these microsomes effected the oxidation of carbamates, pyrethrins, rotenone, and the 1,3-benzodioxole synergists (Table 1).

To add to the problem of endogenous inhibitors, equivalent techniques for microsome isolation do not necessarily produce comparable preparations from different insects, or even from different tissues of the same insect, and there are variations in enzyme activity with age in the life cycle, nutritional status, stage of biological rhythms, etc., as in mammals. These difficulties have been discussed in recent reviews (Wilkinson and Brattsten, 1972; Kulkarni and Hodgson, 1975).

Ray (1965, 1967) showed that a CO-binding pigment similar to cytochrome P-450 is present in microsomes from houseflies, German cockroaches (*Blattella germanica*), and American cockroaches (*Periplaneta americana*) and that the CO-inhibition of aldrin (**14**) epoxidation by housefly microsomes is substantially reversible by light of wavelength 450 nm if care is taken to remove free flavins from the preparation. Further support for the role of cytochrome P-450 in insecticide metabolism was afforded by the observation (Lewis, 1967) that appropriate CO/O_2 mixtures inhibited aldrin epoxidation *in vivo* in houseflies and synergized other insecticides that were known to be detoxified by hydroxylation (Lewis, 1967; Brooks, 1968). The housefly microsomes used in these experiments were from whole insects; they usually contained some cytochrome P-420, which increased in content when the preparations were kept or treated with detergents. There has been a proliferation of papers on one aspect or another of the insect microsomal oxidase system since 1970, and Hodgson (1974) lists 15 insect species whose tissues had by that time been shown to contain cytochrome P-450.

Much has been written about the electron transport chain in hepatic microsomes and in view of the now evident similarities between the two, the insect system is usually discussed by reference to the hepatic one. Most information is available for the microsomal preparation from housefly abdomens. In these microsomes both NADPH and NADH are rapidly oxidized in the absence of any substrate and the inhibition of NADPH oxidation by CO, which is partly reversed by cytochrome c, indicates that a CO-binding pigment is involved in electron transfer; stoichiometry between NADPH oxidized and substrate metabolized has not been established (Hodgson and Plapp, 1970; Wilkinson and Brattsten, 1972). The inhibition of NADPH oxidation by SKF 525A or sulfoxide (**11**) is reversed by cytochrome c, whereas that caused by *p*-chloromercuribenzoate is not, indicating that the sulphydryl reagent probably acts at the NADPH-cytochrome c reductase level and the 'drug extenders' at the P-450 level (Hodgson and Plapp, 1970). Cytochrome b_5 is found in insect microsomes; its concentration does not appear to be rate limiting for microsomal enzyme activity and its function is unknown (Wilkinson and Brattsten, 1972).

The NADPH-cytochrome c reductase from housefly abdominal microsomes was solubilized with isobutanol, an ineffective method for mammalian microsomes (Wilson and Hodgson, 1971a, b), and substantially purified. Its molecular weight of 57,000 is similar to that of the analogous enzyme from rat liver, and it resembles the flavoproteins from rat and pig liver in that they all transfer electrons to cytochrome c, ferricyanide, and 2,6-dichlorophenolindophenol and do not accept electrons from NADH. The insect enzyme apparently has a lower affinity than the mammalian enzymes for the above electron acceptors and for NADPH; the precise nature of its prosthetic group has not yet been established but both FAD and FMN restore the activity of the housefly apoenzyme.

Current research on insect cytochrome P-450 centres on the methodology of measurement; development of solubilization techniques; interaction with xenobiotics, especially insecticides and insecticide synergists; induction by insecticides; relation between P-450 levels and oxidative detoxication mechanisms conferring resistance; relation between P-450 and microsomal epoxide hydrase. The status of most of these projects has been discussed in recent reviews (Wilkinson and Brattsten, 1972; Hodgson, 1974; Hodgson *et al*, 1974; Hodgson and Tate, 1976) and the following is a summary of the salient findings.

Reported values for P-450 in insect tissue lie typically between 0·2–0·5 nmol/mg protein, about one-fifth of those reported for hepatic microsomes, although values from 0·004 to 0·034 nmol/mg protein were recorded for microsomal preparations from tissues of the cockroach (*Gromphadorhina portentosa*) and 1·48 nmol/mg protein for the particularly active preparation from southern armyworm gut (Wilkinson and Brattsten, 1972). The specific activity of this last preparation for aldrin epoxidation is about 6-fold higher than that of rabbit liver microsomes (Krieger and Wilkinson, 1969) expressed on an equivalent basis. The above measurements of cytochrome P-450 were based on the extinction coefficient of 91 cm^{-1}mM^{-1} derived from rabbit liver microsomes and measurement of ΔOD/mg protein is clearly more appropriate until the respective cytochromes have been solubilized. Extinction coefficients of 97–110 cm^{-1} mM^{-1} and 83–86 cm^{-1} mM^{-1}, respectively, have recently been reported for the cytochromes P-450 and P-448·5 solubilized from F$_c$ housefly microsomes using Triton X-100 or cholate (Capdevila *et al*, 1975; Agosin, 1976).

The P-450 of housefly microsomes is readily converted into P-420 by trypsin, sodium cholate, and phospholipase A; it is more stable to *Crotalus* venom, sodium deoxycholate, subtilisin, and phospholipase C, although *Crotalus* venom inhibited NADPH oxidation and oxygen uptake (Folsom *et al*, 1971). The microsomal systems of lepidopterous larval gut may be more amenable to these techniques and further progress on the solubilization problem is likely in the near future.

Interaction with Xenobiotics

Hodgson and colleagues (Hodgson, 1974; Hodgson and Tate, 1976) examined the interaction of a number of xenobiotics and insecticides with the cytochrome P-450 in microsomes from the abdomens of insecticide susceptible (S-) houseflies and resistant houseflies (F$_c$ strain) having an oxidative detoxication mechanism for DDT. As yet unexplained is the observation that compounds which gave typical type I binding spectra with oxidized microsomes from mammals and F_c houseflies gave no measurable interaction with microsomes of the S-strain (many are known to be substrates for its MFO), although recognized type II substrates generally gave type II spectra for both housefly preparations. A recent report indicates, however, that S-microsomes do give a type I interaction with certain 1,3-benzodioxole synergists (Kulkarni and Hodgson, 1976). Type I binding (F_c strain) was noted with chlorinated insecticides, pyrethrins, carbamates, and several organophosphorus insecticides. Type II binding (both strains) was noted with a variety of nitrogenous compounds (excluding carbamates) including pyridine, pyrrolidine, piperidine, amines, amides, aliphatic and aromatic nitriles, imidazoles, benzothiadiazoles, and with various phenols and alcohols. Although compounds in which the sp^2 or sp^3 non-bonded electrons of nitrogen atoms are sterically accessible appear to be the best type II ligands, the electrons of accessible oxygen atoms can evidently participate to give modified type II spectra in which the maxima and minima are at lower intensity and wavelength. The interactions with housefly P-450 are clearly basically similar to those seen with mammalian P-450.

Nevertheless, the comparison between mouse liver microsomes and the microsomes of the two housefly strains previously referred to (Hodgson, 1974; Kulkarni *et al*, 1974; Mailman *et al*, 1974) revealed some differences between mammal and insect and between the two insect strains. For example, several pyrethrins gave typical type I spectra with mouse liver microsomes but an unusual spectrum with a peak at 415–418 nm and a trough at 443–445 nm with those from either housefly strain. The phosphorodithioate aphicide menazon, which contains a triazine ring, gave a type II spectrum with mouse liver microsomes but a type I spectrum with F_c microsomes, whereas *s*-butanol and 1-cyclohexenyl pyrrolidine were type I with mouse microsomes and type II with housefly microsomes. The apparent lack of type I binding with S-housefly P-450 has been mentioned previously. Thus, 1-cyclohexyl-2-pyrrolidone gave a type I spectrum with F_c-P-450 but type II with S-P-450, while 2,6-lutidine gave a mixed type I and II interaction with F_c-P-450 but type II with S-P-450.

These differences await explanation, although Hodgson (1974) was led to speculate that the haem iron of housefly P-450 is more accessible to type II ligands than is the haem iron of mouse P-450. Also, fragments of evidence from studies of phospholipid content and from solubilization experiments indicate differences between the housefly and mammalian microsomal membranes (Hodgson, 1974). The relation between metabolism and substrate binding to P-450 is not an obvious one; studies on various strains of insecticide-resistant houseflies (see below) show that P-450 is not necessarily rate limiting, since high oxidase activity (as compared with susceptible strains) is not always associated with a higher than normal level of the cytochrome.

An interaction of long-standing interest is that between insecticide synergists, themselves non-toxic by definition, and insect enzyme systems. The insect microsomal mixed function oxidase system involving cytochrome P-450 has been implicated in the biotransformations of insecticides which involve, for example, aromatic, aliphatic, and alicyclic hydroxylation; dealkylation of ethers and substituted amines; oxidation of thioethers to sulphoxides and sulphones; epoxidation of double bonds, oxidation of phosphorothionates (PS) to phosphates (PO), and most of these conversions are inhibited by synergists (sometimes behaving as antagonists, depending on the situation) of the 1,3-benzodioxole type (e.g. **8–13**). The 1,3-benzodioxoles have been most studied, but the well-known 'drug extenders' SKF 525A and Lilly 18947 can also act as insecticide synergists (Table 1), and in recent years the search for new structural types has produced several other groups of compounds that are effective carbamate synergists. Examples are shown below (Wilkinson, 1976a):

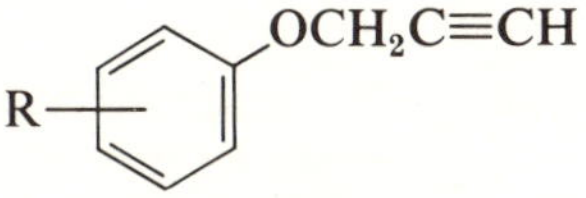

aryl 2-propynyl
ethers
(**20**)

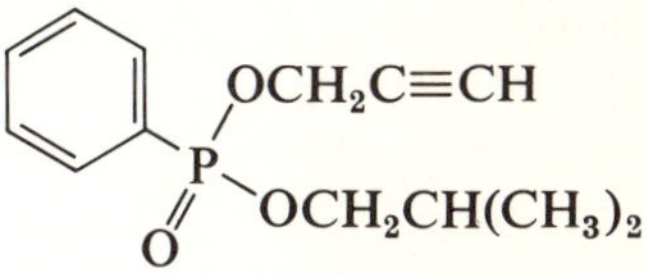

propynyl phosphonates
(NIA 16824)
(**21**)

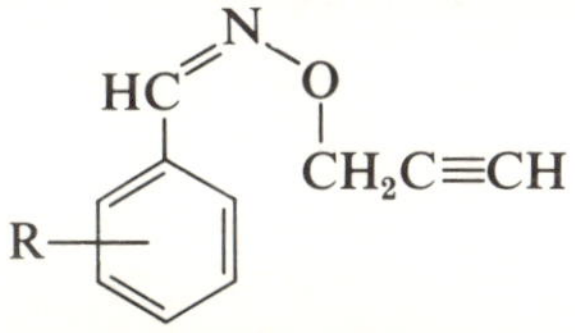

oximino-propynyl
ethers
(**22**)

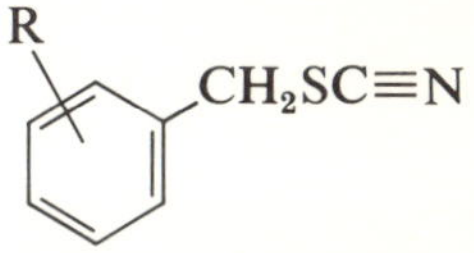

benzyl thiocyanates
(**23**)

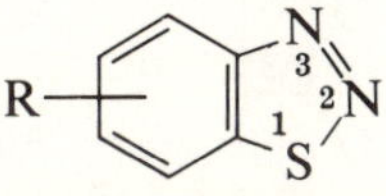

1,2,3-benzothiadiazoles
(**24**)

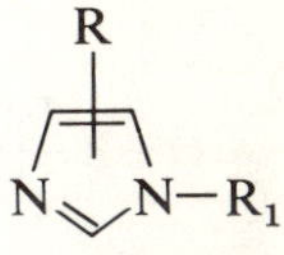

imidazoles
(**25**)

A recent review (Hodgson and Philpot, 1974) gives a comprehensive list of literature citations of the inhibition of mixed function oxidases from both mammals and insects by 1,3-benzodioxoles. Since the unsubstituted 1,3-dioxole moiety appears to be essential for synergist activity and is itself cleaved to the free catechol and formate by microsomal oxidases of both mammals and insects, it was suggested that these compounds inhibit by acting as alternative high affinity substrates for MFO (Casida *et al*, 1966a). The possibilities for reactive fragment formation leading to non-competitive inhibition are shown in figure 1 and all of these have been considered.

It was noticed in 1970 that when houseflies (Perry and Buckner, 1970; Matthews and Casida, 1970) and mice (Matthews *et al*, 1970) were treated with piperonyl butoxide (PB) *in vivo*, there was at first a significant reduction in the P-450 measurable *in vitro*, followed by a return towards normal levels after about 12 hours for mice and 24 hours for houseflies. For mice, NIA 16824 (**21**) and 5,6-dichloro-1,2,3-benzothiadiazole (WL 19255) had similar effects, which were initially accompanied by a reduction in ability to metabolize hexobarbitone *in vitro*. In the case of PB and NIA 16824, a peak of P-450 induction developed after 36 hours and was followed by a return to normal enzyme activity and P-450 level; both suppression and subsequent induction of P-450 levels lasted longer following pretreatment of mice with WL 19255. With houseflies, carbamate synergism was measurable for up to 48 hours following the application of either PB or sesamex (**13**); the approach to normal P-450 levels was complete after 72 hours. It is also interesting to note that the synergistic effect of sesamex (**13**) with certain biodegradable cyclodienes applied to houseflies persisted for about 24 hours after synergist application (Brooks and Harrison, 1964a).

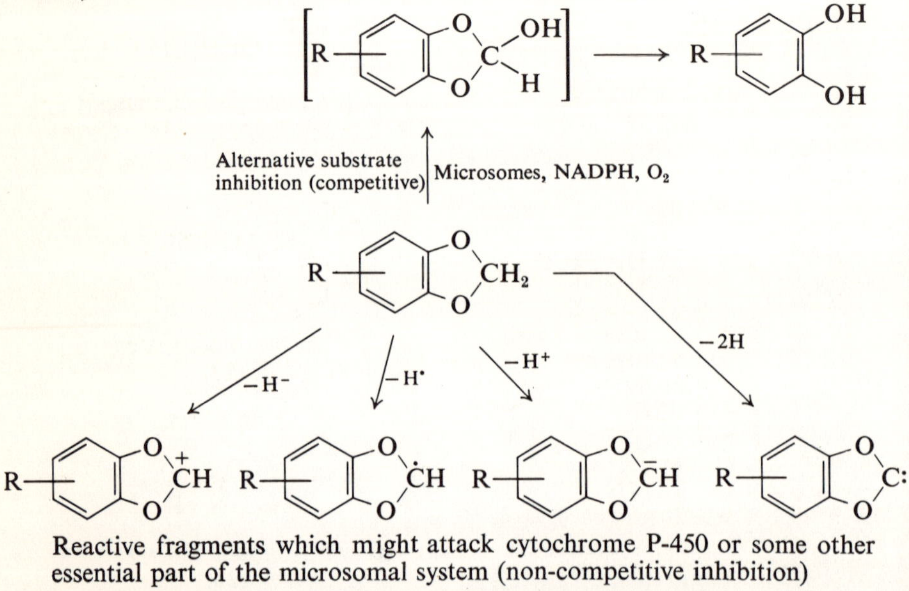

Reactive fragments which might attack cytochrome P-450 or some other essential part of the microsomal system (non-competitive inhibition)

Figure 1 Theories of mode of action of 1,3-benzodioxole synergists (Casida *et al*, 1966a ; Hennessy, 1965; Hansch, 1968; Ullrich and Schnabel, 1973)

Later experiments showed that while PB gives a typical type I binding spectrum with both mammal (Matthews *et al*, 1970) and insect microsomes (Hodgson and Plapp, 1970), the addition of NADPH results in an optical difference spectrum called type III, with peaks at 455 nm and 427 nm (existing in pH-dependent equilibrium) and the non-competitive blockade of CO-binding to a portion of the P-450. The complex is stable and reverts not to the type I spectrum but to an oxidized form (single peak at 437 nm) when NADPH is exhausted; additional NADPH regenerates the reduced form, findings which suggest that a metabolite of PB is responsible for complex formation (Franklin, 1971; other references in Hodgson and Tate, 1976). The formation of this stable complex preventing CO-binding to a portion of P-450 accounts (Philpot and Hodgson, 1971) for the aforementioned effect of PB treatment *in vivo*, and it has since been shown (for mice) that the spectral dissociation constant (K_s) for inhibition of CO-binding by PB is the same as that for formation of the type III complex from PB (Philpot and Hodgson, 1972). Although variations have been observed, the type I→type III conversion is the most common one for 1,3-benzodioxoles.

The formation of a tightly bound complex with P-450 supports the possible involvment of reactive fragments such as those shown in figure 1. However, no more than about 50% of the P-450 is complexed in this way, indicating the possibility of more than one form of the cytochrome; the remainder is apparently free to participate in oxidative reactions and may possibly be subject to alternative substrate inhibition by 1,3-benzodioxoles. The nature of the interaction of the other types of synergists with the microsomal complex remains in question. Some of the aryl 2-propynyl ethers (e.g. **20–22**) are highly effective carbamate synergists (see Table 2); like 1,3-benzodioxoles, they depress P-450 levels *in vivo* (up to 50% when given in housefly diet for 24 hours) and inhibit microsomal oxidase activity (Perry *et al*, 1971). Information about their binding to housefly P-450 is scanty, although Kulkarni and Hodgson (1976) reported no spectral interactions for 2-nitrophenyl propargyl ether. Matthews *et al* (1970) reported a strong type I binding with oxidized mouse P-450.

Table 2 Synergism of carbaryl towards susceptible houseflies by compounds representing different synergist groups (data of Wilkinson, 1976a*)

Synergist	Topical LD_{50} of carbaryl in 1 : 5 ratio with synergist (μg/g)	Synergistic ratio
None	900	—
Piperonyl butoxide	12·5	72
1,2-Methylenedioxynaphthalene	4·0	225
p-Nitrobenzylthiocyanate	77·5	12
2-Propynyl-4-chloro-2-nitrophenyl ether	4·2	214
2-(Diethylamino)ethyl 2,2-diphenyl pentanoate (SKF 525A)	58·5	15
5,6-Dichloro-1,2,3-benzothiadiazole	14·5	62
1-(2,3-Dimethylphenyl) imidazole†	2·5	360

* From Metcalf and McKelvey (eds) (1976), *The future of insecticides: needs and prospects*, p. 202, Wiley, New York.

† Houseflies pretreated with 50 μg of synergist 1 hour prior to treatment with carbaryl.

The 1,2,3,-benzothiadiazoles (**24**) and substituted imidazoles are generally recognized as type II substrates. The 432 nm peak of the type II difference spectrum observed for benzothiadiazoles with both insect and mammalian microsomes is shifted to 444 nm if the cytochrome is reduced (Matthews *et al*, 1970; Wilkinson and Brattsten, 1972) but the new peak is displaced to 450 nm by CO and it is not clear whether the shift on reduction represents metabolite formation or merely reflects a change of conformation of the reduced ligand complex. Imidazoles (**25**) with a single aryl substituent (R or R_1) are likewise powerful inhibitors of microsomal oxidases and are synergists for carbamates against houseflies (when R = H, R_1 = alkyl or aryl). Their type II spectra formed with oxidized armyworm gut or housefly microsomes are unchanged by reduction (Kulkarni and Hodgson, 1976; Wilkinson, 1976), and CO readily displaces the peak in the reduced spectrum to 450 nm as expected; the unusually low spectral dissociation constants (K_s) are quantitatively similar to the molar I_{50} values for microsomal enzyme inhibition, which are therefore considered to result mainly from a high affinity for cytochrome P-450 (Wilkinson *et al*, 1974; Wilkinson, 1976a).

Numerous applications of classical enzyme kinetics to the interaction between insect microsomes and several classes of synergists have not been particularly helpful in elucidating the mode of action, indicating sometimes competitive, sometimes mixed, and sometimes non-competitive inhibition for a particular synergist, depending on the system. This is not surprising in view of the particulate nature of the enzyme system and the complexities just discussed.

Several 1,3-benzodioxoles inhibited aldrin epoxidation in a modified Fenton's reagent generating $OH^{\bullet}$ and were simultaneously converted into the corresponding catechols at a rate strongly correlated with inhibiting capacity. Lineweaver–Burk plots indicated 'competitive inhibition', suggesting that 1,3-benzodioxoles compete with aldrin for $OH^{\bullet}$. While 5-nitro-1,3-benzodioxole and 6-nitro-1,2,3-benzothiadiazole inhibited the reaction and were both degraded, neither compound inhibited the low level of epoxidation by the Udenfriend or mercaptobenzoate systems (generating $O_2H^{\bullet}$ or $^{\bullet}O_2{}^{-}$) or epoxidation by peracetic acid (OH^{+}) or pertrifluoracetic acid systems. Titanous chloride/O_2 (generating $^{\bullet}O_2H$) effected no epoxidation, and epoxidation by titanous chloride/H_2O_2 ($OH^{\bullet}$) was inhibited by the 1,3-benzodioxoles (Marshall and Wilkinson, 1973). These limited results suggest that the two types interfere only with reactions that generate OH radicals. The great theoretical interest of these synergists will undoubtedly ensure that further answers to some of the puzzling features of their action will emerge as detailed knowledge of the mechanism of oxygen activation by cytochrome P-450 develops.

Induction and Resistance

It is generally accepted that classical insect resistance arises through 'Darwinian selection'. The insecticide selects an insect population over several generations for those few individuals already possessing genes that confer resistance; thus, the resistant survivors form the new resistant population. In contrast, enzyme induction occurs within the lifetime of the individual, is normally expected to decline if individual exposure to the toxicant ceases, and is non-inheritable, although an individual might inherit an exceptional capacity for enzyme induction. The relation between 'induction' and 'resistance' has interested insect toxicologists for some time.

It is evident that exposure of normal insects to non-toxic inducers of enzymes, especially microsomal oxidases, might give them some temporary tolerance towards classes of insecticides that are susceptible to detoxication by such enzymes, while insects already resistant to one class might acquire temporary cross-tolerance to others. Induction by an insecticide, on the other hand, usually requires levels of toxicant that would kill normal insects and can therefore be demonstrated only in insects already resistant to the insecticide chosen; the inductive effect might therefore be evident as an enhanced level of resistance to that insecticide or as some additional cross-tolerance to others, due to its temporary presence in the tissues. However, such cross-tolerance might be difficult to differentiate from that already produced by the Darwinian selection for resistance, since resistant strains frequently have elevated levels of microsomal oxidases that confer cross-tolerance to other toxicants. Only in the case of true resistance, however, should such cross-tolerance persist indefinitely (i.e. in successive generations), when exposure to the inducing insecticide ceases.

Although the induction of mammalian liver MFO was observed in 1954 (Brown *et al*, 1954), no similar phenomenon was indicated for insects until Morello (1964) showed that following treatment with 3-methylcholanthrene and then DDT, the blood sucking bug *Triatoma infestans* became more tolerant to the insecticide and produced a higher proportion of polar metabolites from it. Other investigations showed that the treatment with phenobarbitone *in vivo* increased the ability of isolated *Triatoma* microsomes to metabolize DDT (Agosin *et al*, 1969) and that DDT itself induced an increase in protein synthesis in *Triatoma* nymphs and resistant houseflies (Ilevicky *et al*, 1964; other references cited in Wilkinson and Brattsten, 1972). Houseflies already resistant to both DDT and dieldrin showed substantial increases in both heptachlor (**16**) epoxidase and naphthalene hydroxylase activity and were protected against carbaryl (**7**) following pretreatment with dieldrin; these effects were abolished when the flies were preinjected with a non-toxic dose of cycloheximide, an inhibitor of protein synthesis (Walker and Terriere, 1970).

More recent reports indicate induction of insect microsomal oxidases by such diverse structures as phenobarbitone, butylated hydroxytoluene (BHT) and triphenylphosphate (Perry *et al*, 1971), insect juvenile and moulting hormones (Yu and Terriere, 1971), and methylbenzenes (Brattsten and Wilkinson, 1973b). Several of these investigations indicated that an increased level of P-450 was associated with the elevated microsomal oxidase activity. In the last investigation cited, pentamethylbenzene in the diet of the southern armyworm produced rapid (within 8 hours) and significant increases in the aldrin epoxidase, *p*-chloro-N-methylaniline demethylase, NADPH-cytochrome c reductase, and P-450 of midgut tissue which returned quickly to normal when exposure ceased. The 11-fold increase in tolerance to carbaryl (**7**) which resulted from this treatment demonstrates the possibility that seemingly inert compounds in the diet (e.g. various additives used in insecticide formulations) may have a significant effect on the control of such pests in the field.

Some resistant housefly strains with high oxidase activity contain an apparently normal cytochrome P-450, whereas others have a cytochrome resembling that found in 3-methylcholanthrene-induced livers; insecticide-susceptible strains appear to possess only the normal cytochrome. For example, microsomes from the DDT-resistant F_c strain mentioned earlier exhibited type I binding spectra (not demonstrable in S-houseflies) and a peak absorbance at 450 nm in the CO-difference spectrum which was shifted to 448 nm by dietary exposure to naphthalene or phenobarbitone (Capdevila *et al*, 1973). Phenobarbitone (or BHT) also increased the 'normal' P-450 content of both S-houseflies and strains resistant to DDT or malathion, respectively, as well as the 'normal' P-448 of a diazinon-resistant strain (Perry *et al*, 1971). Changes in microsomal oxidase activity do not necessarily parallel changes in cytochrome level; in the first two resistant strains, oxidase activity increased relatively more than cytochrome level, whereas the converse was true for the diazinon-resistant strain (Perry *et al*, 1971). It seems to be generally true that the capacity for induction is greater in strains already having a high basic level of MFO activity. Several synergists of the 1,3-benzodioxole and phenyl 2-propynyl ether types caused a peak shift from 448 nm to 450–452 nm in the CO-difference spectrum of this last strain when fed on the diet, besides reducing the cytochrome measurable *in vitro*. These observations await detailed explanation and some of the changes may reflect alterations in the haemoprotein environment rather than qualitative changes in the haemoprotein itself.

Hodgson and colleagues (Hodgson *et al*, 1974; Hodgson and Tate, 1976) considered the difference between the P-450 of susceptible and resistant housefly strains in terms of size and peak position of the CO, types I, II, III, *n*-octylamine, and ethyl isocyanide (EtNC) difference spectra and concluded that the resistant cytochrome differs in that:

1. The CO-difference peak is moved several nanometres to lower wavelengths and increased in size.
2. Type I binding spectra can be measured.
3. Type II binding spectra are increased in intensity relative to the CO-difference peak.
4. The *n*-octylamine spectrum has a single trough at 390 nm, in contrast to the double trough (394 nm and 410 nm) seen with susceptible cytochrome.
5. The type III EtNC difference spectrum is decreased relative to the CO-difference spectrum.

A qualitative difference between the cytochromes is also indicated by the fact that the interstrain ratios for these various parameters (resistant compared with the susceptible houseflies) are different, contrary to expectation if an increase in a single, common cytochrome was being measured.

The biochemical genetics of resistance in houseflies is fairly well understood and susceptible strains are available that carry visible mutant characteristics associated with specific chromosomes. One well-known composite susceptible strain has distinct visible characters associated with chromosomes II, III, and V and the P-450 level and characteristics normally associated with an S-strain. Major oxidative resistance mechanisms in houseflies are associated with chromosome V (F_c strain) and chromosome II (e.g. R-Baygon strain). By crossing these strains individually with the composite S-strain and examining the progeny, those phenotypes can be identified in which one or more of the S-marker chromosomes are replaced by the (unmarked) chromosomes of the resistant strain. Thus, a substrain from the F_c cross that carries the visible markers for chromosomes II and III must have S-chromosomes II and III and resistant chromosome V. This substrain exhibited type I binding spectra but had susceptible P-450 characteristics, despite the fact that the resistance of the original F_c strain is due to high oxidase activity associated with chromosome V. Only those substrains containing chromosome II of the F_c strain had the high P-450 levels of this strain, so that high P-450 and high oxidase activity are separable. Likewise, a substrain from the R-Baygon cross that combined S-chromosomes III and V with the R-Baygon chromosome II (conferring resistance due to high oxidase activity) had susceptible P-450 characteristics. These and other genetic studies (Hodgson *et al*, 1974; Hodgson and Tate, 1976) suggest that the only P-450 characteristic that is regularly associated with resistance is type I binding; the level of the cytochrome is not necessarily rate limiting for oxidative metabolism and other factors must be sought.

Capdevila *et al* (1975) solubilized cytochromes P-450 and P-448 from F_c housefly microsomes and the P-448 appears to differ in its catalytic properties from the P-448 found in a diazinon-resistant strain (Perry *et al*, 1971; Capdevila *et al*, 1974). The situation is further complicated by a recent report (Schonbrod and Terriere, 1975) that susceptible houseflies also contain more than one form of P-450 and the assignment of chromosomes to these different forms has become controversial.

NON-OXIDATIVE METABOLISM AND CONJUGATION

The term 'non-oxidative' is used for convenience but needs to be regarded with caution; in the past few years, for example, certain of the detoxification products of organophosphorus esters that were thought to arise by hydrolysis have been shown to result from an initial oxidative attack mediated by micro-somal enzymes.

Hydrolytic Conversions

The esterases and amidases that hydrolyse pesticides are widely distributed in nature, may be either membrane bound or soluble, vary considerably between species and tissues in their substrate specificity, and have been particularly well examined in relation to the behaviour of organophosphorus insecticides in mammals and insects (O'Brien, 1967). Taking parathion (**4**) and paraoxon (**18**) as examples, the 'hydrolytic' reactions that can occur, in principle, are (a) cleavage to *p*-nitrophenol and diethyl phosphorothioic acid or diethyl phosphoric acid, respectively (arylester hydrolysis), (b) removal of one or more alkyl groups to give the corresponding *p*-nitrophenyl dealkylated esters of these acids. These possibilities are shown below.

It is well known that the A-esterases in a variety of mammalian tissues effect reaction (a) for paraoxon, but there is also considerable evidence for its oxidative dearylation. For parathion, microsomal oxidation leads to activation to para-oxon, and concurrently to O-aryl bond cleavage. A common oxygenated intermediate has been invoked to account for these two reactions but proof is lacking (Ptashne *et al*, 1971; Wustner *et al*, 1972). Both dearylation and mono-deethylation of parathion are effected by soluble enzymes of rat liver that

$$CH_3CHO \quad C_2H_5SG \quad C_2H_5OH \Big\} + C_2H_5O-\overset{\overset{\displaystyle S(O)}{\uparrow}}{\underset{\displaystyle OH}{P}}-O-\!\!\!\left\langle\!\!\!\bigcirc\!\!\!\right\rangle\!\!\!-NO_2$$

(2) Microsomes, NADPH, O_2 | Soluble fraction, GSH | Soluble fraction: hydrolase

$$\underset{C_2H_5O}{\overset{C_2H_5O}{>}}\!\!\overset{\overset{\displaystyle S(O)}{\uparrow}}{P}-O-\!\!\!\left\langle\!\!\!\bigcirc\!\!\!\right\rangle\!\!\!-NO_2$$

Parathion (paraoxon)

(1) Microsomes, NADPH, O_2 | Soluble fraction, GSH | Hydrolases

p-Nitrophenol

$$GS-\!\!\!\left\langle\!\!\!\bigcirc\!\!\!\right\rangle\!\!\!-NO_2 \qquad \textit{p}\text{-Nitrophenol} \Big\} + (C_2H_5O)_2\overset{\overset{\displaystyle S(O)}{\uparrow}}{P}-OH$$

require GSH but there is little evidence for hydrolysis. The situation is generally similar for insects (Nakatsugawa *et al*, 1968) but there is also some evidence that phosphothioates such as parathion may be hydrolysed directly (for reviews see: Brooks, 1972; Dauterman, 1976). Although paraoxon has been reported to suffer hydrolytic monodeethylation in houseflies (Nolan and O'Brien, 1970), the evidence is mainly in favour of oxidative or GSH-mediated dealkylation for

$$\begin{array}{c} (O)\,(activation) \\ \nearrow \\ \underset{CH_3O}{\overset{CH_3O}{>}}\!\overset{\overset{\displaystyle S}{\parallel}}{P}SCHCOOC_2H_5 \\ CH_2COOC_2H_5 \end{array}$$

malathion
(26)

[↑ Main points of attack
↑ Further hydrolysis leading to the di-acid]

phosphates and GSH-mediated dealkylation for the P→S analogues, and this probably applies to both insects and mammals.

Malathion (26) is an outstanding example of an organophosphorus insecticide that combines low toxicity to mammals with broad spectrum toxicity to insects. The selectivity appears to be due to carboxylesterase (EC 3.1.1.1) activity in mammals which leads to extensive hydrolysis of the secondary ester group and probably also to the di-acid. Insects generally degrade malathion much less readily and mainly by enzymic attack at the O-methyl or P—S—C linkages (Krueger and O'Brien, 1959; O'Brien, 1967). The acquired resistance of some insects and natural tolerance of others is related to the possession of carboxylesterase activity; chemicals that block this activity *in vivo* frequently reduce or abolish the tolerance of both insects and mammals to malathion (O'Brien, 1967). A large number of chemicals have been evaluated as synergists for malathion against malathion-resistant houseflies and mosquitoes. The most active in this respect are triphenyl phosphate (TPP), tri-*n*-butyl phosphorotrithiolate (DEF), tri-*n*-propyl phosphorotrithiolate, and a number of non-insecticidal carbamates (Plapp *et al*, 1963; Plapp and Tong, 1966; Plapp and Valega, 1967); TPP in particular has been used with malathion as a diagnostic tool in the detection of carboxylesterase-linked resistance to this widely used insecticide.

The natural pyrethrins are esters of secondary alcohols that are not very susceptible to hydrolysis in the tissues of either insects or mammals and for these compounds, detoxication is mediated mainly by the microsomal oxidases. Many of the new synthetic pyrethroids, on the other hand, are esters of primary alcohols, a change which reduces the possibilities for optical isomerism and also introduces vulnerability to carboxylesterase attack (see p. 196). With these molecules a balance between oxidative and hydrolytic detoxication is possible and its significance for selective toxicity will be discussed in a later section. As in the case of organophosphorus insecticides, non-toxic inhibitors of both esterases and microsomal oxidases have proved to be invaluable as aids in exploring the metabolic pathways of pyrethroids.

Despite their structural simplicity, the metabolism of carbamate insecticides is evidently rather complex. Enzymic hydrolysis of the carbamate ester group leading to the parent phenol is an obvious route and a plasma albumin fraction from various vertebrate sources was found to hydrolyse carbaryl (7) and other carbamates (Casida and Augustinsson, 1959; Casida *et al*, 1960). Many of the metabolites of carbamates produced by insects and mammals are now known to result from oxidative attack on the intact molecules and, following a comparative study between insects, mice, and rabbits, Douch *et al* (1971) questioned whether the activity of hydrolases would be sufficient to account for the amounts of phenols present in the urine of mammals treated with carbamates. They did not detect a cofactor-independent aryl methylcarbamate esterase activity in any of these species and concluded that an NADPH-dependent microsomal enzyme accounted for the formation of phenolic metabolites in both insects and mice. The mouse liver microsomal enzyme was inhibited by both piperonyl butoxide and metyrapone, whereas only metyrapone inhibited the housefly enzyme. Thus, both mammalian and insect enzymes had the major characteristics of mixed function oxidases but the insect enzyme clearly merits further examination.

A number of the metabolites of naphthalene and the related insecticide carbaryl (7) in insects (and mammals) clearly point to the formation of an epoxide as the primary product of oxidation of the aromatic system. Thus, the intermediate formation of naphthalene 1,2-epoxide accounts for the formation of 1-naphthol (by rearrangement), 1,2-dihydroxy-1,2-dihydronaphthalene (by epoxide hydration), and the various conjugation products that are formed by insects and mammals. The aromatic epoxide hydrases of liver and other mammalian tissues have been widely studied in recent years (see Chapter 5) but their presence in insects is recognized only by inference from the nature of the metabolic products of aromatic compounds.

In contrast to aromatic epoxides, the epoxides of chlorinated, reduced polycyclic insecticides such as aldrin (**14**) are quite stable, and although the addition of water to dieldrin (**15**), followed by conjugation of the resultant diol, appears to be an obvious detoxication mechanism for this compound, diol formation *in vivo* was not noticed in either insects or mammals until some 16 years after its introduction as an insecticide (Oonnithan and Miskus, 1964; Korte and Arent, 1965). At about the same time an epoxide hydrase that rapidly converts the related compound HEOM (**27**) into the corresponding *trans*-diol was discovered in microsomes from houseflies and mammalian liver (references in Table 1). Only the mammalian liver enzyme significantly hydrated the isomer HCE (**28**).

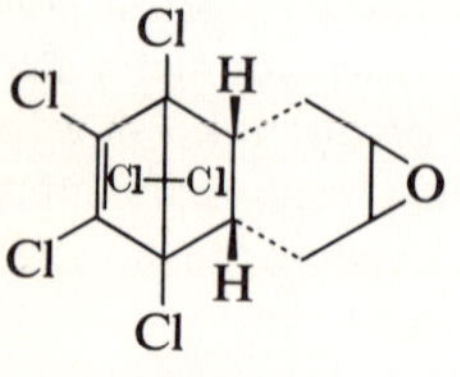

HEOM
(27)

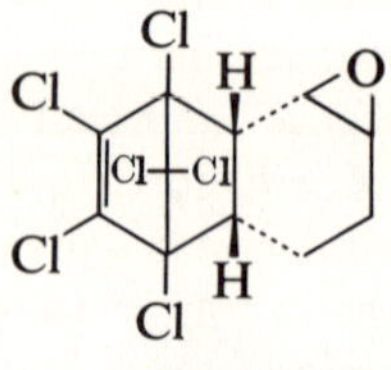

HCE
(28)

Subsequent surveys showed that HEOM was enzymically hydrated by homogenates of tissues from blowflies (*Calliphora erythrocephala*), fleshflies (*Sarcophaga barbata*), mosquitoes (by *Culex fatigans* and *Aedes aegypti* but not readily by *Anopheles stephensi*), various lepidopteran larvae (by *Galleria mellonella* homogenates and *Philosamia ricini* and *Manduca sexta* gut but not readily by *Pieris brassicae* gut), bed bugs (*Cimex lectularius*), and cattle ticks (*Boophilus decoloratus*); from larvae of the yellow mealworm beetle (*Tenebrio molitor*) but not adult mustard beetles (*Phaedon cochleariae*). The low conversions in some of the above cases may have been due to the liberation of endogenous inhibitors but are apparently genuine in the case of stable fly (*Stomoxys calcitrans*), tsetse fly (*Glossina austeni*), and a triatomid bug (*Rhodnius prolixus*), as indicated by experiments *in vivo* (Brooks, unpublished results). Some of these results are discussed in relation to selective toxicity in a later section.

The enzymic hydration of HEOM by the microsomes of various species required no added cofactors, was not inhibited by CO/O_2 mixtures, and proceeded under anaerobic conditions; the optimum pH (8·0–9·0) for hydration was higher than for oxidative metabolism. Hydration occurs more slowly in the case of HCE (**28**) and oxidation products are formed simultaneously when NADPH is added (Brooks *et al*, 1970). In this case hydration is favoured by raising the pH and oxidation by lowering it (towards pH 7·0). The hydration process is inhibited *in vitro* by a variety of compounds, including 1,3-benzodioxoles, SKF 525A, and various non-toxic phosphorus esters such as triphenyl phosphate and tri-*o*-cresyl phosphate at 10^{-5} M to 10^{-3} M, depending on the species examined. A search for epoxide hydrase inhibitors that might act as synergists for HEOM in insects *in vivo* has shown that, as in the case of the aromatic epoxide hydrase of mammalian liver, the best inhibitors are themselves epoxides (Brooks, 1973a, b, 1974a; Slade *et al*, 1975; Craven *et al*, 1976). Only transient synergism has been observed to date, which is explained by the probability that most of the better inhibitors are alternative substrates for the enzymes.

The mechanism of cyclodiene epoxide ring opening remains to be elucidated but deserves some comment in the light of recent findings. Chemically, epoxide ring opening may be initiated by 'backside' attack of OH^- (alkaline conditions) on one carbon atom, followed by ring opening to give usually a *trans*-diol. Alternatively, the oxygen atom may be protonated (acid hydrolysis) so that hydrative ring opening is initiated with the formation of a *trans*-diol. The addition of water to a double bond may be viewed similarly.

There is evidence that both reactions may be catalysed by the same enzyme. Thus, fumarase, which catalyses the reversible interconversion of fumarate and L-malate, also stereospecifically hydrates *trans*-2,3-epoxysuccinate; only the L-epoxide is hydrated, to give mesotartaric acid, and the epoxide hydrase and olefin hydrase activites are inseparable (Hill and Teipel, 1971). A mechanism involving enzyme-facilitated protonation followed by spontaneous ring opening has some attractions, since the intermediate in a hydrolase mechanism involving, for example, ring opening initiated by a serine hydroxyl might be further hydrolysed only with difficulty and then with formation of the *cis*-diol.*

Matthews and Matsumura (1969) detected the formation of the *trans*-diol from dieldrin in rat liver microsomes plus supernatant and the conversion was evidently stimulated by NADPH but not inhibited by sesamex. Brooks *et al* (1970) found that hepatic microsomes of pig and rabbit very slowly hydrated dieldrin (**15**) to the *trans*-diol. No cofactors were added, and although no attempt was made to measure endogenous NADPH, its rapid exhaustion would appear extremely likely under these conditions. More recently Matthews and McKinney (1974) demonstrated that rat liver microsomes produced steady-state amounts of the *cis*-diol (**29**) from dieldrin, while the amount of *trans*-diol

---

* DuBois *et al* (1978), *J. Biol. Chem.*, **253**, 2932 suggest that a histidine residue catalyses the nucleophilic addition of water.

176

(**31**) steadily increased. Furthermore, epimerization of the synthetic *cis*-diol (to *trans*-diol) occurred in these microsomes and was stimulated by NADPH. The ketol (**30**), an obvious intermediate, was synthesized and in both washed microsomes and soluble fraction gave a mixture of *cis*- and *trans*-diols by a reduction that did not require NADPH and was unaffected by CO or nitrogen. These observations are summarized below:

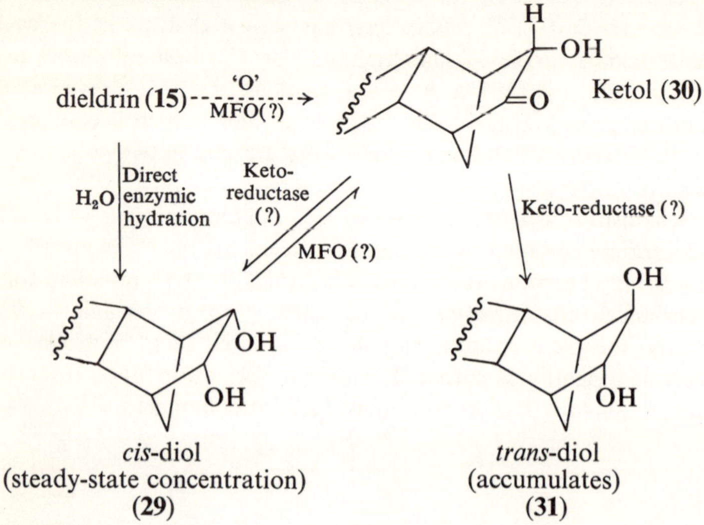

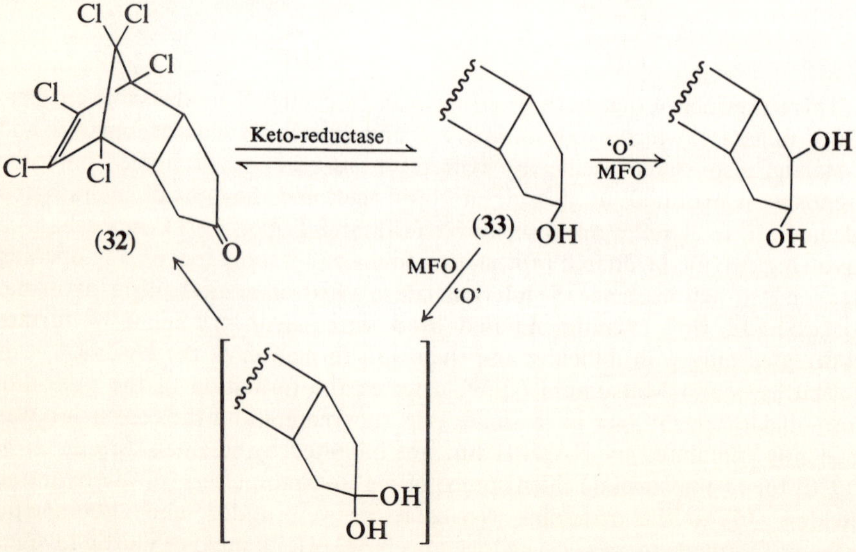

An enzyme of the steroid alcohol dehydrogenase/keto-reductase type would seem most likely to mediate the *second* stage of this NADPH-stimulated epimerization. The overall conversion (i.e. *cis*- to *trans*-diol) was apparently inhibited by CO and metyrapone but not greatly by nitrogen or piperonyl butoxide. These properties are only partly those expected for a mixed function oxidase and the system clearly requires close examination. A somewhat similar situation was noticed for the reversible oxidation of a dihydrochlordene alcohol (**33**) to the corresponding ketone (**32**) by housefly microsomes and pig liver microsomes. In this case ketone formation was stimulated by NADPH, but not by NAD or NADP, and was inhibited by sesamex (**13**); the synthetic ketone was reduced to the alcohol by pig liver microsomes plus NADPH, and sesamex (**13**) blocked further hydroxylation of the alcohol but had little effect on its formation from the ketone (Brooks and Harrison, 1967a, b).

As an alternative to hydrative *cis*-diol formation direct from dieldrin, Bedford (1975) has suggested that the ketol (**30**) might be formed directly by MFO-mediated hydroxylation of the epoxide ring. It may be that more than one mechanism is possible for such stable epoxides and that there are species differences in metabolism.

Nelson and Matsumura (1973) found that American cockroaches produced mainly the *cis*-diol plus a little *trans*-diol from dieldrin *in vivo*. Microsomes plus supernatant from fat body gave both the *cis*- and the *trans*-diol. In this case the addition of NADPH stimulated the formation of other, oxidative, metabolites; *trans*-diol formation was unaffected but *cis*-diol formation was reduced by 57%. Thus, oxidation appears to be competing with diol formation, as found with dieldrin analogues in other systems (Brooks *et al*, 1970), and the hydrative mechanism for diol production appears to operate in this insect. The nerve cords of these cockroaches contain an epimerase that converts the *cis*-into the *trans*-diol (Brooks, 1977; Schroeder *et al*, 1977) but the requirements for this conversion have not yet been explored. The *cis*- and the *trans*-diol from dieldrin are neuroactive when applied to nerve preparations from both insects and vertebrates, as are the diols from certain analogues, so that diol formation, whatever its mechanism, continues to be of considerable theoretical interest.

Several of the natural juvenile hormones of insects, and numerous synthetic analogues thereof, contain both a carboxyl ester group and an epoxide ring. It is therefore to be expected that both epoxide hydration and ester hydrolysis may be significant processes for the deactivation of such molecules in insect tissues. This has been found to be the case and the relative significance of the two pathways differs between insect species. Thus, methyl 10,11-epoxyfarnesoate (**35**) suffered both ester hydrolysis and epoxide hydration in fifth instars of locusts (*Schistocerca gregaria*) and triatomid bugs (*Rhodnius prolixus*) (White, 1972). Slade and Zibitt (1972) compared the metabolism of cecropia juvenile hormone (**34**) in prepupae and fifth instar larvae of the tobacco hornworm (*Manduca sexta*), pupae of the silk-moth (*Hyalophora cecropia*), fourth instar nymphs of a locust (*Schistocerca vaga*), and third instar larvae of the fleshfly (*Sarcophaga bullata*) and found differing patterns of deactivation. *Manduca* prepupae produced epoxy-acid (**37**) and diol-acid (**38**) but no diol-ester (**36**); ester hydrolysis occurred in blood and several other tissues of larvae, but epoxide ring hydration occurred mainly in fat body. *Hyalophora* gave the epoxy-acid (**37**), diol-ester (**36**), and diol-acid (**38**), whereas *Sarcophaga* gave mainly

178

the diol-ester (**36**) and the diol-acid (**38**) was not detected. Like *Manduca*, the locust gave the epoxy-acid (**37**) and diol-acid (**38**), without much evidence of diol-ester formation.

In insects, the two hydrolytic routes appear to be overriding and there is little evidence for MFO attack on these molecules. Clearly, enzyme inhibitors able to block one, or preferably both hydrolytic mechanisms, might function as stabilizers (and hopefully synergists) of exogenous natural juvenile hormone or its synthetic analogues applied to insects *in vivo*, depending on both hormone

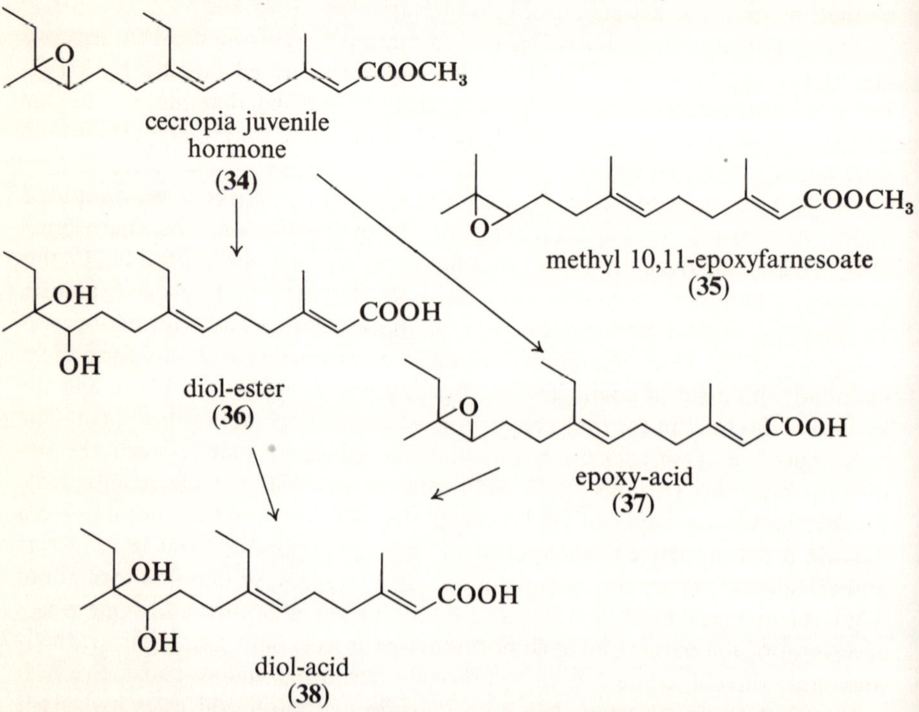

.COOCH₃

cecropia juvenile
hormone
(**34**)

methyl 10,11-epoxyfarnesoate
(**35**)

.COOH

diol-ester
(**36**)

.COOH

epoxy-acid
(**37**)

.COOH

diol-acid
(**38**)

structure and the metabolic pathway involved (Brooks, 1973b, 1974a; Slade and Wilkinson, 1973). Since, for example, *Manduca* appears to metabolize the cecropia hormone mainly by ester hydrolysis rather than epoxide hydration, non-toxic esterase inhibitors (some of which may also inhibit epoxide hydrase) might function well in this case and Ajami (1975) found this to be so. On the other hand, epoxide hydrase inhibitors cannot be expected to be synergists for juvenile hormone in this species (unless they are also inhibitors of the esterase) and this also appears to be true. If *both* hydrolytic routes are present, the selective inhibition of one of them may serve only to provide more substrate for the second; therefore, no synergism may be seen unless the metabolic capacity of the second mechanism is exceeded. In such cases, multifunctional synergists, or 'cocktails' of specific inhibitors are necessary. Many juvenile hormone analogues or mimics have been made in which one or both of the sites of hydrolytic attack have been eliminated by structural modification. The limited information available indicates that when this is done, oxidative mechanisms may become significant and can be blocked by appropriate inhibitors, with synergistic (sometimes antagonistic) consequences (Solomon and Metcalf, 1974).

Some of the pathways of chlorinated insecticide metabolism described in the literature indicate an apparent hydrolytic replacement of chlorine atoms by hydroxyl groups and it is possible that this may occur when the chlorine atom is reactive. For example, some replacement of the allylic chlorine atom of heptachlor (**16**) by a hydroxyl group probably occurs enzymically in the tissues of mosquito larvae but there is also chemical hydrolysis in the water containing them (Bowman *et al*, 1964). Although evidence for the true hydrolytic mechanism is generally lacking, there is evidence (Brooks and Harrison, 1967b; Khan *et al*, 1970) for an oxidative mechanism in houseflies and mosquitoes that involves hydroxylation of the carbon carrying a chlorine atom to give an intermediate α-chlorohydrin (*gem*-chlorohydrin). The ketone formed spontaneously from this chlorohydrin may then be reduced to the alcohol by keto-reductase activity, as indicated previously for dihydroheptachlor metabolism (Brooks and Harrison, 1967b):

$$\ce{>CHCl ->[\text{'O'}] [>C(OH)Cl] -> >C=O ->[2H][\text{Keto-reductase}] >CHOH}$$

This type of dechlorination, which is inhibited by sesamex (**13**), also occurs in rats and is clearly mediated by a mixed function oxidase. It is probably the most common mechanism for chlorinated alicyclic compounds.

Reductive Conversions

The nitroreductase activity of housefly microsomes (J. W. Ray, 1967, cited in Brooks, 1972) was not affected by MFO inhibitors but was inhibited by CO, suggesting some involvement of the cytochrome P-450 complex. Partial destruction of P-450 did not alter reductase activity, however, so the cytochrome was apparently not rate limiting. According to Lichtenstein and Fuhremann (1971), the 10,000 **g** supernatant from housefly abdomens reduced parathion (**4**) to its *p*-amino-derivative; the 150,000 **g** 'microsome' pellet had no nitroreductase activity but activity was found in the supernatant. The reduction was stimulated by NADPH, indifferent to oxygen, and inhibited by sesamex (**13**) and SKF 525A.

Nitrobenzene reductase activity occurs in fat body, gut, and Malpighian tubules of the Madagascar cockroach (*Gromphadorhina portentosa*). All subcellular fractions of these tissues contained activity, which was apparently NADH linked in the soluble fractions but NADPH linked in microsomes. As found by Ray (1967, see Brooks, 1972) for housefly microsomes, these activities were stimulated by FAD, FMN, or riboflavin and partly inhibited by CO (especially the microsomal fractions). Much of the activity appeared to result from non-enzymic reduction of the nitro-group by reduced flavins that are

180

probably produced by NADH or NADPH-linked flavoproteins. The azo-group in azofuchsin is reduced by a stoichiometrically equivalent amount of FMN produced by pyridine-nucleotide-linked flavin reductases; FMN reduction is linked to NADPH in microsomes but to either NADH or NADPH in the soluble fraction of *G. portentosa* midgut tissue (Rose and Young, 1973; R. G. Young, cited in Dauterman, 1976).

The replacement of one chlorine atom in the CCl_3 group of DDT (**1**) by hydrogen to give DDD occurs in many living organisms, including insects. Much of the previous discussion on nitroreductase applies also to this transformation, which can certainly occur non-enzymically. In general, the transformation requires anaerobic conditions, but Morello (1965) reported that liver microsomes produced DDD from DDT with a requirement for NADPH and oxygen. The mechanism of this conversion in insects is unknown.

As indicated in the previous discussion on epoxide hydrase, keto-reductases may play a significant part in the metabolism of appropriate xenobiotics in insects, as in mammals.

Desaturation

The metabolism of lindane (γ-HCH) in mammals and insects is complex because several different types of primary enzymic attack on the molecule are possible. This problem has been under discussion ever since insect resistance to lindane first arose nearly thirty years ago, the difficulty being to identify as many of the large number of metabolic products as possible and then to devise a rational scheme (or schemes) to explain their formation (Brooks, 1974b; Yang, 1976).

A desaturation reaction leading to γ-hexachlorocyclohexene (γ-HCCH (**39**)) was recently reported for the first time for lindane in rats (Chadwick *et al*, 1975) and this has been corroborated for houseflies by Tanaka *et al* (1976b). In both species the activities were microsomal, required NADPH and oxygen, and were inhibited by piperonyl butoxide, SKF 525A, and appropriate CO/O_2 mixtures but not by cyanide (in contrast to cytochrome-b_5-mediated desaturases). Rats given synthetic HCCH metabolized it more rapidly than lindane and excreted all the previously identified lindane metabolites for which adequate analytical procedures are available. γ-PCCH (**40**) has previously been considered to be a primary metabolite in several organisms but its formation does not readily account for the variety of metabolites subsequently produced. According to Tanaka *et al* (1976b), the housefly microsomes produce not only γ-HCCH (**39**) but also γ-PCCH (**40**) and an isomeric PCCH (**41**), the last two reactions requiring a *trans*- and a *cis*-dehydrochlorination, respectively. The further metabolism of lindane and of DDT is discussed later in the context of glutathione-mediated reactions.

Conjugations

Most research on the conjugation of xenobiotics in insects has involved identification of the conjugates rather than detailed examination of the enzymic mechanisms involved and conjugation reactions are generally assumed to follow the pathways established for mammals. Yang (1976) has listed (for insects and mammals) the types of conjugation that have been reported for metabolites of insecticides, insecticide synergists, insect hormones, and related compounds. Many of these primary metabolites are simple aliphatic or aromatic compounds whose metabolism and conjugation can be investigated separately. This approach was adopted by Smith and colleagues (Table 1), who established that in insects various simple phenols are converted into conjugates with glucose, sulphate, and phosphate and that glutathione and cysteine are also involved in conjugation.

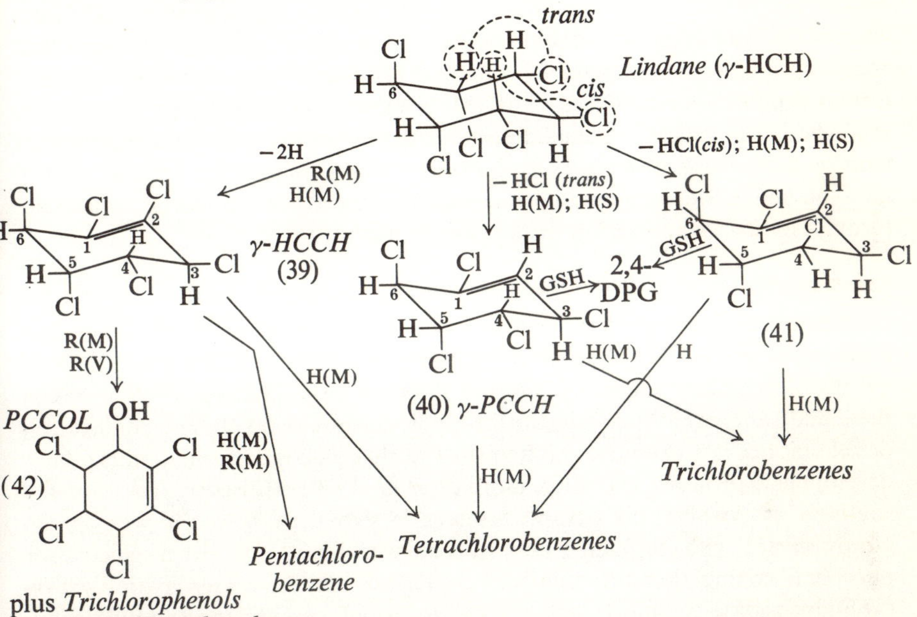

Figure 2 Pathways of lindane metabolism suggested by recent metabolism studies *in vivo* and *in vitro*. R = rat; H = housefly; M = microsomes; S = soluble fraction; V = *in vivo*; GSH = glutathione; 2,4-DPG = 2,4-dichlorophenylglutathione (Chadwick *et al*, 1975; Tanaka *et al*, 1976a, b)

Glucose

Glucose conjugation is widespread. Smith (1968) listed 52 species of insects of which some 46, including 5 species of lepidoptera, were indicated to effect this conjugation. Glucuronide formation does not appear to occur (Binning *et al*, 1967), and it seems likely that some reports have confused glucuronide conjugation with phosphate conjugation. El-Shourbagy and Dorough (1974) examined the glucosylation of 1-naphthol in 5,000 g supernatants from homogenates of whole bodies and selected tissues of houseflies, American cockroach, larvae of Alfalfa weevil (*Hypera postica*), tobacco hornworm (*Manduca sexta*) and Indian meal moth (*Plodia interpunctella*). In these experiments, 1-naphthyl glucoside was the only water-soluble product. In the presence of UDPG, the conjugating activity was high and similar in all the preparations examined. More detailed studies of tissue distribution indicate that insect fat body has the highest enzyme titres, although for *M. sexta* the midgut is quite active when 1-naphthol is used for the assay. Patterns of subcellular localization seem to differ between species; maximum activity was associated with the soluble fraction in *M. sexta* but with the particulate fractions of houseflies (Kuhr and Dorough, 1976).

The glucosylation of 1-naphthol (apparent K_m 5–7×10^{-5} M) by housefly microsomes utilized UDPG with an apparent K_m of 2×10^{-4} M at an optimum pH of 8·5. Competitive inhibition was shown by *p*-nitrophenol and non-competitive inhibition by monoamine oxidase inhibitors such as harmaline and tranylcypromine (Kumar and Dorough, 1974). The effects of inhibitors merit further exploration since other work (Mehendale and Dorough, 1971) indicates that when conjugation of the oxidative metabolites of carbaryl (7) is suppressed, there is a feedback effect which results in reduced oxidation. In insects, this kind of action on conjugation mechanisms might lead to useful synergism through indirect stabilization of the parent insecticide.

Sulphate

Sulphate conjugation has been demonstrated in a number of insects and other arthropods. The presence of sulphate conjugation in the two primitive groups of peripatus and scorpions and the absence of glucose conjugations in these and some other non-insect arthropods suggests that sulphate conjugation of xenobiotics is a primitive mechanism and that glucoside formation is a later development in insect evolution (Jordan *et al*, 1970). However, larvae of the southern armyworm, an advanced insect in evolutionary terms, conjugated *p*-nitrophenol with sulphate; no evidence was found for either glucose or phosphate conjugation although such conjugates may have been hydrolysed by the β-glucosidase and phosphatase of gut tissue and faeces (Yang and Wilkinson, 1971). Sulphotransferases in the gut tissues of the southern armyworm were later found to conjugate cholesterol, α-ecdysone, β-sitosterol, and *p*-nitrophenol. Similar enzymes were found in the tissues of several other lepidopteran larvae, housefly, honeybee, and Madagascar cockroach. The insect sulphotransferases resemble the mammalian enzymes in their subcellular localization, cofactor requirements, and pH optima (Yang, 1976).

Phosphate

Phosphate conjugation, although rarely encountered in nature, has been demonstrated either *in vivo* or *in vitro* for the housefly, blowfly (*Lucilia sericata*), fruit fly (*Drosophila melanogaster*), Madagascar cockroach, tobacco hornworm, and grass grub (*Costelytra zealandica*). In grass grubs and houseflies, phosphate conjugates are often the major products from phenols but smaller amounts of sulphates and glucosides are also formed (Binning *et al*, 1967). The supernatant (100,000 **g**) from gut tissue homogenates of tobacco hornworm and Madagascar cockroach and whole body homogenates of houseflies contains a phospho-transferase that mediates the phosphorylation of *p*-nitrophenol in the presence of Mg^{2+} and ATP. Phenobarbitone treatment induced the cockroach phospho-transferase, which may therefore have some toxicological significance when the insect is stressed with xenobiotics (Yang and Wilkinson, 1973; Gil *et al*, 1974).

Amino acids

Amino acids, principally glycine, are conjugated with foreign aromatic and some aliphatic carboxylic acids in all terrestial animals. Among arthropods, the arachnids (ticks and spiders) and myriapods (millipedes and centipedes) are well supplied with arginine and use it for conjugation. Arachnids also form glutamine and glutamic acid conjugates (e.g. with benzoic acid) and a scorpion (*Palamnaeus* sp) formed an agmatine conjugate. Peripatus (*Peripatoides novazealandiae*) produced substantial amounts of a histidine conjugate from benzoic acid, with smaller amounts of agmatine, arginine, and glutamic acid derivatives. The conjugates with agmatine and glutamate are believed to arise from the arginine, glutamine, and histidine conjugates by secondary reactions (Parke, 1968; Jordan *et al*, 1970). Piperonylic acid derivatives, formed *in vivo* by the side-chain cleavage of several 1,3-benzodioxole synergists, are conjugated with glycine, serine, alanine, glutamine, and glutamate in houseflies. Piperonyl alcohol is formed from some of these compounds *in vivo* and is converted into the β-glucoside (Esaac and Casida, 1969).

Glutathione

Glutathione (GSH) has a special significance in detoxication reactions since in addition to its involvement in the conjugation of primary metabolites formed by other enzymes, it may itself generate primary metabolites (as in the case of organophosphorus insecticides) or attack toxicants that contain labile halogens, etc., to give conjugation products directly. The various glutathione S-trans-ferases (EC 2.5.1.18) that mediate the interaction of glutathione with alkenes, epoxides, alkyl groups, aralkyl groups, aryl groups, etc. in mammals have been discussed in recent reviews (Hutson, 1972, 1975; Arias and Jakoby, 1976), and there is much evidence that similar detoxication mechanisms occur in insects. Examples from the organophosphate and organochlorine groups of insecticides are instructive.

Fukami and Shishido (1966) noted that the high speed supernatants from homogenates of rat liver and various tissues of silk worms and horn beetle larvae removed one methyl group of methyl parathion (**43**) in the presence of GSH, to give methyl *p*-nitrophenyl phosphorothioate (**44**). The horn beetle preparation slowly removed a single ethyl group from parathion (**4**) also, and it was suggested that GSH might act as an alkyl group acceptor in these O-dealkylation reactions. Lewis (1969) later found a high rate of single O-deethylation of both diazinon (**45**) and diazoxon (**46**) in the soluble fraction

184

(plus GSH) of housefly homogenates. The reaction has been completely confirmed for houseflies (Oppenoorth *et al*, 1972) and for mammals by the isolation of the appropriate S-alkylglutathiones and the generally greater reactivity of dimethyl compared with higher alkyl phosphates accounts for much of the favourable mammalian toxicity of the former type of insecticide.

The GSH-dependent dearylation of diazinon and diazoxon by homogenates of cockroach fat body was demonstrated by Fukami and Shishido (1966) and the expected S-arylglutathione subsequently isolated from the corresponding high speed supernatant fortified with GSH (Shishido *et al*, 1972). Activities for O-dealkylation and O-dearylation are frequently present together and the relative importance of each pathway may depend on the species investigated and the structure of the toxicant under attack; thus, a dimethyl phosphate may be preferentially attacked by the GSH S-transferases at an alkyl moiety, whereas attack by these enzymes at the aryl moiety may become significant when dealkylation is more difficult, as in the case of diethyl phosphates.

$$(CH_3O)_2P(S)-O-\!\!\left\langle\;\right\rangle\!\!-NO_2 \quad \xrightarrow[\substack{\text{soluble}\\\text{enzyme}}]{\text{GSH}} \quad (CH_3O)(OH)P(S)-O-\!\!\left\langle\;\right\rangle\!\!-NO_2$$

methyl parathion
(**43**)

(**44**)

diazinon
(**45**)

diazoxon
(**46**)

The first evidence for GSH involvement in the conjugation of aromatic compounds in insects was provided when Kikal and Smith (1958) showed that locusts (*Schistocerca gregaria*) injected with *p*-chlorobenzene excreted *p*-chlorophenylcysteine and its N-acetyl-derivative (*p*-chlorophenylmercapturic acid). It was then shown that the isomeric chlorophenylcysteines and chlorophenylmercapturic acids were present in locust excreta as acid-labile precursors and that *p*-nitrobenzyl chloride gave first S-(*p*-nitrobenzyl) glutathione, which was then hydrolysed in locust gut, Malpighian tubules, and excreta to S-(*p*-nitrobenzyl) cysteine. The GSH S-transferase activity for this and several other benzene derivatives with reactive halogens was highest in locust fat body, Malpighian tubules, and gut, with lower activity in other tissues. Similar activity towards 1-chloro-2,4-dinitrobenzene was found in homogenates of housefly, flour beetle (*Tenebrio molitor*), turnip beetle (*Phaedon cochleariae*), cockroach (three species), cotton stainer (*Dysdercus*), and cattle tick (*Boophilus*). In contrast to the enzymes in mammalian liver and cattle tick, the insect enzymes were strongly inhibited by various phthaleins (Gessner and Smith, 1960; Cohen and Smith, 1964; Cohen *et al*, 1964).

Nakatsugawa and Dahm (1965) noted that while houseflies had highly active GSH-dependent enzymes that degraded α-HCH, γ-HCH, γ-PCCH (**40**), and δ-PCCH, the metabolizing ability of several other species was much lower and rather variable. Enzymes of the fruit fly (*Drosophila melanogaster*) degraded δ-PCCH much faster than γ-PCCH but did not attack α- or γ-HCH. Those of stable fly (*Stomoxys calcitrans*), three species of cockroach (*Periplaneta americana*, *Blatella germanica* and *Leucophaea maderae*) and European corn borer (*Ostrinia nubilalis*) had low activity towards γ-PCCH but little activity towards the other compounds, while honey bee (*Apis mellifera*), corn rootworm (*Diabrotica virgifera*), and bark louse (*Lachesilla pedicularia*) preparations apparently had no activity towards any of these substrates.

The conversion of DDT into DDE by DDT-dehydrochlorinase (EC 4.5.1.1) in houseflies requires GSH, which is not depleted by the reaction. In contrast, lindane is converted into various chlorinated benzenes and precursors of dichlorothiophenols by complex pathways which consume GSH and are still not clearly understood. γ-PCCH (**40**) had been implicated as a metabolic intermediate in houseflies (Sternburg and Kearns, 1956), and the available information led to the suggestion that the enzymic detoxication of both DDT and lindane might be initiated by a GSH conjugation involving replacement of one chlorine atom. Decysteinylation of a subsequently formed cysteine conjugate could then give DDE or γ-PCCH (Gessner and Smith, 1960). Further dehydrochlorination of γ-PCCH would lead to the various chlorinated benzenes identified as lindane metabolites, whereas replacement of an allylic (reactive) chlorine atom by GSH, then dehydrochlorination, would explain the isolation of sulphur-containing benzene derivatives (Bradbury and Standen, 1959). An unproven alternative (Clark *et al*, 1966) is the formation of S-pentachlorocyclohexylglutathione followed by aromatization. For DDT, the objection that GSH would be depleted by the proposed mechanism (Lipke and Chalkley, 1962) would be overcome if an initially formed GSH conjugate dissociated directly to DDE with regeneration of GSH.

The nature of these enzymes and the possible relationship between them have been the subject of much research during the past decade (see Brooks, 1972, 1974b; Yang, 1976 for extensive discussions). In summary, homogenates of cattle ticks, houseflies, or locust fat body converted lindane into 2,4-dichlorophenylglutathione when fortified with GSH (Clark *et al*, 1966), and enzymes in the postmicrosomal soluble fraction from houseflies (plus GSH) degraded lindane into unspecified products (Ishida and Dahm, 1965a, b; Sims and Grover, 1965). However, Sims and Grover (1965) also reported that anaerobic housefly supernatant liberated one molecule of HCl from lindane with no enzymic depletion of GSH and without conjugate formation, whereas γ-PCCH (**40**) formed a conjugate 'identical with' that formed by a crude rat liver GSH S-transferase preparation. Using a similar supernatant, Tanaka *et al* (1976a, b) found that hexadeuterolindane (lindane-d$_6$) was degraded 6-fold more slowly than lindane, demonstrating an isotope effect expected if elimination of a proton from lindane is rate limiting, but not if direct nucleophilic attack by

GSH is involved. Thus, γ-PCCH and γ-PCCH-d$_5$ were rapidly degraded by the supernatant in the presence of GSH and there was virtually no isotope effect, in accordance with the nucleophilic replacement of an allylic chlorine by GSH; replacement of the chlorine at C$_6$ (see figure 2), followed by two dehydrochlorinations, gives 2,4-dichlorophenylglutathione. Several questions remain unanswered but the above results partly support the view that an enzyme-mediated removal of a proton by GS$^-$ might initiate the first dehydrochlorination of lindane. Conjugation of γ-PCCH (or an isomer) with GSH would then be followed by dehydrochlorinations mediated again by GS$^-$, or by some other mechanism.

Tanaka *et al* (1976b) have indicated that an MFO system in housefly microsomes desaturates lindane to γ-HCCH (**39**) and also dehydrochlorinates it to γ-PCCH (**40**) and the isomeric PCCH (**41**). Houseflies given lindane convert it *in vivo* into γ-HCCH, γ-PCCH, and pentachlorobenzene, together with tri- and tetrachlorobenzenes; the isomeric PCCH (**41**) does not appear and is known to react much more rapidly with GSH than either γ-HCCH or γ-PCCH in the postmicrosomal fraction. Assuming that conjugation must occur at C-6 for all three compounds, then the γ-HCCH and γ-PCCH conjugates each require one *cis*- and one *trans*-dehydrochlorination for aromatization, whereas (**41**) requires two *trans*-dehydrochlorinations and might well react more rapidly. It seems likely that a second approach of GS$^-$, to C-3, would lead to proton removal (followed by C-3–C-4 double bond formation and conjugation) rather than replacement of chlorine by GS$^-$; the final elimination of HCl required for aromatization might then occur spontaneously. The total system is clearly quite versatile and may explain most of the metabolites formed from lindane in houseflies. The presence in rat liver microsomes of a similar desaturase that produces γ-HCCH explains the formation of PCCOL (**42**) and a number of recently characterized rat metabolites (Chadwick *et al*, 1975).

Ishida and Dahm (Ishida and Dahm, 1965a, b; Ishida, 1968) found that DDT was readily converted into DDE by partly purified housefly enzymes that convert γ-HCH into water-soluble products and speculated on the relationship between these enzymes and the GSH S-transferases (EC 2.5.1.18). Housefly DDT-ase is a phospholipoprotein said to have a molecular weight of 36,000 (Lipke and Kearns, 1960) or to exist as a monomer (molecular weight 30,000), which in the presence of DDT aggregates to an active tetramer requiring GSH for stabilization and catalytic activity (Dinamarca *et al*, 1971, 1975a, b). Other work has also indicated that more than one form of DDT-ase is present in houseflies (Goodchild and Smith, 1970) and distinguished it from the GSH S-transferases (Ishida, 1968; Balabaskaran and Smith, 1970; Goodchild and Smith, 1970) which have similar physical characteristics.

The housefly enzymes investigated by Balabaskaran and Smith (1970) that metabolized γ-HCH, the PCCH-isomers, and DDT, and the GSH S-transferases that conjugated 1-chloro-2,4-dinitrobenzene with GSH were all inhibited by bromophenol blue. DDT-ase and the GSH S-transferases were inhibited by bis(3,5-dibromo-4-hydroxyphenyl)methane, whereas compounds related to bis(N-dimethylaminophenyl)methane inhibited only DDT-ase. The inhibition of the GSH S-transferases appears to involve competition with GSH for its binding site on the enzymes and such inhibitors might inhibit DDT-ase by competing for an analogous site on this enzyme; their structural resemblance to DDT might also result in competition at the DDT binding site on the enzyme, although dual competition was not observed by Balabaskaran and Smith (1970). Bis(N-dimethylaminophenyl)methane inhibited the metabolism of γ-PCCH but not γ-HCH in blowflies (Clark *et al*, 1969) whereas another DDT-ase inhibitor, N,N-di-*n*-butyl *p*-chlorobenzene sulphonamide, had no effect on the metabolism of γ-PCCH. The latter is converted into S-2,4-dichlorophenyl-glutathione, and presumably the GSH-binding site on the S-transferases involved has quite different affinities for these two inhibitors.

The term GSH S-aryltransferase that was used in these investigations is confusing. If such an enzyme system transiently attacks the $-CCl_3$ group of DDT, it is strictly an S-alkyltransferase system, whereas if the attack is on the benzylic carbon atom (proton removal by GS^- followed by elimination of Cl^-) the enzyme system is an S-aralkyltransferase or, more realistically, an S-proton-transferase. Similarly, the GSH S-transferase system for γ-PCCH could be regarded strictly as an S-cycloalkenyltransferase. In fact, the discovery that mammalian GSH S-transferases have broad and overlapping second substrate specificities (see Arias and Jakoby, 1976), may also apply in the insect situation and makes terms such as GSH S-aryltransferase redundant. The degree of analogy between the GSH binding sites of the GSH S-transferases (assayed, for example, using 1-chloro-2,4-dinitrobenzene) and the DDT and γ-PCCH metabolizing enzymes is debatable and more appropriate model substrates than activated chlorobenzenes might be preferable for comparison.

DDT-dehydrochlorinase activity in houseflies is increased by electron-with-drawing and decreased by electron-donating *p*-substituents, and when the α-hydrogen atom is replaced by deuterium, there is an isotope effect on both the enzymic and OH^- catalysed dehydrochlorinations, indicating that they each involve an E_2-type elimination of HCl initiated by removal of the α-proton (Metcalf, 1976). An enzyme-mediated removal of this proton by GS^-, as suggested above for the initial dehydrochlorination of γ-HCH, then seems a likely explanation for the fact that GSH is required for, but not consumed during, DDT-dehydrochlorination.

DETOXICATION AND THE DESIGN OF SELECTIVE INSECTICIDES

It will be evident from the above summary of detoxication mechanisms in insects that they show considerable qualitative similarity with mammals. This is also generally true between different insect species. Natural tolerance and resistance to insecticides are both frequently associated with quantitative differences in the titre of a particular detoxifying enzyme or enzymes, and qualitative differences are uncommon. Certain cases of tolerance (or resistance) do arise which apparently involve differences in intrinsic toxicity due to changes in the structure of the site of action and these are probably unrelated to the metabolism of the toxicant. There is, however, an obvious difference in morphology between mammals and insects. Insects have a large surface to volume ratio and consequently their nervous system and internal organs are rather accessible to toxicants applied on the cuticle or ingested with the food. It is therefore fortunate that although an insecticide may show little difference between insect and mammal in its intrinsic toxicity, the overall pharmacodynamic process may still confer advantages in favour of the mammal (Winteringham, 1969; Brooks, 1976a, b).

Detoxication is most readily prevented or modified by changes in molecular structure of the toxicant. Alternatively, an enzyme inhibitor may be used that is effective in a target insect but ineffective in a non-target insect or mammal, and this approach has been employed successfully by combining pyrethrins with 1,3-benzodioxole synergists which inhibit their microsomal oxidation.

Two general approaches to chemical modification have arisen out of comparative metabolic studies of xenobiotics in insects and mammals. In one of these, which relates particularly to interspecies selectivity, a derivative of an existing insecticide is synthesized that readily reverts to the parent toxicant in the target species but not in a non-target one. When a chemical requires such bioactivation to produce its toxic effect, 'opportunity' is provided for other metabolic processes which may lead to overall detoxication (O'Brien, 1967). The other approach involves chemical modification of a toxicant to increase its vulnerability to recognized detoxicative conversions such as oxidation, hydrolysis, etc. This approach has the advantage that since biotransformations (e.g. biological oxidations) frequently resemble chemical conversions (e.g. photooxidations) that occur in the abiotic environment, modifications to enhance biotransformations are also likely to increase general environmental degradability. Although such modification may be beneficial for non-target insects and other organisms, it may well be accompanied by a loss in the broad spectrum activity towards pest insects that was shown by the original chemical and by reduced toxicity to those the modified chemical still controls. Thus, although these modified insecticides are more desirable from the environmental standpoint, the economics of their use may not be encouraging. Some developments in the design of selective and biodegradable insecticides are discussed for the major chemical classes in the following sections.

Organophosphorus Insecticides

The greatest scope for molecular modification to improve selectivity exists when a group of compounds have high intrinsic toxicity due to rapid interaction with some function that is absolutely critical for survival. This situation means that various opportunity factors for detoxication can be incorporated with the assurance that the small amount of toxicant finally available at the site of action (target) will still be highly efficient. The best examples are found among the anticholinesterases.

The use of phosphorothioates (PS) rather than phosphates (PO) as practical toxicants provides an opportunity for the degradation of both compounds before the phosphate can attain damaging levels in the nervous system. Fortunately this opportunity frequently favours mammal more than insect and the mammalian selectivity ratio (MSR: mammal oral LD_{50}/insect topical LD_{50}) is usually (although not invariably) higher for the phosphorothioate than the phosphate. The use of methyl phosphorothioates or phosphates rather than the ethyl or higher alkyl esters favours the GSH S-transferase detoxication mechanism discussed earlier and with suitable substitution of the aromatic ring, methyl parathion (Table 3, R = H; X = S) can be converted into compounds having remarkably favourable MSR's. In addition to enhanced vulnerability to detoxication mechanisms, as compared with paraoxon, there appears to be a much higher affinity of insect (e.g. housefly-head) cholinesterase than of mammalian (e.g. bovine erythrocyte) cholinesterase for the phosphates derived from these PS analogues, several of which show relatively moderate mammalian toxicity.

Table 3 Selective toxicity of analogues of methyl parathion and methyl paraoxon (data of Metcalf and Metcalf, 1973)

		LD_50 (mg/kg)		
R	X	Mouse (oral)	Housefly (topical)	MSR*
H	S	99 ± 17	$1 \cdot 4 \pm 0 \cdot 1$	71
H	O	$15 - 20$	$3 \cdot 4 \pm 0 \cdot 2$	$5 \cdot 3$
3-Cl	S	$> 1{,}500$	$10 \cdot 6 \pm 0 \cdot 7$	> 140
3-Cl	O	130 ± 41	$5 \cdot 0 \pm 0 \cdot 2$	26
3-CF$_3$	S	$> 2{,}000$	$3 \cdot 1 \pm 0 \cdot 1$	> 650
3-CF$_3$	O	291 ± 153	$3 \cdot 1 \pm 0 \cdot 1$	92
3-CH$_3$	S	$1{,}500$	$2 \cdot 4 \pm 0 \cdot 1$	630
3-CH$_3$	O	$150 - 200$	$11 \cdot 5 \pm 0 \cdot 7$	15
2-F	S	500	$6 \cdot 0 \pm 0 \cdot 2$	83
2-F	O	$12 \cdot 3 \pm 2 \cdot 7$	$1 \cdot 4 \pm 0 \cdot 05$	$8 \cdot 8$
2-Cl	S	$> 1{,}500$	$1 \cdot 7 \pm 0 \cdot 1$	> 880
2-Cl	O	99 ± 7	$2 \cdot 7 \pm 0 \cdot 1$	37

* Mouse LD_{50}/housefly LD_{50} (mammalian selectivity ratio).

Malathion (**26**) was discussed in an earlier section in connection with carboxylesterase-mediated detoxication. The evident value of the ethoxycarbonyl group in conferring selective toxicity in favour of mammals led to its incorporation into several other structures. Of these, acethion (**47**) shows generally more favourable mammalian toxicity than malathion but has found no favour commercially on account of its narrow spectrum of insecticidal activity (O'Brien,

1967). The mammalian toxicity of phenthoate (**48**) is less favourable but this compound has shown promise as a replacement for DDT in house-spraying for malaria control. Dimethoate (**49**) has various valuable uses in agriculture and for the control of public health pests, especially diptera. The effect of the amide group is not clear-cut as there are sensitive and insensitive species among both insects and vertebrates. In insects a number of factors evidently contribute to

$$CH_3O \diagdown \overset{S}{\underset{\parallel}{P}} SCHCOC_2H_5$$
$$CH_3O \diagup \ \ \beta CH_2COC_2H_5$$
$$O$$

malathion
(**26**)

$$C_2H_5O \diagdown \overset{S}{\underset{\parallel}{P}} SCH_2COOC_2H_5$$
$$C_2H_5O \diagup$$

acethion
(**47**)

$$CH_3O \diagdown \overset{S}{\underset{\parallel}{P}} SCH(C_6H_5)COOC_2H_5$$
$$CH_3O \diagup$$

phenthoate
(**48**)

$$CH_3O \diagdown \overset{S}{\underset{\parallel}{P}} SCH_2CONHCH_3$$
$$CH_3O \diagup$$

dimethoate
(**49**)

the observed toxicity, whereas for several vertebrate species O'Brien (1967) established a clear positive correlation between total hydrolysis (amidase plus phosphatase attack) by liver homogenates and tolerance for dimethoate.

The evolution of relativity safe organophosphorus insecticides is well illustrated by the vinyl phosphate series, of which dichlorvos (**50**) is an early example. Trichlorfon (**51**) is said to be converted into dichlorvos *in vivo* and so is butonate (**52**) which is effectively a derivatized form of these compounds. All three compounds have similar insecticidal activity but butonate is much less toxic to mammals (Arthur and Casida, 1958) and clearly offers opportunity factors that favour them over insects.

Further exploration in this area has led to the interesting series of compounds which includes chlorfenvinphos (**53**) and tetrachlorvinphos (**55**). The parent compound of the series, 2-chlorovinyl diethyl phosphate, is toxic to both mammals and insects, but is effectively deactivated by conversion into its 2-chloro-1-phenylvinyl analogue. Anticholinesterase activity is restored when this analogue is converted into chlorfenvinphos (**53**), which exhibits the biological stability associated with diethyl phosphates and, due to its persistence in soil, is useful in the control of soil pests. There is a progressive reduction in mammalian toxicity through the series chlorfenvinphos, 'ethyl' tetrachlorvinphos (**54**), and tetrachlorvinphos (**55**) without much change in insect toxicity (Whetstone *et al*, 1966). It appears that the additional chlorine confers distribution properties that favour mammals, besides which there is a progressive reduction in affinity for mammalian cholinesterase. Tetrachlorvinphos (**55**) combines these favourable properties with an increased susceptibility to GSH-dependent dealkylation; it has an LD_{50} for mice greater than 5,000 mg/kg but is as toxic as chlorfenvinphos to houseflies. In contrast to chlorfenvinphos, tetrachlorfenvinphos is rapidly degraded in soil and is therefore ineffective against soil insects but is valuable in situations involving contact with food commodities and livestock.

Sun (1972) found the MSR (mouse/housefly) to vary between 19 to 1,060 (mean 376) for 14 analogues of tetrachlorovinphos (**55**) and from 0·87 to 56 (mean 19·4) for 15 traditional chlorinated insecticides, which shows that these organophosphates are generally safer than the chlorinated insecticides tested (lindane, cyclodienes, DDT).

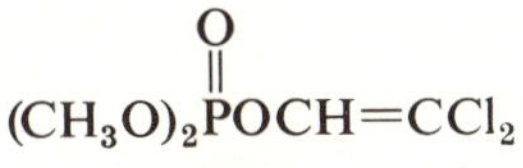

$(CH_3O)_2\overset{O}{\overset{\|}{P}}OCH{=}CCl_2$

dichlorvos
(**50**)

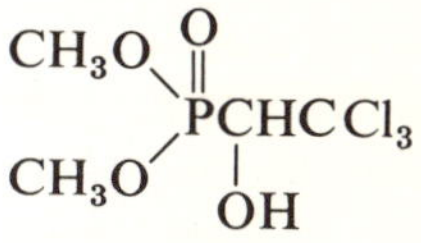

CH_3O, CH_3O — $\overset{O}{\overset{\|}{P}}CHCCl_3$, OH

trichlorfon
(**51**)

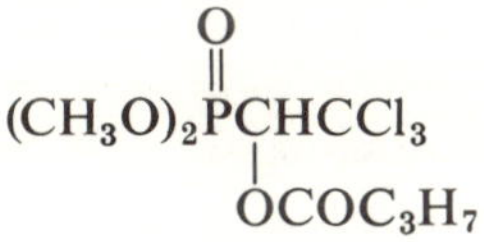

$(CH_3O)_2\overset{O}{\overset{\|}{P}}CHCCl_3$, $OCOC_3H_7$

butonate
(**52**)

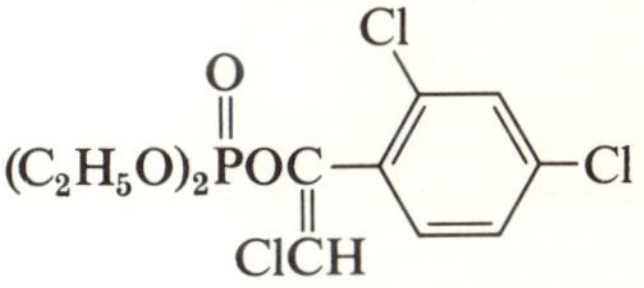

$(C_2H_5O)_2\overset{O}{\overset{\|}{P}}OC$ (2,4-dichlorophenyl), $ClCH$

chlorfenvinphos
(**53**)

$(C_2H_5O)_2\overset{O}{\overset{\|}{P}}OC$ (2,4,5-trichlorophenyl), $ClCH$

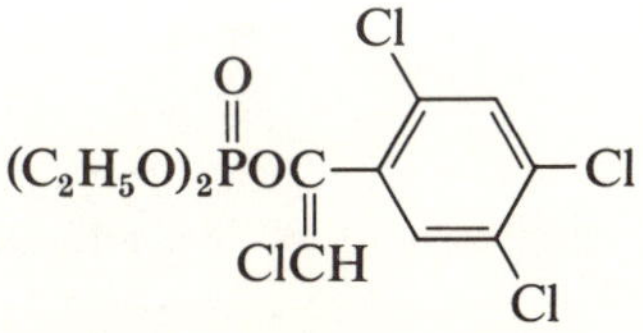

'ethyl' tetrachlorvinphos
(**54**)

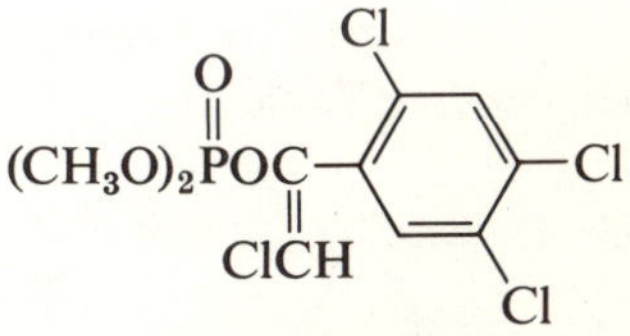

$(CH_3O)_2\overset{O}{\overset{\|}{P}}OC$ (2,4,5-trichlorophenyl), $ClCH$

tetrachlorvinphos
(**55**)

The behaviour of isopropyl parathion (diisopropyl *p*-nitrophenyl phosphorothioate) and its phosphate analogue in housefly, honeybee, and white mouse may be cited as an illustration of the way several factors may combine to confer selectivity (Camp *et al*, 1969). These compounds are >212 and 18-fold more toxic to the housefly than to the honeybee, respectively, and housefly cholinesterase is about 36-fold more sensitive to isopropyl paraoxon than the honeybee enzyme. Thus, selectivity is still apparent with the phosphate analogues that are the direct toxicants. Metabolism studies and enzymology indicate that lower toxicity to honeybee than housefly is related to the lower sensitivity of its cholinesterase to the phosphate analogue, which is also produced more slowly from the phosphorothioate by honeybees. Both insects produced diisopropyl phosphorothioic acid as the only watersoluble metabolite and there was no evidence for enhanced cleavage of isopropoxy-groups by the honeybee. Metabolism of isopropyl parathion in the white mouse (oral LD_{50} 537 mg/kg) was more complex and involved O-dealkylation as well as O-dearylation.

Carbamate Insecticides and Synergists

Carbamate insecticides are particularly vulnerable to attack by the microsomal oxidases and interspecific differences in susceptibility to them appear to be due mainly to differing activities of these enzymes (Metcalf, 1968; Brattsten and Metcalf, 1970). For example, carbaryl (7) and several other aryl methylcarbamates are highly toxic to honeybees and mosquitoes but poorly toxic to housefly, German cockroach, and rat. In contrast, propoxur (Baygon® (56)), which is a favoured, though much more expensive replacement for DDT in malaria control programmes, has a broader spectrum of insect toxicity but retains favourable mammalian toxicity. Another simple carbamate, butacarb (3,5-di-*t*-butylphenyl methylcarbamate), combines remarkably low mammalian toxicity (> 3000 mg/kg) with outstanding persistence on sheep wool and correspondly high efficiency against sheep blowfly.

Carbaryl and propoxur suffer oxidative attack (see earlier section for discussion on 'hydrolysis') at the positions indicated to give the parent phenols and N-methylol derivatives. Also produced from carbaryl are the 5,6-dihydrodiol derivative and the 4- and 5-hydroxy derivatives, and from propoxur the 3-hydroxy derivative, the free carbamate, and the phenol resulting from oxidative isopropyl group cleavage. These patterns, with quantitative and minor qualitative variations, are similar for insects, mammals, and plants (Fukuto, 1972). They result in a topical LD_{50} of 900 mg/kg for carbaryl against the housefly and spectacular synergistic effects when this compound is co-applied with various non-toxic 1,3-benzodioxoles and other types of MFO-inhibiting synergists (see Table 2).

Table 4 Selective synergism of carbaryl against houseflies (data of Metcalf, 1968; Sacher *et al*, 1968, 1969)

Synergist*	Topical LD_{50} of carbaryl to housefly (μg/g) at (ratio to synergist)	Synergistic ratio to housefly†	Oral LD_{50} of carbaryl to mouse (mg/kg) at (ratio to synergist)
None	900	—	> 400
Naphtho (2,3-d)-1,3-dioxole	5·0 (1 : 5)	180	> 750 (1 : 5)
1-Naphthyl-2-propynyl ether	15·5 (1 : 5)	58	> 400 (1 : 5)

* Synergists non-toxic at dosage employed.
† LD_{50} carbaryl/LD_{50} carbaryl plus synergist.

In practical terms, some of these synergistic combinations can be selectively toxic to insects (Table 4), since metabolic studies have shown that 1,3-benzodioxoles and certain aryl 2-propynyl ethers, for example, suffer oxidative cleavage of the critical 1,3-dioxole or 2-propynyl groups much more quickly in mammals than in insects (Metcalf, 1968; Esaac and Casida, 1969; Sacher *et al*, 1969; Casida, 1970). This differential metabolism, together with probable differences in distribution of the components of the synergist/insecticide combination *in vivo*, seems likely to negate the synergistic effect of many such combinations in mammals. Similar selectivity is found when biodegradable DDT analogues are combined with 1,3-benzodioxole synergists (Table 6). The synergism of carbaryl against houseflies is so spectacular (amounting to the generation of a highly toxic mixture from two non-toxic components) that the combination with carbaryl against houseflies is a widely used test for putative synergists. When 1,3-dioxole or propargyloxy-groups are incorporated into metabolically labile carbamates, their metabolism is often inhibited, with correspondingly increased insect toxicity, an effect termed 'autosynergism' by Metcalf (1968).

The high toxicity of carbaryl and other carbamates to the honeybee is associated with this insect's poor ability to metabolize the compounds oxidatively. However, the honeybee is not totally lacking in MFO activity, since it slowly converts isopropyl parathion into the phosphate and methyl parathion (43) into methyl paraoxon at a rate comparable with that found in the housefly (Metcalf, 1968). Insect resistance to carbamates is associated largely with selection for enhanced MFO activity, and in some resistant strains of housefly the resistance factor can be greatly reduced by using the carbamate with a synergist such as piperonyl butoxide. Thus, PB combined with propoxur (in 5 : 1 ratio) was as effective against houseflies completely resistant to this toxicant as propoxur was to a susceptible strain; however, the combination was 4-fold more toxic than propoxur alone to the latter strain, showing that it too had some ability to detoxify the insecticide. Studies of metabolism *in vivo* show that in spite of this spectacular synergism, detoxication is not necessarily completely suppressed and, since the synergists are themselves metabolized, recovery from intoxication may be observed in some circumstances. This may well be explained by the slow recovery of cytochrome P-450 from complexation with such synergists and also by the fact that not all of the P-450 is complexed and the remainder may be free to effect synergist deactivation.

In the case of carbamates, quite small structural alterations may have a profound effect on toxicity. Thus, the aromatic position isomers of dimethoxyphenyl methylcarbamate vary considerably in their toxicity to houseflies and the differences are largely abolished in the presence of PB, indicating that they are caused by differing susceptibilities to attack by MFO. Accordingly, aromatic position isomerism may be used to mask or reveal potential sites of detoxicative attack when something is known of the insect's metabolic preferences.

A number of carbamates which have valuable insecticidal activity also have high mammalian toxicity and attempts have been made to promote the expression of differing metabolic routes in insects and mammals by incorporating opportunity factors for detoxication in the form of derivatizing groups (Fukuto, 1976). The high mouse toxicity of the bis-methylcarbamate of salicylaldoxime was thought to be due to its slow conversion into the moderately toxic (oral LD_{50} 225 mg/kg) 2-cyanophenyl methylcarbamate in the acid stomach of this animal. Replacement of the methylcarbamyl oxime moiety by the more stable alkoxyiminomethyl moiety, as in (57), reduced the mouse toxicity 2-fold and increased the housefly toxicity 8-fold, as compared with the 2-cyano-carbamate (Lee *et al*, 1974; Sanborn *et al*, 1974). The structural change doubtless affords the mammal more time for the familiar types of oxidative attack on the aromatic ring or N-methyl group.

As another example, considerable reductions in mammalian toxicity result when 2-(2-butyl), 3-(2-butyl), and 3-isopropylphenyl methylcarbamates are converted into their N-acyl derivatives (acyl = $COCH_3$, $COCH_2Cl$, $COCHCl_2$), and the chloracetyl and dichloroacetyl derivatives have toxicities similar to those of the parent carbamates toward some insects (Fraser *et al*, 1968). The available evidence indicates that the acyl derivatives are readily hydrolysed to the active parent carbamates in insects, whereas in mammals this conversion is sufficiently slow to allow detoxication to occur by other routes.

Since work on the comparative metabolism of malathion indicated that mammals detoxify it by carboxylesterase attack, whereas insect enzymes more readily attack bonds to phosphorus or sulphur, Fukuto (1976) was led to prepare the N-dimethoxyphosphinothioyl derivatives of various carbamates. It was hoped that insect enzymes might hydrolyse the N—P bond to give the toxic parent carbamate whereas mammalian enzymes would hydrolyse the O—CO bond to give the parent phenol, thereby detoxifying the molecule. These derivatives of carbaryl (7), propoxur (56), carbofuran (58), and 3-isopropylphenyl methylcarbamate are indeed less toxic to mice than the parent carbamates, while their insect toxicities are little changed. Furthermore, houseflies treated with the carbofuran derivative (59) converted it mainly into carbofuran (58) and 3-hydroxycarbofuran, whereas mice and rats given (59) orally excreted 75% of the administered dose as conjugates of the phenols corresponding to carbofuran (58), 3-keto-carbofuran, and 3-hydroxycarbofuran, thereby verifying the original postulate regarding the different metabolic routes in insect and mammal.

A variety of N-arylsulphenyl and N-alkylsulphenyl derivatives of the above carbamates also retain good insecticidal activity and are substantially less toxic to mice than the original insecticides (Fukuto, 1976). In general, the arylsulphenyl moiety reduced mouse toxicity by 10- to 50-fold and the alkylsulphenyl group by 5- to 17-fold, with 4-*t*-butylphenylsulphenyl substitution giving greatest effect. Thus, N-4-*t*-butylphenylsulphenyl propoxur (**60**) is more toxic than propoxur (**56**) to house flies ($\times 2.5$) and mosquitoes *Culex fatigans* ($\times 20$), whereas the mouse toxicity is reduced about 40-fold.

Metabolic studies on N-(2-toluenesulphenyl)-carbofuran (**61**) showed that the housefly produced mainly carbofuran (**58**) and its 3-hydroxy derivative and indicated that the toxicity of (**61**) results from the liberation of carbofuran *in vivo*. In contrast, mice treated orally with (**61**) excreted most of the dose in urine within 24 hours, mainly as conjugates of 3-hydroxycarbofuran and its N-methylol analogue, together with conjugates of the various expected phenols; very little carbofuran was isolated. Rapid conjugation may be a considerable factor in the survival of mice, since 3-hydrocarbofuran is rather toxic to them (oral LD_{50} 7 mg/kg).

The results of these and other studies detailed by Fukuto (1976) show that a judicious increase in the structural complexity of the methylcarbamate molecule can be used to exaggerate pre-existing differences in metabolism between insects and mammals that may not be very evident from the behaviour of the parent unsubstituted compounds. There appears to be considerable scope for such innovation in the carbamate series and it is certain that this group will continue to make valuable contributions to insect control.

Pyrethroids

The recent development (Elliott, 1976) of synthetic pyrethroids combining the traditional low mammalian toxicity and high insecticidal efficiency of the

196

natural materials with increased environmental stability gives much promise
for the future of these insecticides, especially if their cost can be reduced.
Increased environmental stability is especially necessary in order that they can
be used economically in agriculture, horticulture, and forestry. The lipophilicity
of the more recent pyrethroids is similar to that of the chlorinated insecticides
but the pyrethroids are more insecticidal. Also, their susceptibility to both
oxidative and hydrolytic metabolism in mammals favours rapid elimination
from tissues rather than storage, and the mammalian toxicities are rather
favourable (Table 5).

Table 5 Comparative toxicities of pyrethroids (data of Verschoyle and Barnes, 1972;
Elliott *et al*, 1974; Barnes and Verschoyle, 1974)

| Compound | Relative toxicities* | | Toxicity to rats (mg/kg) | |
	Houseflies	Mustard beetles	Oral	Approx. lethal intravenous dose
Pyrethrin I	2·0	160	260–420	5
Bioresmethrin	100†	100‡	8,000	340
Cismethrin	41	52	168	6–7
Allethrin	3	1	—	—
Bioallethrin	10	4	1,030	4
RU 11679	130	170	100	5–10
NRDC 143	60	120	1,500	270
NRDC 161	2,300	1,600	25–63	2–2·5
Parathion	37	7	13§	—
DDT	4–15	1·1	113§	—
Dieldrin	35	4–10	46§	—

* Insect toxicities by topical application.

† LD_{50} *c.* 0·006 μg/insect.

‡ LD_{50} *c.* 0·005 μg/insect.

§ Data from Martin, H. (ed.) (1972), Pesticide Manual, 3rd edn., British Crop Protection
Council.

Natural pyrethrins such as pyrethrin I (**62**) are susceptible to both atmospheric
and biological oxidations, but the ester link to the secondary alcohol moiety is
stable. In insects and in rats and mice, the synthetic pyrethroid bioresmethrin
(**63**) is attacked by microsomal oxidases at the positions indicated, but the ester
link to the primary alcohol is now vulnerable and in mammals especially its
hydrolysis becomes an important additional route of detoxication (Miyamoto
et al, 1971; Abernathy and Casida, 1973). Synergistic effects with esterase
inhibitors indicate that cleavage of primary alcohol esters occurs to a variable
degree in insects, depending on the species and isomer tested. For example, it is
significant for tetramethrin (**67**) in houseflies and more so in milkweed bugs
(Jao and Casida, 1974; Suzuki and Miyamoto, 1974).

Ester hydrolysis is markedly reduced by the *trans-* to *cis*-isomerization that
converts bioresmethrin (**63**) into cismethrin (**65**) and mammalian toxicity is

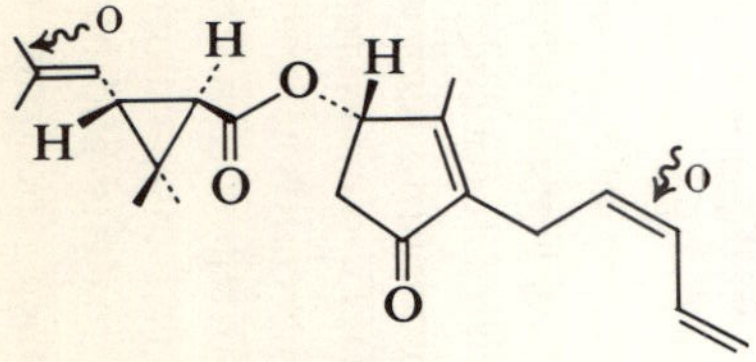

NRDC 143
(64)
tetramethrin
(67)
bioresmethrin
(63)
Est
Is
RU 11679
(66)
NRDC 161
(68)
pyrethrin I
(62)
cismethrin
(65)

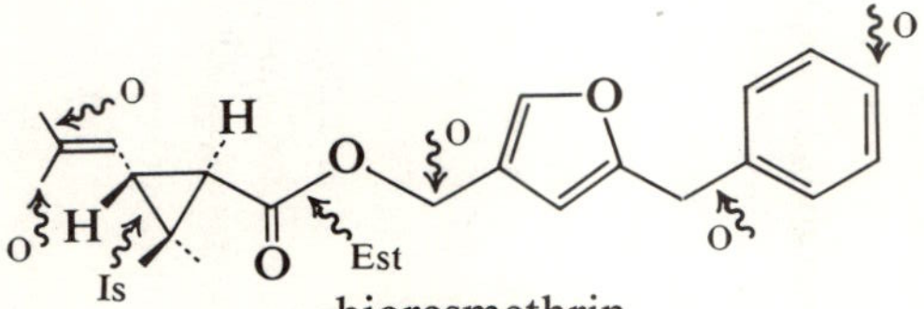

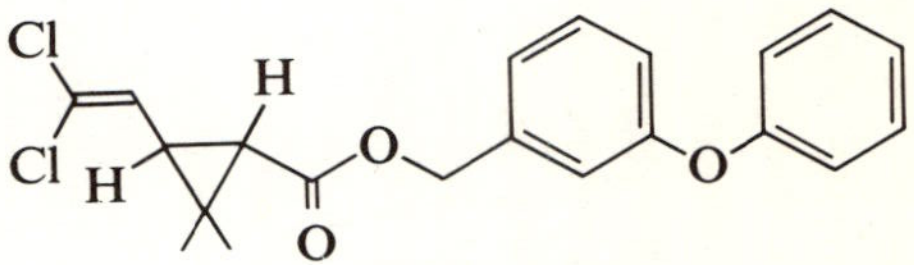

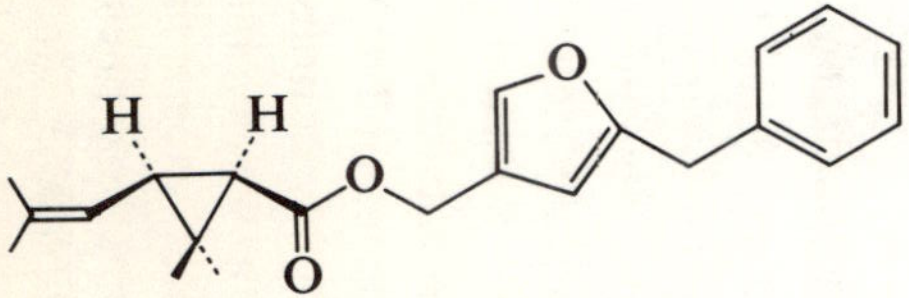

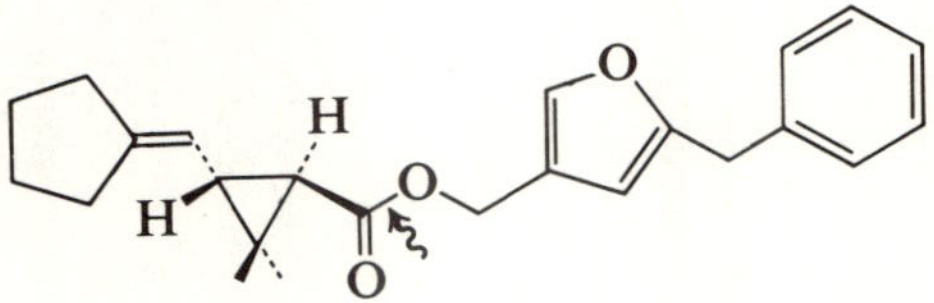

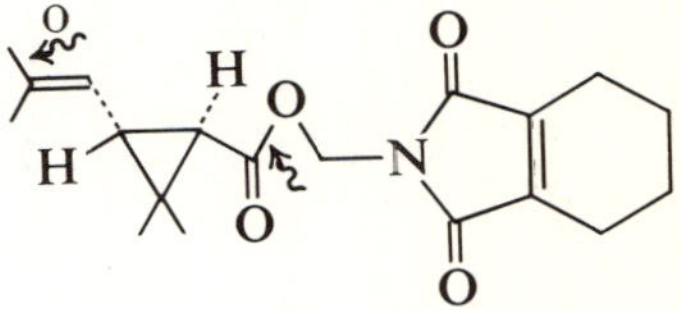

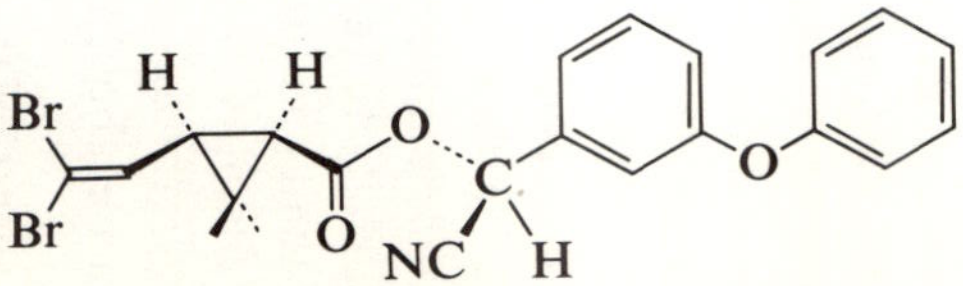

greatly increased, with a slightly adverse effect on toxicity to houseflies and mustard beetles (Table 5) that is probably due in part to a less favourable interaction with the site of action. Consequently, the MSR (rat/insect) is much less favourable for cismethrin (**65**) than for bioresmethrin (**63**). The detoxification of bioresmethrin becomes mainly dependent on ester cleavage if oxidation of the isobutenyl side-chain is inhibited, as in the cyclopentylidene analogue Ru 11679 (**66**); insect and mammalian toxicity are both increased by this change. MFO inhibitors (sesamex, PB) do not alter the toxicities of bioresmethrin or RU 11679 to mice and the esterase inhibitor DEF (tributyl phosphorotrithioate) synergizes only the latter, although it inhibits the hydrolysis of both *in vivo* (Abernathy and Casida, 1973). Thus, it appears that if either the oxidative or the hydrolytic detoxification of bioresmethrin is separately inhibited, the remaining route is still adequate for protection. In RU 11679, however, the oxidative route is suppressed by the structural change: ester hydrolysis becomes vital for detoxication and its inhibition results in marked synergism. The *trans*- to *cis*-isomerization for RU 11679 retards ester hydrolysis, as for bioresmethrin, and there is a corresponding increase in mammalian toxicity. The insect toxicity of these compounds is generally high regardless of metabolic possibilities.

The stability of these pyrethroids to both biotic and abiotic transformations is greatly increased by replacing the labile furan ring and the isobutenyl moiety, as in NRDC 143 (**64**) and NRDC 161 (**68**) and these compounds are promising agricultural insecticides. In NRDC 161, most of the structural features that favour oxidative and hydrolytic detoxication have been removed. Although this compound is much more toxic to insects than bioresmethrin, and the increase in toxicity to rats is relatively even greater (Table 5), it is still no more toxic to rats than dieldrin. It is apparent that, as with other classes of insecticides, the availability of both oxidative and hydrolytic pathways of detoxication in the new pyrethroids increases the possibility for expression of interspecific differences in metabolism and provides a basis for improved selectivity.

Chlorinated Insecticides and their Analogues

A great many analogues of DDT have been made and various aspects of their structure–activity relationships have been reviewed recently (Brooks, 1973a; Metcalf, 1976). The most obvious molecular modifications for DDT involve the replacement of biologically stable functional groups such as halogens by labile groups of similar size, the electronic properties of the substituted groups being immaterial if molecular size is of paramount importance. Potentially more biodegradable analogues of DDT have existed for a long time but were overshadowed by the seemingly desirable persistence (and high efficiency) of DDT itself. The group as a whole, including DDT, shows remarkable selectivity in favour of vertebrates, except fish. Commercially used analogues, such as methoxychlor (1,1-bis(*p*-methoxyphenyl)-2,2,2-trichloroethane), Prolan® (1,1-bis(*p*-chlorophenyl)-2-nitropropane, and DDD (1,1-bis(*p*-chlorophenyl)-2,2-dichloroethane) have very favourable mammalian toxicity and have found valuable applications against particular pests, but their spectrum of insect toxicity is inevitably narrower than that of DDT. Of the structures shown **(69–74)** (housefly toxicities relative to DDT = 1·0 are in italics), methylchlor **(69)** was once considered as a practical insecticide and dianisyl neopentane **(70)**, which dates from 1950, is the first example of a non-chlorinated DDT isostere having measurable insecticidal activity.

The methyl- and methoxy-groups in these compounds are, of course, vulnerable to biological oxidation, which produces the corresponding aromatic

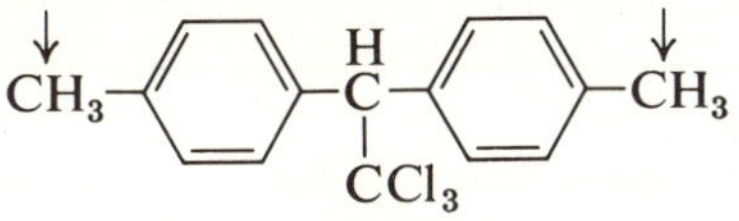

CH_3—⟨ring⟩—$\overset{\displaystyle H}{\underset{\displaystyle CCl_3}{C}}$—⟨ring⟩—$CH_3$

methylchlor; *0·14*
(69)

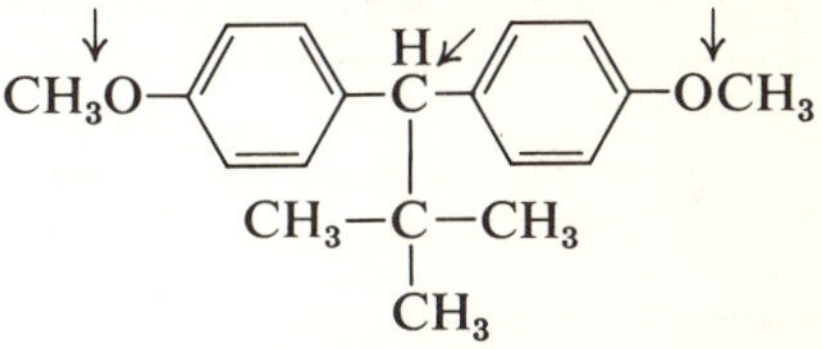

CH_3O—⟨ring⟩—$\overset{\displaystyle H}{C}$—⟨ring⟩—$OCH_3$; CH_3—$\overset{\displaystyle}{\underset{\displaystyle CH_3}{C}}$—$CH_3$

DANP *0·08*
(70)

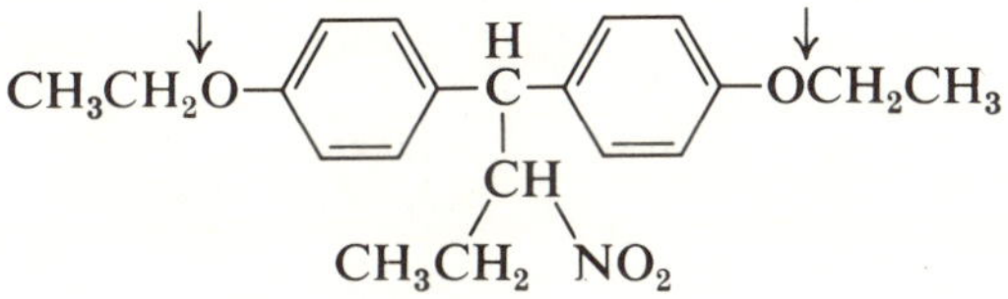

CH_3CH_2O—⟨ring⟩—$\overset{\displaystyle H}{\underset{\displaystyle \overset{CH}{CH_3CH_2\ \ NO_2}}{C}}$—⟨ring⟩—$OCH_2CH_3$

0·5
(71)

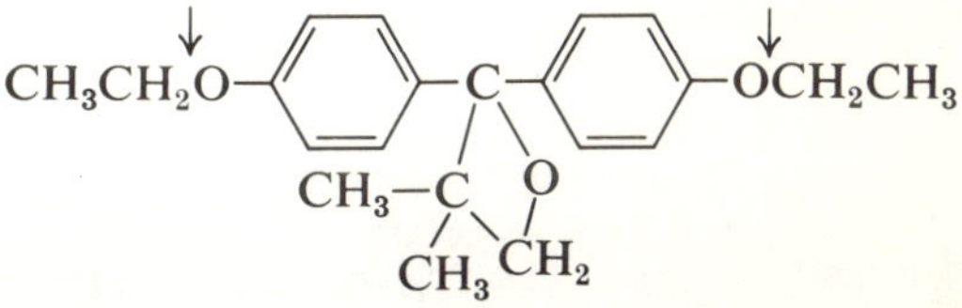

CH_3CH_2O—⟨ring⟩—$\overset{\displaystyle}{\underset{\displaystyle CH_3-\overset{}{\underset{CH_3}{C}}\ \overset{O}{CH_2}}{C}}$—⟨ring⟩—$OCH_2CH_3$

0·5
(72)

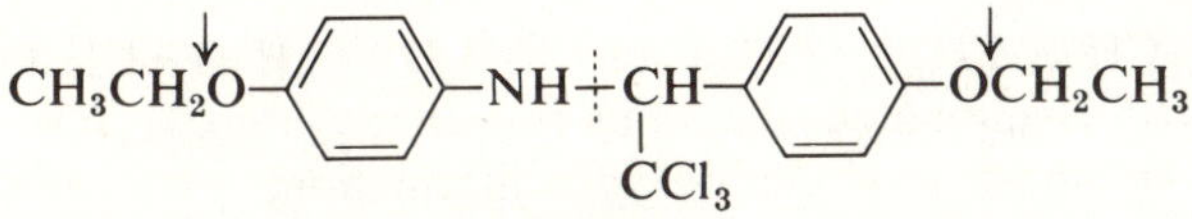

CH_3CH_2O—⟨ring⟩—NH—$\overset{\displaystyle}{\underset{\displaystyle CCl_3}{CH}}$—⟨ring⟩—$OCH_2CH_3$

0·77
(73)

Cl—⟨ring⟩—$O\overset{\displaystyle}{\underset{\displaystyle CCl_3}{CH}}$—⟨ring⟩—$OCH_2CH_3$

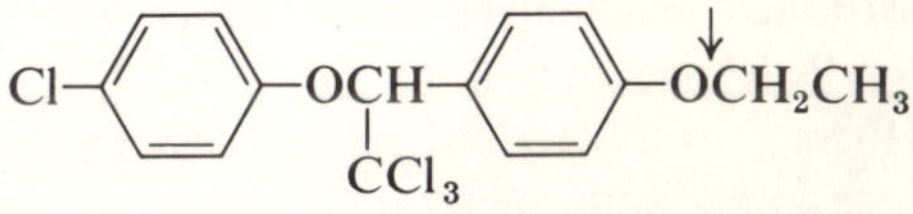

0·64
(74)

carboxylic acids and phenols, respectively. Also, electron-withdrawing *p*-substituents on the aromatic rings enhance enzymic dehydrochlorination, whereas *p*-alkyl- or alkoxy-groups suppress it, and these biodegradable analogues tend to be as toxic to resistant insects that have this mechanism as they are to susceptible ones. In recent years, the renewed interest in analogues of this type as possible replacements for DDT has led to various new structures (Holan, 1971a, b; Metcalf *et al*, 1971; Hirwe *et al*, 1972; Metcalf, 1976). As anticipated, some of these compounds are subject to MFO attack and are therefore synergized by inhibitors of the 1,3-benzodioxole type, use of which therefore provides some indication of their intrinsic toxicity (Table 6). The data of Table 6 also indicate synergism in mice in some cases, but the effect is so much greater in houseflies that the MSR (mouse/housefly) is actually improved when the synergized mixture is used.

Experience with DDT analogues in which the p-Cl atoms of DDT are replaced by other groups indicates an approximate order of biodegradability in

Table 6 Selective toxicity of biodegradable DDT analogues (data of Holan, 1971a, b)

| | Housefly LD$_{50}$ (μg/fly) | | Mouse LD$_{50}$ | |
Compound	Alone	Synergist*	(mg/kg)	MSR†
DDT	0·24	0·25	570	47
1-(p-Ethylthiophenyl)-1-(p-ethoxyphenyl)-2-nitropropane	0·16	0·015	1,040 (360)	130 (480)
1-(3,4-Methylenedioxy-phenyl)-1-(p-ethoxy-phenyl)-2-nitropropane	0·14	0·019	>2,000 (>2,000)	286 (>2,000)
1,1-*bis*(p-Ethoxyphenyl)-2-nitrobutane	0·55	0·061	1,160 (980)	42 (326)
2,2-*bis*(p-Ethoxyphenyl)-3,3-dimethyloxetane	0·52	0·01	1,200 (380)	46 (760)

* Synergist $= +5$ μg sesamex/fly.

† MSR is mouse LD$_{50}$ (i.p.)/housefly LD$_{50}$ (topical in acetone) in mg/kg; figures in parentheses are MSR derived from synergized LD$_{50}$s.

‡ Plus synergist at 1 : 1 or 2 : 1 ratio with insecticide.

houseflies to be $Cl < H < CH_3 < CH_3O < CH_3S$ and $C_2H_5O < C_3H_7O < CH_3O < iso\text{-}C_3H_7O < CH_3S$; CH_3S is anomalous due to its conversion into CH_3SO— and CH_3SO_2—, which enhances enzymic dehydrochlorination, when this resistance mechanism exists. Thus, the p,p'-diethoxy-analogue of DDT has slightly less acute oral toxicity than DDT to mice and is a good housefly toxicant (Hirwe *et al*, 1972). Differences between insect species are evident, since many of these compounds are strongly synergized in the housefly but scarcely synergized in the blowfly (*Phormia regina*). In contrast to the housefly, this blowfly has a generally low titre of MFO activity and so the toxicities measured without synergist give a reasonable measure of intrinsic toxicity in this insect.

Besides the possibility of O-alkyl cleavage in the nitropropane analogue (**71**), the nitro-group may be eliminated, with eventual loss of the alkyl chain leading to derivatives of benzophenone (Metcalf, 1976). The analogue (**72**) in which a —CCl_3 group has been replaced by 2,2-dimethyloxetane (Holan, 1971a, b) shows good housefly toxicity, especially when synergized (Table 6) and readily loses formaldehyde under environmental conditions to give the innocuous 2,2-dimethylethylene derivative, a conversion which can be inhibited by suitable formulation. Compounds with an additional nitrogen or oxygen atom in the molecule retain DDT-like insecticidal activity (Hirwe *et al*, 1972); (**73**) suffers oxidation of its p,p'-substituents but may also be dehydrochlorinated, followed by rearrangement and cleavage to p-ethoxyaniline and p-ethoxydichloroaceto-phenone, which are significant metabolites in housefly and salt marsh caterpillar (*Estigmene acrea*). Since these two fragments should be readily degradable by microorganisms, molecules of this type have an obvious advantage from an environmental standpoint. In contrast, ethers such as (**74**) are more stable and suffer only oxidative O-dealkylation.

Several of the compounds discussed above no longer contain chlorine and therefore can no longer be classed as chlorinated insecticides, although their biological action is similar to that of DDT. It must be recognized that although some of them are quite active against diptera, their increased biodegradability, as compared with DDT, carries with it the economic disadvantage of a narrower spectrum of insecticidal activity.

Lindane (γ-HCH; **2**) combines excellent insecticidal properties with inter-mediate acute- and low chronic toxicity to mammals, and moderate environ-mental persistence (Ulmann, 1973). Because insecticidal activity resides specifically in the γ-isomer, it is difficult to devise structural modifications that retain activity. There is a long-recognized similarity between lindane and the cyclodiene group in molecular structure and mode of action, a resemblance which is emphasized by the cross-resistance to both that follows insect selection with one or the other. In principle, isosteric replacement of some of the chlorine atoms by other biodegradable groups should be possible in both lindane and

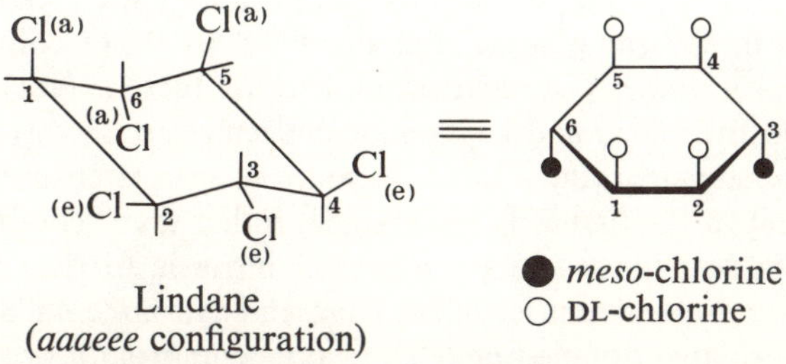

$$\text{lindane} > 3\text{-}SCH_3 > 3\text{-}OCH_3 > 1\text{-}CH_3 > 1\text{-}OCH_3 > 1\text{-}H > 1\text{-}OCH_2CH_3 > 1,4\text{-di-}CH_3 > \text{hexa-}OCH_3$$

Figure 3 Order of mosquito toxicity in lindane analogues having one or more chlorines replaced by biodegradable groups at the indicated positions (Nakajima, 1976)

the cyclodiene insecticides (Brooks, 1973a), and Nakajima (1976) has described various analogues of lindane in which the γ-configuration is retained and one or more chlorine atoms are replaced by CH_3, CH_3O, or CH_3S. As described previously (see glutathione conjugations), lindane is biodegradable in insects and mammals. However, some of the chlorinated benzenes and phenols produced may themselves be undesirable environmental contaminants. There-fore, replacement of chlorine by biodegradable groups should increase both the degradability of lindane itself in higher organisms and, hopefully, the degradability of its metabolic residues in the environment.

In general, analogues in which one of the *meso*-chlorines at C-3 or C-6 is replaced by a biodegradable group are more toxic than those in which a *dl*-chlorine is replaced and indeed some of the *meso*-analogues approach lindane in toxicity to mosquitoes. The housefly toxicities of these analogues are rather variable but more uniform toxicities are obtained by cotreatment with piperonyl butoxide (PB); factors of synergism up to 120-fold (for the 3-CH_3S-analogue), as well as metabolite identification, confirm that the instability is due to attack by MFO. For this insect the order of biodegradability (Nakajima, 1976) appears to be $1,2$-$H,OCH_3 \doteqdot 1$-$H \doteqdot$ lindane < 1-$OC_2H_5 < 1,4$-di-$CH_3 \doteqdot 1$-$OCH_3 \doteqdot 1$-$CH_3 < 3$-$OCH_3 < 3$-SCH_3.

On the other hand, the variations in toxicity to mosquitoes (*Culex pipiens pallens*) and German cockroaches appear to be due to more fundamental causes; the synergistic ratios with PB are low and uniform, except that the 3-CH_3S-analogue is again strongly synergized (120-fold) against the cockroach. The low insect toxicity of the hexamethoxy-analogue and lack of significant synergism by PB suggest that this compound lacks intrinsic toxicity. However, this conclusion requires the confirmatory evidence that the compound is extensively metabolized and that PB actually suppresses its metabolism *in vivo*, but such confirmation has not been reported. This lipophilic derivative of mucoinositol (*aaaeee* configuration), an approximate isostere of lindane, is of some interest in relation to the early theory that lindane is an antagonist of inositol *in vivo*.

The conversion of aldrin (**14**) and heptachlor (**16**) to their stable and toxic epoxides occurs in the majority of living organisms and these epoxidations are excellent examples of microsomal oxidations that produce toxic products. They are not activations in the same sense that the $P{=}S$ to $P{=}O$ conversion of insecticidal phosphorothioates is an activation, because there is much evidence (Brooks, 1973a) that the aldrin and heptachlor molecules are themselves toxic. However, the conversion to rather stable epoxides in insects ensures that the total level of toxicant in the tissues is maintained, rather than reduced. Nevertheless, the epoxides do appear to have a greater intrinsic toxicity than their precursors, which are preferable insecticides from an environmental standpoint because their unchlorinated double bonds allow opportunities for chemical and biological reactions that lead to detoxication, as well as epoxidation.

Cyclodiene insecticides can be made increasingly vulnerable to detoxication, although such changes usually result in loss of their broad-spectrum insecticidal activity. A remarkable exception is the change in stereochemistry between dieldrin (**15**) and its stereoisomer endrin. This change (to endrin) results in slightly reduced toxicity in some insects (e.g. houseflies) but insecticidal efficiency is largely retained. The change also makes endrin much more vulnerable to MFO attack in mammals and the molecule is considerably less persistent in the tissues than dieldrin (Bedford and Hutson, 1976). Unfortunately, endrin is more toxic to mammals, despite this reduced persistence.

A simple way to exchange detoxicative for toxicative metabolism is to reduce the double bond in heptachlor (**16**) or aldrin (**14**). The products, α-dihydroheptachlor (**75**) and dihydroaldrin (**77**) are less toxic to insects and mammals because they are hydroxylated rather than epoxidized (Brooks and Harrison,

1967b, 1969). Of the three known dihydroheptachlor isomers, the β-isomer (**76**) combines significant toxicity to houseflies, mosquito larvae, cabbage butterfly larvae (*Pieris brassicae*), and bedbugs (*Cimex lectularius*) with remarkably low toxicity (2,000–9,000 mg/kg) to mice, rats, dogs, and hens (Büchel *et al*, 1964). Microsomal preparations from houseflies and from pig liver hydroxylate the dihydroheptachlor isomers (chlorohydrin formation) and replace the isolated chlorine atom by hydroxyl (apparently via the α-chlorohydrin and the ketone; see p. 179) with further hydroxylation to give diols. Sesamex suppresses these hydroxylations, and the associated 10-fold increase in housefly toxicity makes the combination as insecticidal as heptachlor epoxide (Brooks and Harrison, 1967b).

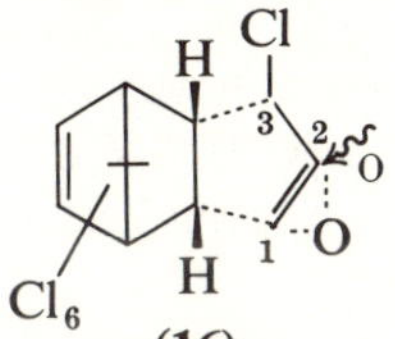

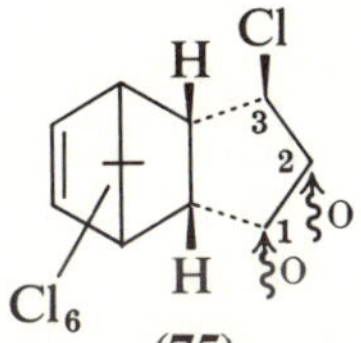

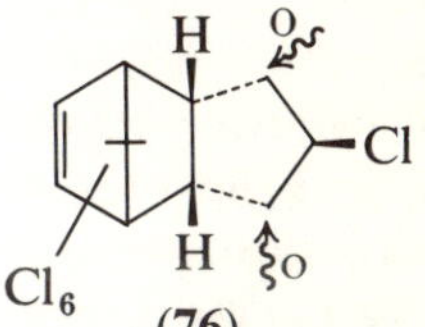

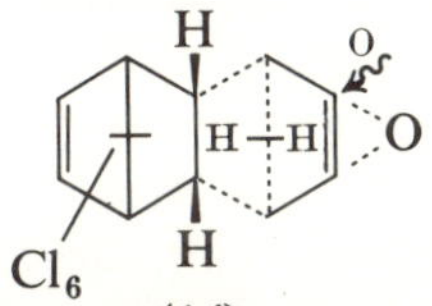

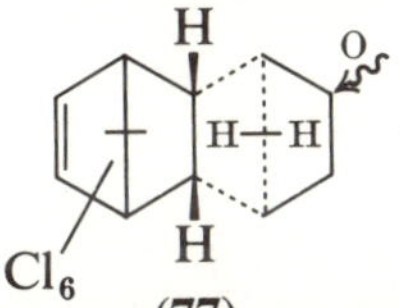

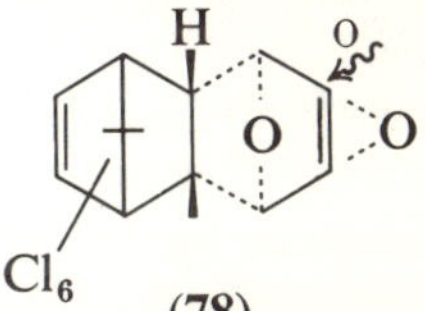

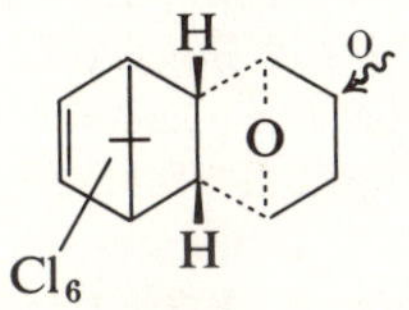

Oxa-aldrin (**78**) is epoxidized *in vivo*, but hydroxylated instead if the double bond is reduced, as in oxadihydroaldrin (ODA; **79**). The housefly toxicities of dihydro-compounds (**77**) and (**79**) are increased 10-fold and 20-fold, respectively by sesamex. ODA is particularly interesting because it combines the apparently stable 1,4-oxide system and a polarity similar to that of dieldrin with the susceptibility to detoxicative hydroxylation shown by dihydroaldrin (**77**). In contrast, isomers of ODA having a 1,2-epoxide ring are vulnerable to both cyclohexane ring hydroxylation and attack by epoxide hydrase; HCE (**80**) and HEOM (**81**) show interesting interspecies differences in biodegradability that arise from variations in the balance between attack by MFO and epoxide hydrase.

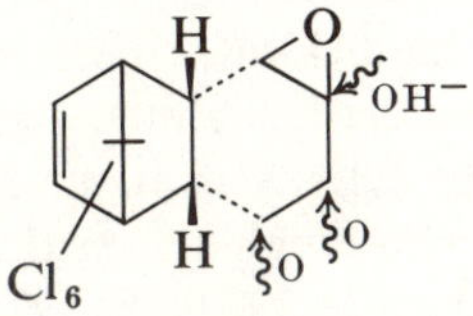

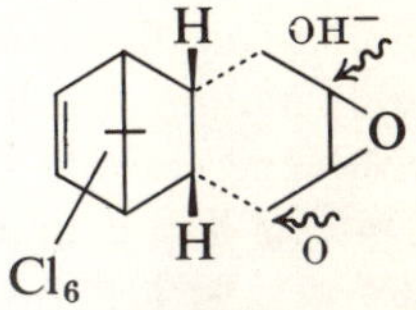

The epoxide ring in HCE (**80**) is stable in many insects but cyclohexane ring hydroxylation occurs to an extent that is species dependent. Vertebrates, generally speaking, hydroxylate the ring and also show species-dependent levels of epoxide hydrase activity, so that both oxidative and hydrolytic routes of detoxication are available to them (Brooks *et al*, 1970; Brooks, 1972; El Zorgani *et al*, 1970; Walker and El Zorgani, 1973; Walker *et al*, 1973). The capacity for enzymic hydration is in the order fish < birds < mammals, although the rat and the rook (*Corvus frugilegus*) are exceptional in having lower and higher hydrase activity, respectively, than is typical of their classes.

The symmetrical epoxide HEOM (**81**) is readily hydrated by mammals (less readily by birds and fish) and, unlike HCE (**80**), by several insects (see section on hydrolytic metabolism). This hydration is a detoxication, as indicated by the lack of toxicity of HEOM to houseflies or blowflies, which hydrate it readily, and a toxicity approaching that of DDT against tsetse flies, which have poor hydrative ability. HEOM is measurably toxic to the stable fly (*Stomoxys calcitrans*), which is also deficient in epoxide hydrase, and these specialized insects provide rather extreme examples of selectivity (Table 7). HCE (**80**), which is hydroxylated but not hydrated by houseflies, approaches dieldrin in toxicity when synergized by sesamex (50-fold synergism). Tsetse flies and stable flies appear to be deficient in microsomal oxidases, and, as anticipated, both HCE and ODA (**79**) are quite toxic to them in the absence of any synergist (Table 7).

The metabolism of HCE has been extensively studied in vertebrates, which metabolize it mainly by cyclohexane ring hydroxylation, but the *trans*-diol is also excreted by rat, rabbit, and quail (Walker and El Zorgani, 1974). The half-lives of elimination of HCE following intraperitoneal injection (10–30 mg/kg) are 5, 2, 4, and 8 days, respectively, for rat, rabbit, quail, and pigeon, and these values compare favourably with dieldrin, especially for the birds. Since HEOM is readily hydrated, it has been used as a model substrate for the measurement of cyclodiene epoxide hydrase activity in tissue and microsomal preparations from insects and mammals, with emphasis on the search for inhibitors which might synergize it in insects (Brooks 1973a, b, 1974a; Slade *et al*, 1975; Craven *et al*, 1976). The best inhibitors are themselves epoxides and the inhibition is mainly competitive, as with mammalian aromatic epoxide hydrase (Oesch *et al*, 1971). Therefore, it is not surprising that only transient synergistic effects have been obtained so far. Added interest in inhibitors arises from the observation (Brooks, 1973b) that the cecropia juvenile hormone (see non-oxidative detoxication, p. 178) competitively inhibits the cyclodiene epoxide hydrase in pupal homogenates of blowfly (*Calliphora erythrocephala*) and yellow mealworm (*Tenebrio molitor*). Although a specific inhibitor for the juvenile hormone epoxide hydrase might be expected to resemble it structurally, there is some hope that really powerful inhibitors of the cyclodiene epoxide hydrase might also inhibit the enzyme and act as synergists for exogenous juvenile hormone or its analogues in cases where epoxide hydration is a significant deactivation mechanism.

It is now clear that the unchlorinated ring systems of even rather stable molecules such as dieldrin can be attacked by detoxifying enzymes and that biodegradability may be enhanced by structural modification. The further

Table 7 Toxicities of some chlorinated insecticides to various insects

Compound or mixture‖	LD$_{50}$(µg/insect)*,†				
	Housefly (*Musca domestica*)	Blowfly (*Calliphora erythrocephala*)	Mosquito (*Anopheles stephensi*)	Tsetse fly (*Glossina austeni*)	Stable fly (*Stomoxys calcitrans*)
HCE‡	2·0	12·0	0·055	0·042	0·14
HCE : sesamex	0·04	1·7	0·013	0·024	0·07
HEOM	>10	>20	0·12	0·16	0·67
HEOM : sesamex	>10	>20	0·05	0·10	0·45
ODA	0·60	1·82	0·03	0·01	0·03
ODA : sesamex	0·03	0·07	0·01	NT§	0·02
Dieldrin	0·02	0·02	0·004	0·01	0·03
Dieldrin + sesamex	0·02	0·02	0·004	NT	0·03
DDT	0·24	NT	0·025	0·09	0·12

* 5 µg sesamex preapplied with housefly and blowfly; simultaneous application at 5 : 1 ratio (synergist : toxicant) for other insects (Brooks and Harrison, 1964a; Brooks, 1975; Barlow and Hadaway, unpublished results).
† Mixed sexes for tsetse fly; other insects female.
‡ Mouse oral LD$_{50}$, 200–400 mg/kg; rat oral LD$_{50}$ > 400 mg/kg.
§ NT =not tested.
‖ Structures on p. 203.

possibility that certain chlorine atoms in the hexachloronorbornene nucleus might be replaced by more biodegradable groups, as in the case of lindane, has not been systematically examined. Replacement of vinylic chlorine atoms in dieldrin results in a 5-fold increase in insect toxicity, despite the fact that such replacement is expected to increase the chance of enzymic attack. Therefore, the possibility is currently being explored (Brooks, 1975) that analogous chlorine atoms in the more biodegradable molecules previously discussed might be replaced by hydrogen without much loss in insect toxicity.

INSECT METABOLISM AND ENVIRONMENTAL PROBLEMS

In recent years, attempts have been made to examine the insect metabolism of insecticides as part of the environmental complex as a whole. This is a most difficult task but a method of predicting the environmental biodegradability of putative commercial insecticides, especially in relation to their transport in food webs, would obviously be of great value. In pursuit of this aim, Metcalf (Lu *et al*, 1975; Metcalf, 1976) has developed 'model ecosystems' in which to study the metabolism and transport of insecticides. Thus, in a model aquatic ecosystem, radiolabelled insecticide is added at about 0·1 ppm to water containing plankton, daphnia (*Daphnia magna*), mosquito larvae, fish (*Gambusia affinis*), algae, and snails. After a predetermined period the balance of radiolabel is measured for water and samples of organic material and the identities of metabolites etc. are determined as far as possible. This gives a measure of accumulation of the unchanged insecticide and its metabolites in the various elements of the model aquatic food chain.

Another type of model ecosystem incorporates a terrestial portion (sand) on which *Sorghum vulgare* is grown, in addition to an aquatic portion containing the organisms previously mentioned. The plants, previously treated with radiolabelled insecticide in a simulated agricultural application, are then infested with larvae of the salt marsh caterpillar (*Estigmene acrea*), so that radiolabelled insecticide and its conversion products enter the terrestrial portion as faecal products, leaf debris, etc. Radiolabelled products eventually enter the aquatic portion and become distributed through the food web as before, and after several weeks a careful balance is made of the radiolabel in the various elements of the system. Since the amount of polar metabolites within an organism is usually a measure of its ability to degrade the insecticide, the ratio of polar/nonpolar products is called the biodegradability index of the insecticide for that organism. For *Gambusia*, for example, this value is 60-fold greater for methoxychlor (*p,p'*-chlorines of DDT replaced by methoxyl) than for DDT. Further, the 'ecological magnification' (concentration of parent compound in organism/concentration in water) for *Gambusia* is 84,500 for DDT and 1,545 for methoxychlor. These values indicate the much greater biodegradability of methoxychlor, which is replacing DDT for the control of blackfly (*Simulium* sp.; vectors of river blindness) in various parts of the world. It seems likely that increasingly elaborate developments of this technique will be used to forecast the environmental behaviour of insecticides and other xenobiotics.

Another example of the value of insects in environmental studies is provided by the use of *Drosophila melanogaster* in tests for the mutagenic effects of xenobiotics. Much is known about the formal genetics of this insect and the history of its resistance to insecticides, particularly organochlorines, has been recorded by Brown and Pal (1971). The benzylic hydroxylation of DDT was first observed in *D. melanogaster* (Tsukamoto, 1959, 1960), and the widespread existence of microsomal oxidase and other metabolizing activities among insects supports the view that *Drosophila* will be capable of effecting other enzymic transformations of xenobiotics. In view of the difficulties with the housefly, discussed previously, it is not surprising that metabolism in the smaller insect has not been widely studied. However, indirect evidence for the metabolic capacity of *Drosophila* is provided by the observation that numerous indirect mutagens and carcinogens that are ineffective unless activated by hepatic microsomes give positive responses for the induction of sex-linked recessive lethals in *Drosophila* but negative responses in microbial test systems (Sobels and Vogel, 1976; Vogel and Sobels, 1976). The presence of a well-developed endoplasmic reticulum in *Drosophila* spermatids and spermatocytes suggests, as is found, that these stages of sperm development should be most sensitive to the effects of mutagens that require enzymic activation.

Thus, present indications are that the *Drosophila* test can detect the formation of even short-lived mutagenic metabolic products, since these may actually be formed within the cells most sensitive to their effects. Such effects may well be missed in other tests that require the transport of labile proximate mutagens from the site of activation to the site of action.

REFERENCES

Abernathy, C. O. and Casida, J. E. (1973), *Science*, **179**, 1235.

Agosin, M. (1976), *Mol. Cell Biochem.*, **12**, 33.

Agosin, M., Michaeli, D., Miskus, R., Nagasawa, S. and Hoskins, W. M. (1961), *J. Econ. Entomol.*, **54**, 340.

Agosin, M., Scaramelli, N., Gil, L. and Letelier, M. E. (1969), *Comp. Biochem. Physiol.*, **29**, 785.

Ajami, A. M. (1975), *J. Insect Physiol.*, **21**, 1017.

Arias, I. M. and Jakoby, W. B. (eds), (1976), *Glutathione: metabolism and function*, Raven, New York.

Arias, R. O. and Terriere, L. C. (1962), *J. Econ. Entomol.*, **55**, 925.

Arthur, B. W. and Casida, J. E. (1958), *J. Agr. Food Chem.*, **6**, 360.

Arthur, B. W. and Casida, J. E. (1959), *J. Econ. Entomol.*, **52**, 20.

Asperen, K. van and Oppenoorth, F. J. (1959), *Entomol. Exp. Appl.*, **2**, 48.

Balabaskaran, S. and Smith, J. N. (1970), *Biochem. J.*, **117**, 989.

Barker, R. J. (1960), *J. Econ. Entomol.*, **53**, 35.

Barnes, J. M. and Verschoyle, R. D. (1974), *Nature*, **248**, 711.

Bedford, C. T. (1975), in Hathway, D. E. (ed.), *Foreign compound metabolism in mammals*, vol. 3, p. 405, Chemical Society, London.

208

Bedford, C. T. and Hutson, D. H. (1976), *Chem. Ind. (London)*, **440**.
Benke, G. M. and Wilkinson, C. F. (1971), *Pestic. Biochem. Physiol.*, **1**, 19.
Beroza, M. and Barthel, W. F. (1957), *J. Agr. Food Chem.*, **5**, 855.
Binning, A., Darby, F. J., Heenan, M. P. and Smith, J. N. (1967), *Biochem. J.*, **103**, 42.
Boose, R. B. and Terriere, L. C. (1967), *J. Econ. Entomol.*, **60**, 580.
Bowman, M. C., Acree, F., Lofgren, C. S. and Beroza, M. (1964), *Science*, **146**, 1480.
Bradbury, F. R. (1957), *J. Sci. Food Agr.*, **8**, 90.
Bradbury, F. R. and Standen, H. (1956), *J. Sci. Food Agr.*, **7**, 389.
Bradbury, F. R. and Standen, H. (1959), *Nature*, **183**, 983.
Brattsten, L. B. and Metcalf, R. L. (1970), *J. Econ. Entomol.*, **63**, 102.
Brattsten, L. B. and Wilkinson, C. F. (1973a), *Comp. Biochem. Physiol.*, **45B**, 59.
Brattsten, L. B. and Wilkinson, C. F. (1973b), *Pestic. Biochem. Physiol.*, **3**, 393.
Brooks, G. T. (1960), *Nature*, **186**, 96.
Brooks, G. T. (1966), *World Rev. Pest Control*, **5**, 62.
Brooks, G. T. (1968), *Mededel. Landbouwhogeschool. Opzoekingsta. Staat Gent*, **33**, 629.
Brooks, G. T. (1972), in Coulston, F. and Korte, F. (eds), *Environmental quality and safety*, vol. 1, p. 106, Thieme, Stuttgart; Academic, New York, London.
Brooks, G. T. (1973a), in Ariens, E. J. (ed.), *Drug design*, vol. IV, p. 379, Academic, New York.
Brooks, G. T. (1973b), *Nature*, **245**, 382.
Brooks, G. T. (1974a), *Pestic. Sci.*, **5**, 177.
Brooks, G. T. (1974b), *Chlorinated insecticides*, vols I and II, CRC, Cleveland.
Brooks, G. T. (1975), *Proc. 8th Brit. Insectic. Fungic. Conference*, **2**, 381.
Brooks, G. T. (1976a), in Metcalf, R. L. and McKelvey, J. J. (eds), *The future for insecticides: needs and prospects*, p. 97, Wiley, New York.
Brooks, G. T. (1976b), in Wilkinson, C. F. (ed.), *Insecticide biochemistry and physiology*, Plenum, New York.
Brooks, G. T. (1977), *Gen. Pharmacol.*, **8**, 221.
Brooks, G. T. and Harrison, A. (1963), *Nature*, **198**, 1169.
Brooks, G. T. and Harrison, A. (1964a), *Biochem. Pharmacol.*, **13**, 827.
Brooks, G. T. and Harrison, A. (1964b), *J. Insect Physiol.*, **10**, 633.
Brooks, G. T. and Harrison, A. (1966), *Life Sci.*, **5**, 2315.
Brooks, G. T. and Harrison, A. (1967a), *Life Sci.*, **6**, 681.
Brooks, G. T. and Harrison, A. (1967b), *Life Sci.*, **6**, 1439.
Brooks, G. T. and Harrison, A. (1969), *Biochem. Pharmacol.*, **18**, 557.
Brooks, G. T., Harrison, A. and Cox, J. T. (1963), *Nature*, **197**, 311.
Brooks, G. T., Harrison, A. and Lewis, S. E. (1970), *Biochem. Pharmacol.*, **19**, 255.
Brooks, G. T., Lewis, S. E. and Harrison, A. (1968), *Nature*, **220**, 1034.
Brown, A. W. A. (1969), in *Farm Chemicals*, issues of September, October, November, 1969, and February, 1970.
Brown, A. W. A. and Pal, R. (1971), *Insecticide resistance in arthropods*, WHO Monograph Series, No. 38, WHO, Geneva.
Brown, R. R., Miller, J. A. and Miller, E. C. (1954), *J. Biol. Chem.*, **209**, 211.
Büchel, K. H., Ginsberg, A. E., Fischer, R. and Korte, F. (1964), *Tetrahedron Lett.*, **33**, 2267.
Camp, H. B., Fukuto, T. R. and Metcalf, R. L. (1969), *J. Agr. Food Chem.*, **17**, 243.
Capdevila, J., Ahmad, N. and Agosin, M. (1975), *J. Biol. Chem.*, **250**, 1048.
Capdevila, J., Morello, A., Perry, A. S. and Agosin, M. (1973), *Biochemistry*, **12**, 1445.
Capdevila, J., Perry, A. S. and Agosin, M. (1974), *Chem.-Biol. Inter.*, **9**, 105.
Casida, J. E. (1970), *J. Agr. Food Chem.*, **18**, 753.
Casida, J. E. (ed.) (1973), *Pyrethrum, the natural insecticide*, Academic, New York.
Casida, J. E. and Augustinsson, K. B. (1959), *Biochem. Biophys. Acta*, **36**, 411.

Casida, J. E., Augustinsson, K. B. and Jonsson, G. (1960), *J. Econ. Entomol.*, **53**, 205.

Casida, J. E., Engel, J. L., Esaac, E. G., Kamienski, F. X. and Kuwatsuka, S. (1966a), *Science*, **153**, 1130.

Casida, J. E., Fukami, J. and Yamamoto, I., (1966b), *Bull. Entomol. Soc. Amer.*, **12**, 293.

Chadwick, R. W., Chuang, L. T. and Williams, K. (1975), *Pestic. Biochem. Physiol.*, **5**, 575.

Chakraborty, J. and Smith, J. N. (1964), *Biochem. J.*, **93**, 389.

Chakraborty, J. and Smith, J. N. (1967), *Biochem. J.*, **102**, 498.

Chamberlain, R. W. (1950), *Amer. J. Hyg.*, **52**, 153.

Clark, A. G., Hitchcock, M. and Smith, J. N. (1966), *Nature*, **209**, 103.

Clark, A. G., Murphy, S. and Smith, J. N. (1969), *Biochem. J.*, **113**, 89.

Cohen, A. J. and Smith, J. N. (1961), *Nature*, **189**, 600.

Cohen, A. J. and Smith, J. N. (1964), *Biochem. J.*, **90**, 449.

Cohen, A. J., Smith, J. N. and Turbert, H. (1964), *Biochem. J.*, **90**, 457.

Corbett, J. R. (1974), *The biochemical mode of action of pesticides*, Academic, New York.

Craven, A. C. C., Brooks, G. T. and Walker, C. H. (1976), *Pestic. Biochem. Physiol.*, **6**, 132.

Dachauer, A. C., Cocheo, B., Solomon, M. G. and Hennessey, D. J. (1963), *J. Agr. Food Chem.*, **11**, 47.

Dauterman, W. C. (1976), in Wilkinson, C. F. (ed.), *Insect biochemistry and physiology*, ch. 4, Plenum, New York.

Davison, A. N. (1954), *Nature*, **174**, 1056.

Dinamarca, M. L., Levenbook, K. and Valdés, E. (1971), *Arch. Biochem. Biophys.*, **147**, 374.

Dinamarca, M. L., Ramirez, A., Ballester, E., Del Villar, E., Capdevila, J. and Maccioni, R. (1975a), *Int. J. Biochem.*, **6**, 405.

Dinamarca, M. L., Ramirez, A., Valdés, E. and Poblete, P. (1957b), *Int. J. Biochem.*, **6**, 413.

Dorough, H. W. and Casida, J. E. (1964), *J. Agr. Food Chem.*, **12**, 244.

Douch, P. G. C., Smith, J. N. and Turner, J. C. (1971), *Life Sci.*, **10** (II), 1327.

Dutton, G. J. and Ko, V. (1964), *Comp. Biochem. Physiol.*, **11**, 269.

El Bashir, S. and Oppenoorth, F. J. (1969), *Nature*, **223**, 210.

Eldefrawi, M. E. and Hoskins, W. M. (1961), *J. Econ. Entomol.*, **54**, 401.

Elliott, M. (1976), in Metcalf, R. L. and McKelvey, J. J. (ed.), *The future for insecticides: needs and prospects*, Wiley, New York.

Elliott, M., Farnham, A. W., Janes, N. F., Needham, P. and Pulman, D. A. (1974), *Nature*, **248**, 710.

El-Shourbagy, N. and Dorough, H. W. (1974), *J. Econ. Entomol.*, **67**, 344.

El Zorgani, G. A., Walker, C. H. and Hassall, K. A. (1970), *Life Sci.*, **9** (II), 415.

Esaac, E. G. and Casida, J. E. (1969), *J. Agr. Food Chem.*, **17**, 539.

Eto, M. (1974), *Organophosphorus pesticides: organic and biological chemistry*, CRC, Cleveland.

Fahmy, M. A. and Gordon, H. T. (1965), *J. Econ. Entomol.*, **58**, 451.

Fenwick, M. L. (1958), *Biochem. J.*, **70**, 373.

Fenwick, M. L., Barron, J. R. and Watson, W. A. (1957), *Biochem. J.*, **65**, 58.

Fernando, H. E., Roan, C. C. and Kearns, C. W. (1951), *Ann. Ent. Soc. Amer.*, **44**, 551.

Folsom, M. D., Philpot, R. M. and Hodgson, E. (1971), *Comp. Biochem. Physiol.*, **39B**, 589.

Franklin, M. R. (1971), *Xenobiotica*, **1**, 581.

Fraser, J., Harrison, I. R. and Wakerley, S. B. (1968), *J. Sci. Food Agr. Suppl.*, p. 8.

Fukami, J. and Shishido, T. (1963), *Botyu-Kagaku*, **28**, 77.

Fukami, J. and Shishido, T. (1966), *J. Econ. Entomol.*, **59**, 1338.

Fukuto, T. R. (1972), *Drug Metab. Rev.*, **1**, 117.

Fukuto, T. R. (1976), in Metcalf, R. L. and McKelvey, J. J. (eds), *The future for insecticides: needs and prospects*, Wiley, New York.

Georghiou, G. P. and Metcalf, R. L. (1961), *J. Econ. Entomol.*, **54**, 231.

Georghiou, G. P., Metcalf, R. L. and March, R. B. (1961), *J. Econ. Entomol.*, **54**, 132.

Gessner, T. and Smith, J. N. (1960), *Biochem. J.*, **75**, 165.

Giannotti, O., Metcalf, R. L. and March, R. B. (1956), *Ann. Entomol. Soc. Amer.*, **49**, 588.

Gil, D. L., Rose, H. A., Yang, R. S. H., Young, R. G. and Wilkinson, C. F. (1974), *Comp. Biochem. Physiol.*, **47B**, 657.

Goodchild, B. and Smith, J. N. (1970), *Biochem. J.*, **117**, 1005.

Guthrie, F. E., Ringler, R. L. and Bowery, T. G. (1957), *J. Econ. Entomol.*, **50**, 821.

Hadaway, A. B., Barlow, F. and Duncan, J. (1963), *Bull. Entomol. Res.*, **53**, 769.

Haller, H. L., La Forge, F. B. and Sullivan, W. N. (1942), *J. Org. Chem.*, **7**, 185.

Hansch, C. (1968), *J. Med. Chem.*, **11**, 920.

Hennessey, D. J. (1965), *J. Agr. Food Chem.*, **13**, 218.

Hennessey, D. J., Frantantoni, J., Hartigan, J., Moorefield, H. H. and Weiden, M. J. H. (1961), *Nature*, **190**, 341.

Hewlett, P. S., Lloyd, C. J. and Bates, A. N. (1961), *Nature*, **192**, 1273.

Hewlett, P. S. and Wilkinson, C. F. (1967), *J. Sci. Food Agr.*, **18**, 279.

Hill, R. L. and Teipel, J. W. (1971), in Boyer, P. D. (ed.), *The enzymes*, vol. V, p. 539, 3rd edn, Academic, New York.

Hirwe, A. S., Metcalf, R. L. and Kapoor, I. P. (1972), *J. Agr. Food Chem.*, **20**, 818.

Hodgson, E. (1974), in Khan, M. A. Q. (ed.), *Survival in toxic environments*, Academic, New York.

Hodgson, E. and Philpot, R. M. (1974), *Drug Metab. Rev.*, **3**, 231.

Hodgson, E. and Plapp, F. W. (1970), *J. Agr. Food Chem.*, **18**, 1048.

Hodgson, E. and Tate, L. G. (1976), in Wilkinson, C. F. (ed.), *Insecticide biochemistry and physiology*, Plenum, New York.

Hodgson, E., Tate, L. G., Kulkarni, A. and Plapp, F. W. (1974), *J. Agr. Food Chem.*, **22**, 361.

Holan, G. (1971a), *Nature*, **232**, 644.

Holan, G. (1971b), *Bull. W. H. O.*, **44**, 355.

Hook, G. E. R. and Smith, J. N. (1967), *Biochem. J.*, **102**, 504.

Hook, G. E. R., Jordan, T. W. and Smith, J. N. (1968), in E. Hodgson (ed.), *Enzymatic oxidation of toxicants*, p. 27, North Carolina State University, Raleigh.

Hopkins, T. L. and Robbins, W. E. (1957), *J. Econ. Entomol.*, **50**, 684.

Hutson, D. H. (1972), in Hathway, D. E. (ed.), *Foreign compound metabolism in mammals*, vol. 2, p. 328, Chemical Society, London.

Hutson, D. H. (1975), in Hathway, D. E. (ed.), *Foreign compound metabolism in mammals*, vol. 3, p. 449, Chemical Society, London.

Ilevicky, J., Dinamarca, M. L. and Agosin, M. (1964), *Comp. Biochem. Physiol.*, **11**, 291.

Ishaaya, I. and Chefurka, W. (1968), *Riv. Parassit.*, **29**, 289.

Ishida, M. (1968), *Agr. Biol. Chem.*, *Tokyo*, **32**, 947.

Ishida, M. and Dahm, P. A. (1965a), *J. Econ. Entomol.*, **58**, 383.

Ishida, M. and Dahm, P. A. (1965b), *J. Econ. Entomol.*, **58**, 602.

Jacobson, M. and Crosby, D. J. (eds), (1971), *Naturally occurring insecticides*, Dekker, New York.

Jao, L. T. and Casida, J. E. (1974), *Pestic. Biochem. Physiol.*, **4**, 456.

Jordan, T. W. and Smith, J. N. (1970), *Int. J. Biochem.*, **1**, 139.

Jordan, T. W., McNaught, R. W. and Smith, J. N. (1970), *Biochem. J.*, **118**, 1.

Khan, M. A. Q., Sutherland, D. J., Rosen, J. D. and Carey, W. F. (1970), *J. Econ. Entomol.*, **63**, 470.

Kikal, T. and Smith, J. N. (1958), *Biochem. J.*, **69**, 52P.

Kikal, T. and Smith, J. N. (1959), *Biochem. J.*, **71**, 48.

Kok, G. C. and Walop (1954), *Biochem. Biophys. Acta.*, **13**, 510.

Korte, F. and Arent, H. (1965), *Life Sci.*, **4**, 2017.

Korte, F., Ludwig, G. and Vogel, J. (1962), *Ann. Chem.*, **656**, 135.

Krieger, R. I. and Wilkinson, C. F. (1969), *Biochem. Pharmacol.*, **18**, 1403.

Krieger, R. I. and Wilkinson, C. F. (1970), *Biochem. J.*, **124**, 427.

Krueger, H. R. and O'Brien, R. D. (1959), *J. Econ. Entomol.*, **52**, 1063.

Kreuger, H. R., O'Brien, R. D. and Dauterman, W. C. (1960), *J. Econ. Entomol.*, **53**, 25.

Kuhr, R. J. and Dorough, H. W. (1976), *Carbamate insecticides: chemistry, biochemistry and toxicology*, CRC, Cleveland.

Kulkarni, A. P. and Hodgson, E. (1975), *Insect Biochem.*, **5**, 679.

Kulkarni, A. P. and Hodgson, E. (1976), *Pestic. Biochem. Physiol.*, **6**, 183.

Kulkarni, A. P., Mailman, R. B., Baker, R. C. and Hodgson, E. (1974), *Drug Metab. Disp.*, **2**, 309.

Kumar, S. S. and Dorough, H. W. (1974), *Insect Biochem.*, **5**, 265.

Lee, A., Sanborn, J. R. and Metcalf, R. L. (1974), *Pestic Biochem. Physiol.*, **4**, 77.

Leeling, N. C. and Casida, J. E. (1966), *J. Agr. Food Chem.*, **14**, 281.

Lewis, J. B. (1969), *Nature*, **224**, 917.

Lewis, S. E. (1967), *Nature*, **215**, 1408.

Lewis, S. E., Wilkinson, C. F. and Ray, J. W. (1967), *Biochem. Pharmacol.*, **16**, 1195.

Lichtenstein, E. P. and Fuhremann, T. W. (1971), *Science*, **172**, 589.

Lipke, H. and Chalkley, J. (1962), *Biochem. J.*, **85**, 109.

Lipke, H. and Kearns, C. W. (1960), in Metcalf, R. L. (ed.), *Advances in pest control research*, **3**, 253, Wiley–Interscience, New York.

Lu, Po-Yung, Metcalf, R. L., Hirwe, A. S. and Williams, J. W. (1975), *J. Agr. Food Chem.*, **23**, 967.

Mailman, R. B., Kulkarni, A. P., Baker, R. C. and Hodgson, E. (1974), *Drug Metab. Disp.*, **2**, 301.

Marshall, R. S. and Wilkinson, C. F. (1973), *Pestic. Biochem. Physiol.*, **2**, 425.

Mason, H. S., Fowlks, W. L. and Peterson, E. (1955), *J. Amer. Chem. Soc.*, **77**, 2914.

Matsumura, F. (1975), *Toxicology of insecticides*, Plenum, New York.

Matthews, H. B. and Casida, J. E. (1970), *Life Sci.*, **9** (I), 989.

Matthews, H. B. and Matsumura, F. (1969), *J. Agr. Food Chem.*, **17**, 845.

Matthews, H. B. and McKinney (1974), *Drug Metab. Disp.*, **2**, 333.

Matthews, H. B., Škrinjaric-Špoljar, M. and Casida, J. E. (1970), *Life Sci.*, **9** (I), 1039.

Mehendale, H. M. and Dorough, H. W. (1971), *Pestic. Biochem. Physiol.*, **1**, 307.

Mengle, D. C. and Casida, J. E. (1960), *J. Agr. Food Chem.*, **8**, 431.

Menn, J. J. and Beroza, M. (eds), (1971), *Insect juvenile hormones: chemistry and action*, Academic, New York.

Metcalf, R. L. (1968), in Hodgson, E. (ed.), *Enzymatic oxidation of toxicants*, North Carolina State University, Raleigh.

Metcalf, R. L. (1976), in Metcalf, R. L. and McKelvey, J. J. (eds), *The future for insecticides: needs and prospects*, Wiley, New York.

Metcalf, R. L. and March, R. B. (1953), *Ann. Entomol. Soc. Amer.*, **46**, 63.

Metcalf, R. L. and McKelvey, J. (eds) (1976), *The future for insecticides: needs and prospects*, Wiley, New York.

Metcalf, R. A. and Metcalf, R. L. (1973), *Pestic. Biochem. Physiol.*, **3**, 149.

Metcalf, R. L., Fukuto, T. R. and Winton, M. Y. (1960), *J. Econ. Entomol.*, **53**, 828.

Metcalf, R. L., Kapoor, I. P. and Hirwe, A. W. (1971), *Bull. W.H.O.*, **44**, 363.

212

Metcalf, R. L., Maxon, M. and Fukuto, T. R. and March, R. B. (1956). *Ann. Entomol. Soc. Amer.*, **49**, 274.

Miyamoto, J., Nishida, T. and Ueda, K. (1971), *Pestic. Biochem. Physiol.*, **1**, 293.

Moore, B. P. and Hewlett, P. S. (1958), *J. Sci. Food Agr.*, **9**, 666.

Moorefield, H. H. (1958), *Contrib. Boyce Thompson Inst.*, **19**, 501.

Moorefield, H. H. (1960), *Misc. Publ. Entomol. Soc. Amer.*, **2**, 145.

Moorefield, H. H. and Kearns, C. W. (1955), *J. Econ. Entomol.*, **48**, 403.

Moorefield, H. H. and Tefft, E. (1959), *Contrib. Boyce Thompson Inst.*, **20**, 293.

Moorefield, H. H. and Weiden, M. J. H. (1964), *Contrib. Boyce Thompson Inst.*, **22**, 425.

Morello, A. (1964), *Nature*, **203**, 785.

Morello, A. (1965), *Can. J. Biochem.*, **43**, 1289.

Myers, C. M. and Smith, J. N. (1954), *Biochem. J.*, **56**, 498.

Nakajima, M. (1976), in Metcalf, R. L. and McKelvey, J. J. (eds), *The future for insecticides: needs and prospects*, p. 287, Wiley, New York.

Nakatsugawa, T. and Dahm, P. A. (1962), *J. Econ. Entomol.*, **55**, 594.

Nakatsugawa, T. and Dahm, P. A. (1965), *J. Econ. Entomol.*, **58**, 500.

Nakatsugawa, T. and Dahm, P. A. (1967), *Biochem. Pharmacol.*, **16**, 25.

Nakatsugawa, T., Ishida, M. and Dahm, P. A. (1965), *Biochem. Pharmacol.*, **14**, 1853.

Nakatsugawa, T., Tolman, N. M. and Dahm, P. A. (1968), *Biochem. Pharmacol.*, **17**, 1517.

Nelson, J. O. and Matsumura, F. (1973), *Arch. Environ. Contam. Toxicol.*, **1**, 224.

Nolan, J. and O'Brien, R. D. (1970), *J. Agr. Food Chem.*, **18**, 802.

O'Brien, R. D. (1957), *Can. J. Biochem. Physiol.*, **35**, 45.

O'Brien, R. D. (1961), *Biochem. J.*, **79**, 229.

O'Brien, R. D. (1967), *Insecticides, action and metabolism*, Academic, New York.

O'Brien, R. D. and Spencer, E. Y. (1953), *J. Agr. Food Chem.*, **1**, 946.

O'Brien, R. D. and Spencer, E. Y. (1955), *J. Agr. Food Chem.*, **3**, 56.

Oesch, F., Kaubisch, N., Jerina, D. M. and Daly, J. W. (1971), *Biochemistry*, **10**, 4858.

Oonnithan, E. S. and Casida, J. E. (1968), *J. Agr. Food Chem.*, **16**, 28.

Oonnithan, E. S. and Miskus, R. (1964), *J. Econ. Entomol.*, **57**, 425.

Oppenoorth, F. J. (1954), *Nature*, **173**, 1001.

Oppenoorth, F. J. (1955), *Nature*, **175**, 124.

Oppenoorth, F. J. (1956), *Arch. Neerl. Zool.*, **12**, 1.

Oppenoorth, F. J., Rupes, V., El Bashir, S., Houx, N. W. H. and Veerman, S. (1972), *Pestic. Biochem. Physiol.*, **2**, 262.

Parke, D. V. (1968), *The biochemistry of foreign compounds*, Pergamon, Oxford.

Perry, A. S. (1960), *Misc. Publ. Entomol. Soc. Amer.*, **2**, 119.

Perry, A. S. and Buckner, A. J. (1970), *Life Sci.*, **9** (II), 335.

Perry, A. S. and Hoskins, W. M. (1950), *Science*, **111**, 600.

Perry, A. S., Dale, W. E. and Buckner, A. (1971), *Pestic. Biochem. Physiol.*, **1**, 131.

Perry, A. S., Mattson, A. M. and Buckner, A. J. (1958), *J. Econ. Entomol.*, **51**, 346.

Philpot, R. M. and Hodgson, E. (1971), *Life Sci.*, **10** (II), 503.

Philpot, R. M. and Hodgson, E. (1972), *Mol. Pharmacol.*, **8**, 204.

Plapp, F. W. and Casida, J. E. (1958), *J. Econ. Entomol.*, **51**, 800.

Plapp, F. W. and Tong, H. H. C. (1966), *J. Econ. Entomol.*, **59**, 11.

Plapp, F. W. and Valega, T. M. (1967), *J. Econ. Entomol.*, **60**, 1094.

Plapp, F. W., Bigley, W. S., Chapman, G. A. and Eddy, G. W. (1963), *J. Econ. Entomol.*, **56**, 643.

Ptashne, K. A., Wolcott, R. M. and Neal, R. A. (1971), *J. Pharmacol. Exp. Ther.*, **179**, 380.

Ray, J. W. (1965), in *Pest infestation research, 1965*, Report of the Pest Infestation Laboratory, Agricultural Research Council, p. 59, Her Majesty's Stationery Office, London.

Ray, J. W. (1967), *Biochem. Pharmacol.*, **16**, 99.
Rose, H. A. and Young, R. G. (1973), *Pestic. Biochem. Physiol.*, **3**, 243.
Sacher, R. M., Metcalf, R. L. and Fukuto, T. R. (1968), *J. Agr. Food Chem.*, **16**, 779.
Sacher, R. M., Metcalf, R. L. and Fukuto, T. R. (1969), *J. Agr. Food Chem.*, **17**, 551.
Sanborn, J. R., Lee, A. and Metcalf, R. L. (1974), *Pestic. Biochem. Physiol.*, **4**, 67.
Schonbrod, R. D. and Terriere, L. C. (1971), *Pestic. Biochem. Physiol.*, **1**, 409.
Schonbrod, R. D. and Terriere, L. C. (1975), *Biochem. Biophys. Res. Commun.*, **64**, 829.
Schonbrod, R. D., Gillett, J. W. and Terriere, L. C. (1965), *Abstr.* **49**, *Bull. Entomol. Soc. Amer.*, **11**, 157.
Schroeder, M. E., Shankland, D. L. and Hollingworth, R. M. (1977), *Pestic. Biochem. Physiol.*, **7**, 403.
Shishido, T., Usui, K., Sato, M. and Fukami, J. (1972), *Pestic. Biochem. Physiol.*, **2**, 51.
Sims, P. and Grover, P. L. (1965), *Biochem. J.*, **95**, 156.
Slade, M. and Wilkinson, C. F. (1973), *Science*, **181**, 672.
Slade, M. and Zibitt, C. H. (1972), in Menn, J. J. and Beroza, M. (eds), *Insect juvenile hormones: chemistry and action*, p. 155, Academic, New York.
Slade, M., Brooks, G. T., Hetnarski, H. K. and Wilkinson, C. F. (1975), *Pestic. Biochem. Physiol.*, **5**, 35.
Smith, J. N. (1955), *Biochem. J.*, **60**, 436.
Smith, J. N. (1968), *Adv. Comp. Physiol. Biochem.*, **3**, 172.
Smith, J. N. and Turbert, H. B. (1964), *Biochem. J.*, **92**, 127.
Sobels, F. H. and Vogel, E. (1976), *Mutation Res.*, **41**, 95.
Solomon, K. R. and Metcalf, R. L. (1974), *Pestic. Biochem. Physiol.*, **4**, 127.
Sternburg, J. and Kearns, C. W. (1956), *J. Econ. Entomol.*, **49**, 548.
Sternburg, J., Kearns, C. W. and Bruce, W. N. (1950), *J. Econ. Entomol.*, **43**, 214.
Sun, Y. P. (1972), *J. Econ. Entomol.*, **65**, 632.
Sun, Y. P. and Johnson, E. R. (1960), *J. Agr. Food Chem.*, **8**, 261.
Suzuki, T. and Miyamoto, J. (1974), *Pestic. Biochem. Physiol.*, **4**, 86.
Tanaka, K., Kurihara, N. and Nakajima, M. (1976a), *Pestic. Biochem. Physiol.*, **6**, 386.
Tanaka, K., Kurihara, N. and Nakajima, M. (1976b), *Pestic. Biochem. Physiol.*, **6**, 392.
Terriere, L. C. and Schonbrod, R. D. (1955), *J. Econ. Entomol.*, **48**, 736.
Terriere, L. C., Boose, R. B. and Roubal, W. T. (1961), *Biochem. J.*, **79**, 620.
Tsukamoto, M. (1959), *Botyu-Kagaku*, **24**, 141.
Tsukamoto, M. (1960), *Botyu-Kagaku*, **25**, 156.
Ullrich, V. and Schnabel, K. H. (1973), *Drug Metab. Disp.*, **1**, 176.
Ulmann, E. (ed.) (1973), *Lindane, monograph of an insecticide*, revised 2nd edn, Verlag K. Schillinger, Freiburg im Breisgau.
Verschoyle, R. D. and Barnes, J. M. (1972), *Pestic. Biochem. Physiol.*, **2**, 308.
Vogel, E. and Sobels, F. H. (1976), in Hollaender, A. (ed.), *Chemical mutagens: principles and methods for their detection*, vol. 4, Plenum, New York.
Walker, C. H. and El Zorgani, G. A. (1973), *Life Sci.*, **13**, 585.
Walker, C. H. and El Zorgani, G. A. (1974), *Arch. Environ. Contam. Toxicol.*, **2**, 97.
Walker, C. H., El Zorgani, G. A., Craven, A. C. C., Kenny, J. D. R. and Kurukgy, M. (1973), in *Proceedings of the FAO/IAEA symposium on nuclear techniques in comparative studies of food and environmental contamination*, IAEA, Vienna.
Walker, C. R. and Terriere, L. C. (1970), *Entomol. Exp. Appl.*, **13**, 260.
Whetstone, R. R., Phillips, D. D., Sun, Y. P., Ward, L. F. and Shellenberger, T. E. (1966), *J. Agr. Food Chem.*, **14**, 352.
White, A. F. (1972), *Life Sci.*, **11** (II), 201.
Wilkinson, C. F. (1967), *J. Agr. Food Chem.*, **15**, 139.

Wilkinson, C. F. (1976a), in Metcalf, R. L. and McKelvey, J. J. (eds), *The future for insecticides: needs and prospects*, p. 195, Wiley, New York.
Wilkinson, C. F. (ed.) (1976b), *Insecticide biochemistry and physiology*, Plenum, New York.
Wilkinson, C. F. and Brattsten, L. B. (1972), *Drug Metab. Rev.*, **1**, 153.
Walker, C. H. and El Zorgani, G. A. (1974), *Arch. Environ. Contam. Toxicol.*, **2**, 97.
Wilkinson, C. F. (ed.) (1976b), *Insecticide biochemistry and physiology*, Plenum, New York.
Wilkinson, C. F. and Brattsten, L. B. (1972), *Drug Metab. Rev.*, **1**, 153.
Wilkinson, C. F. and Hicks, L. J. (1969), *J. Agr. Food Chem.*, **17**, 829.
Wilkinson, C. F., Hetnarski, K. and Hicks, L. J. (1974), *Pestic. Biochem. Physiol.*, **4**, 299.
Wilkinson, C. F., Metcalf, R. L. and Fukuto, T. R. (1966), *J. Agr. Food Chem.*, **14**, 73.
Wilson, T. G. and Hodgson, E. (1971a), *Insect Biochem.*, **1**, 19.
Wilson, T. G. and Hodgson, E. (1971b), *Insect Biochem.*, **1**, 171.
Wilson, T. G. and Hodgson, E. (1972), *Pestic. Biochem. Physiol.*, **2**, 64.
Winteringham, F. P. W. (1969), *Ann. Rev. Entomol.*, **14**, 409.
Winteringham, F. P. W. (1952), *Nat. Acad. Sci. Nat. Res. Council, Publ.*, 219, p. 61.
Winteringham, F. P. W. and Harrison, A. (1959), *Nature*, **184**, 608.
Winteringham, F. P. W., Harrison, A. and Bridges, P. M. (1955), *Biochem. J.*, **61**, 359.
Winteringham, F. P. W., Loveday, P. M. and Harrison, A. (1951), *Nature*, **167**, 106.
Wustner, D. A., Desmarchelier, J. and Fukuto, T. R. (1972), *Life Sci.*, **11** (II), 583.
Yamamoto, I. and Casida, J. E. (1966), *J. Econ. Entomol.*, **59**, 1542.
Yang, R. S. H. (1976), in Wilkinson, C. F. (ed.), *Insecticide biochemistry and physiology*, ch. 5, Plenum, New York.
Yang, R. S. H. and Wilkinson, C. F. (1971), *Pestic. Biochem. Physiol.*, **1**, 327.
Yang, R. S. H. and Wilkinson, C. F. (1973), *Comp. Biochem. Physiol.*, **46B**, 717.
Yu, S. J. and Terriere, L. C. (1971), *Life Sci.*, **10** (II), 1173.
Zeid, M. M. I., Dahm, P. A., Hein, R. E. and McFarland, R. H. (1953), *J. Econ. Entomol.*, **46**, 324.

CHAPTER 4

The metabolic fate of synthetic pyrethroid insecticides in mammals

D. H. Hutson

INTRODUCTION

Although the earlier volumes of this series seemed to be primarily concerned with processes occurring in the metabolism of drugs, pesticide metabolism is a subject worthy of consideration in these pages. The emphasis is slightly different in the two fields, but the techniques and technology are virtually identical. Indeed, the two subjects have been pursued in a spirit of enthusiastic competition for some years, progress in one being complementary to and aiding that in the other. Problems such as the attempted prediction of unwanted biological effects ('side-effects' with a drug, 'environmental hazards' with a pesticide) are common to both fields. Both types of compound are subjected to short-term and long-term feeding trials in animals, the results of which have to be interpreted with respect to possible hazard to humans. The use-classification will be important in determining the doses and routes of exposure to be used in toxicity tests. However, once the chemical has been absorbed by the test animal, the mechanisms of biotransformation are common. In this first article on pesticide metabolism in mammals, it seemed appropriate to select a discrete class of insecticides and to use it to exemplify the scope, depth, and complexity of metabolism studies carried out during the development of pesticides.

All major insecticide types act on the nervous system of the target organism and, as absolute insect/mammal selectivity has not been achieved, the insecticides generally exhibit bioactivity towards mammals at appropriate dose levels. The insecticides fall into five major classes:

1. The organochlorines (Brooks, 1973), a diverse collection, exemplified by DDT, dieldrin, mirex, and toxaphene, of which some thousands have been synthesized and tested.
2. The organophosphorus compounds (Eto, 1974), exemplified by parathion, of which several hundreds of thousands have been investigated.
3. The carbamates (Kuhr and Dorough, 1976), e.g. Sevin (carbaryl), some recent examples of which are still under active development.
4. A miscellaneous group based on the natural toxins nicotine, rotenone etc.
5. The pyrethroids which, unlike those in group 4, appear to be on the threshold of a dramatic increase in use.

It should be mentioned that another small group of insecticides has emerged from the research phase: the juvenile hormone analogues (JHA's) which are based on interference with a mechanism which is unique to insects. Of these classes, the pyrethroids are in the most interesting situation at the present time. After many years of very restricted (mostly domestic) use, the photolabile natural pyrethrins and early synthetic pyrethroids appear about to be supplemented with highly insecticidally active photostable synthetic analogues suitable for agricultural use. Probably about a thousand pyrethroids have been synthesized and tested to date. The relatively few that have been selected for large-scale development are now under intensive toxicological studies, including metabolism studies. The metabolic fate of these pyrethroids in mammals and its relevance to their toxicology will form the basis of this chapter. Although some of this text will be overtaken by events, an attempt has been made to cover all published work on the subject to November 1977. Thus it is hoped that this review will form a useful summary of the subject as well as an illustration of metabolism studies in pesticide chemistry and development.

THE DEVELOPMENT OF THE SYNTHETIC PYRETHROIDS

Natural pyrethrum is an extract from the dried flower-heads of *Chrysanthemum cinerariaefolium*. The active components are the pyrethrins, the cinerins, and the jasmolins which are shown in figure 1. Although an apparently complex mixture, it can be seen that series I and II differ only in the C-3 substituent on

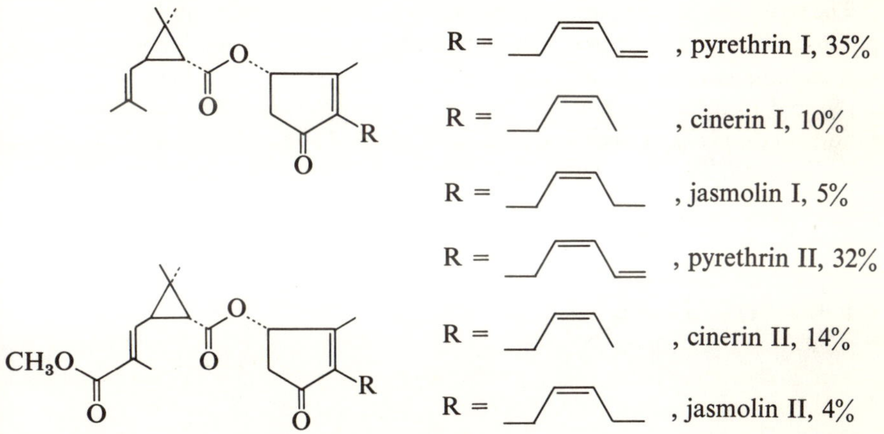

Figure 1   The components of pyrethrum

the cyclopropane carboxylic acid moiety; the difference between pyrethrins, cinerins, and jasmolins lies in the length and number of double bonds of the side-chains on the cyclopentenolone ring. Pyrethrin I is the most important constituent for insecticidal action but pyrethrin II is very effective at rapid 'knock-down'. Knock-down is not synonymous with death but it is very useful in the rapid removal of the nuisance factor—important in a domestic use. In briefly outlining the development of the synthetic pyrethroids it is convenient to use pyrethrin I as a starting point. This compound (figure 1) is an ester of 2,2-dimethyl-3-dimethylvinylcyclopropanecarboxylic acid and 2-pentadienyl-3-methylcyclopentenolone. Features required for maximum activity are: the *gem*-dimethyl groups at C-2 (cyclopropyl), an unsaturated side-chain at C-3 (cyclopropyl), the *R* configuration at C-1 (cyclopropyl), the ester bond, the *S* configuration at C-4 (cyclopentenolone), and a degree of planarity and electron delocalization in the alcohol group. In other words, the bioactivity resides in the molecule as a whole, and its stereochemistry is very important to this reactivity.

218

The advantages of pyrethrum lay in its natural availability, its insecticidal efficiency, and its very low toxicity to mammals. The disadvantage of the material is its photolability and, to a lesser extent, its biodegradability. The points of photoinstability of pyrethrin I are shown in figure 2. Biodegradability is discussed in the section on metabolism below.

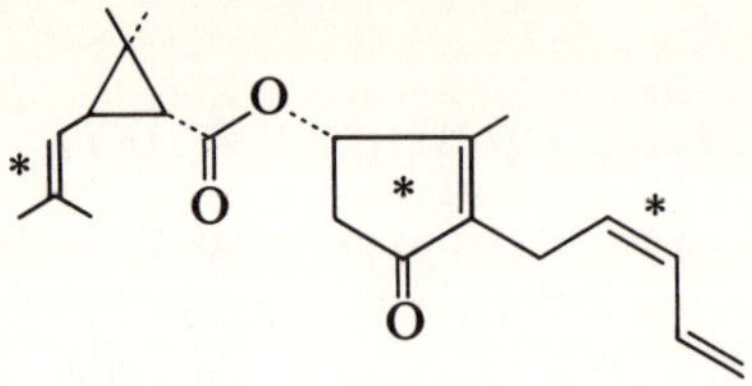

Figure 2   Centres of photolability (∗) in pyrethrin I

The structure–activity studies and chemical modifications leading to increased photostability and increased insecticidal activity while maintaining reasonably low mammalian toxicity will not be discussed in great detail here. The reader is referred to three excellent summaries on the subject (Elliott and Janes, 1973; Elliott, 1976, 1977). However, a brief description of some of the notable advances will illustrate the time-course and trends of events. Allethrin was the first

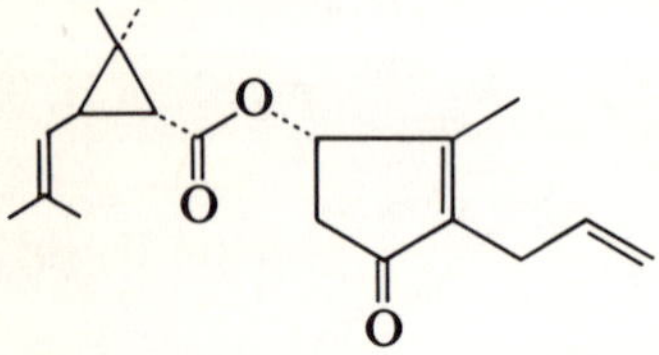

(1) 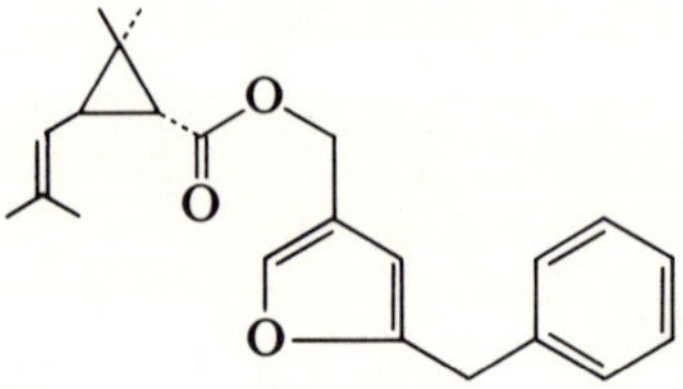   (2)

synthetic analogue; this was developed in 1949 by shortening the pentadienyl side-chain (Schechter et al, 1949). Bioallethrin and S-bioallethrin (1) are specific isomers of allethrin. The replacement of the natural alcohol by 5-benzyl-3-furylmethyl alcohol led to resmethrin and bioresmethrin (2) in 1966 (Elliott et al, 1967). This initiated the start of a rapid phase of development led notably by

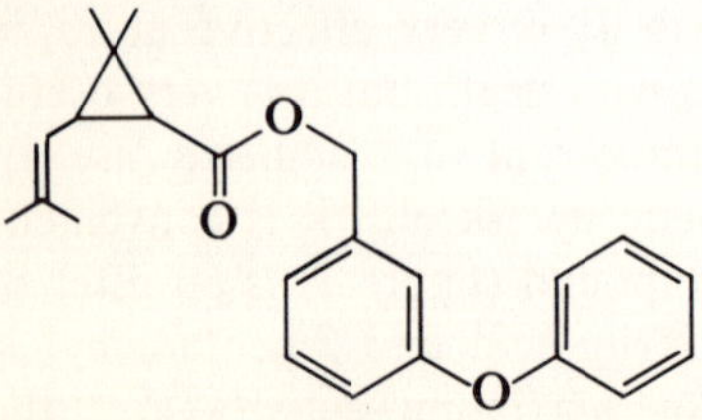

(3) 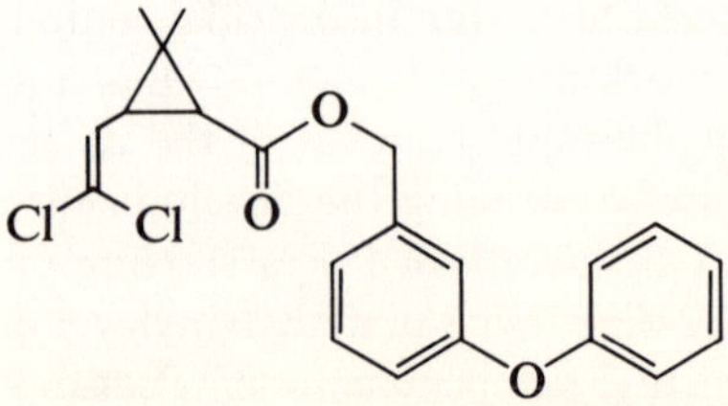   (4)

Elliott and coworkers at the Rothamsted Experimental Station in England. Replacement of the benzylfurylmethyl group of resmethrin by 3-phenoxybenzyl alcohol led to phenothrin (3) (Elliott et al, 1973; Fujimoto et al, 1973). Substitution of the methyl groups of the dimethylvinyl (isobutenyl) side-chain with chlorine afforded permethrin (NRDC 143, **4**), the first photostable pyrethroid, in 1972 (Elliott, 1973). It should be noted how all the weak points shown in pyrethrin I (figure 2) have been removed in permethrin (**4**). Cypermethrin (NRDC 149, **5**) is representative of a further development (Matsuo *et al*, 1976) and involves 3-phenoxybenzaldehyde cyanohydrin as the esterifying alcohol. The presence of the cyano-group reintroduces an asymmetric centre into the alcohol moiety allowing the possibility of further stereochemical refinements. In fact one of the most powerful organic insecticides yet synthesized is a specific

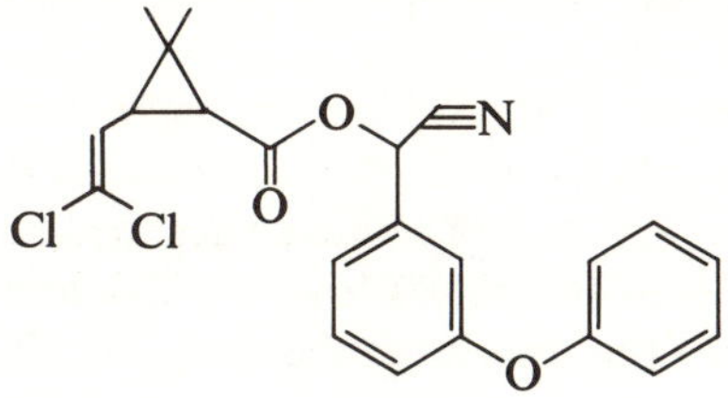

(5)

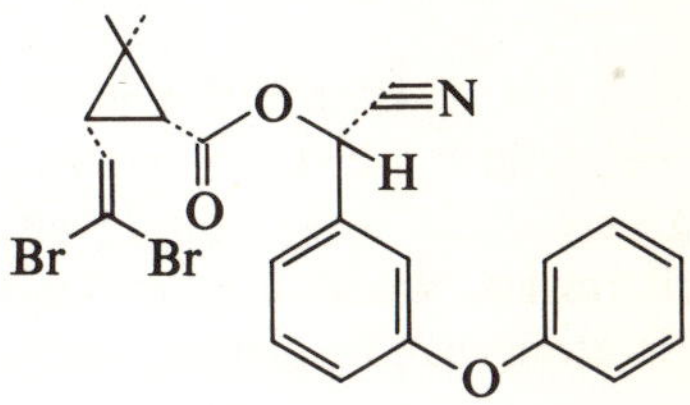

(6)

isomer of this type of structure. This is decamethrin (NRDC 161, **6**) which is a dibromo 1*R cis*-acid esterified with *S*-cyanohydrin (Elliott *et al*, 1974). This compound is more than 1,000 times more active than pyrethrin I (e.g. LD_{50} to houseflies 0·0003 μg) (Elliott, 1977). A further step forward was the discovery by Ohno *et al* (1974, 1976) that esters of 2-(4-chlorophenyl)-3-methylbutyric acid, for example fenvalerate (**7**), afford active photostable insecticides. This shows that even the cyclopropane ring is unnecessary provided an alternative

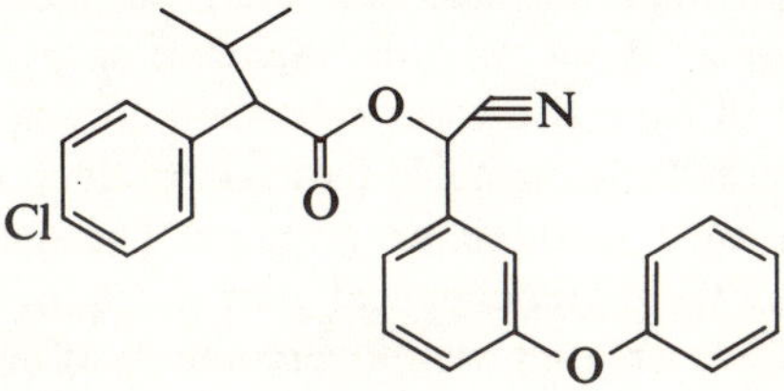

(7)

structure can be found with which to create the necessary stereochemistry. It is noteworthy that fenvalerate (**7**) is virtually unrecognizable as a pyrethroid in the traditional sense and it must point the way to other interesting developments.

Nomenclature

A satisfactory and simple stereochemical nomenclature is important in any discussion on chemical or biochemical aspects of pyrethroids. Cypermethrin (**5**) may be used to exemplify currently accepted nomenclature. The molecule possesses three asymmetric carbon atoms: C-1 (cyclopropane), C-3 (cyclopropane), and α-C (benzyl carbon atom). Considering the acid moiety first, it would be perfectly straightforward to use the Cahn–Prelog–Ingold system and refer to the acid as 1*R*3*R*, 1*R*3*S*, etc. as appropriate. Unfortunately, when the chrysanthemic acid series (as opposed to the halovinyl acid series) is named in this way, the sequence rule gives a different order of precedence at C-3. Thus these acids (dimethylvinyl acids), although of the same stereochemistry as the dihalovinyl acids, have different descriptions. In order to avoid this irritation and possible source of confusion, Elliott and coworkers have consistently used a hybrid nomenclature which is proving very convenient. The configuration at C-1 is defined (*R* or *S*) and the configuration at C-3 is then described by reference to C-1 using *cis* or *trans* as appropriate (if the H atoms at C-1 and C-3 are on opposite sides of the cyclopropane ring, the arrangement is *trans*, and vice versa). The carbon atom attached to the oxygen of the esterifying alcohol is named α and, if asymmetric, is referred to as αR or αS. Thus the eight isomers of cypermethrin are: 1*R trans* αR, 1*R trans* αS, 1*S trans* αR, 1*S trans* αS, 1*R cis* αR, 1*R cis* αS, 1*S cis* αR, and 1*S cis* αS. This system will be used where necessary in this review. Where a compound is referred to only as '*cis*', the C-1 and α-carbon atoms can be assumed to be racemic (or, as is often the case, non-chiral at α).

SUMMARY OF THE METABOLIC FATE OF NATURAL PYRETHRINS

It is a surprising fact that the first reasonable studies on the fate of pyrethrins I and II in mammals were reported as late as 1971 (Casida *et al*, 1971; Yamamoto *et al*, 1971). The delay between the first regular use and the acquisition of metabolic data is much longer than that experienced with the major synthetic insecticide classes. Two major factors contributed to this delay: firstly, a lack of demand for the information, and secondly, the lack of readily available synthetic chemical expertise to provide the necessary radioactively labelled compounds. The lack of expertise was probably a consequence of the industry having developed successfully using a natural product as opposed to using compounds developed by a synthetic programme. The synthetic problems were formidable in view of the stereochemical purity required and the instability of the compounds. However, they were overcome to afford pyrethrins I and II labelled with tritium in the alcohol moiety and carbon-14 in the acid moieties (Elliott *et al*, 1972). Pyrethrins I and II are carboxylic esters and it would be reasonable to predict their rapid hydrolysis to the constituent acids and alcohols in mammals. However, this was not found in practice. When pyrethrin I (figure 3, 3.1) was dosed orally to rats (3–5 mg/kg), the component acid and alcohol were not observed as excretion products. Rather, oxygenation occurred at the *trans*-methyl group of the chrysanthemate isobutenyl group affording (3.3), and at the terminal double bond of the 2,4-pentadienyl side-chain of the alcohol group. The former metabolite (3.3) was further oxidized via the aldehyde (3.4) to the acid (3.5). The (undetected) epoxide (3.6), resulting from oxygenation of the alcohol side-chain, was hydrolysed to the 4,5-*trans*-diol (3.7) which partially conjugated with glucuronic acid or sulphate (to give 3.8) before excretion. One conjugate of this metabolite (after methylation) was thought possibly to contain a *p*-methoxybenzyl group (n.m.r. data); however, it could

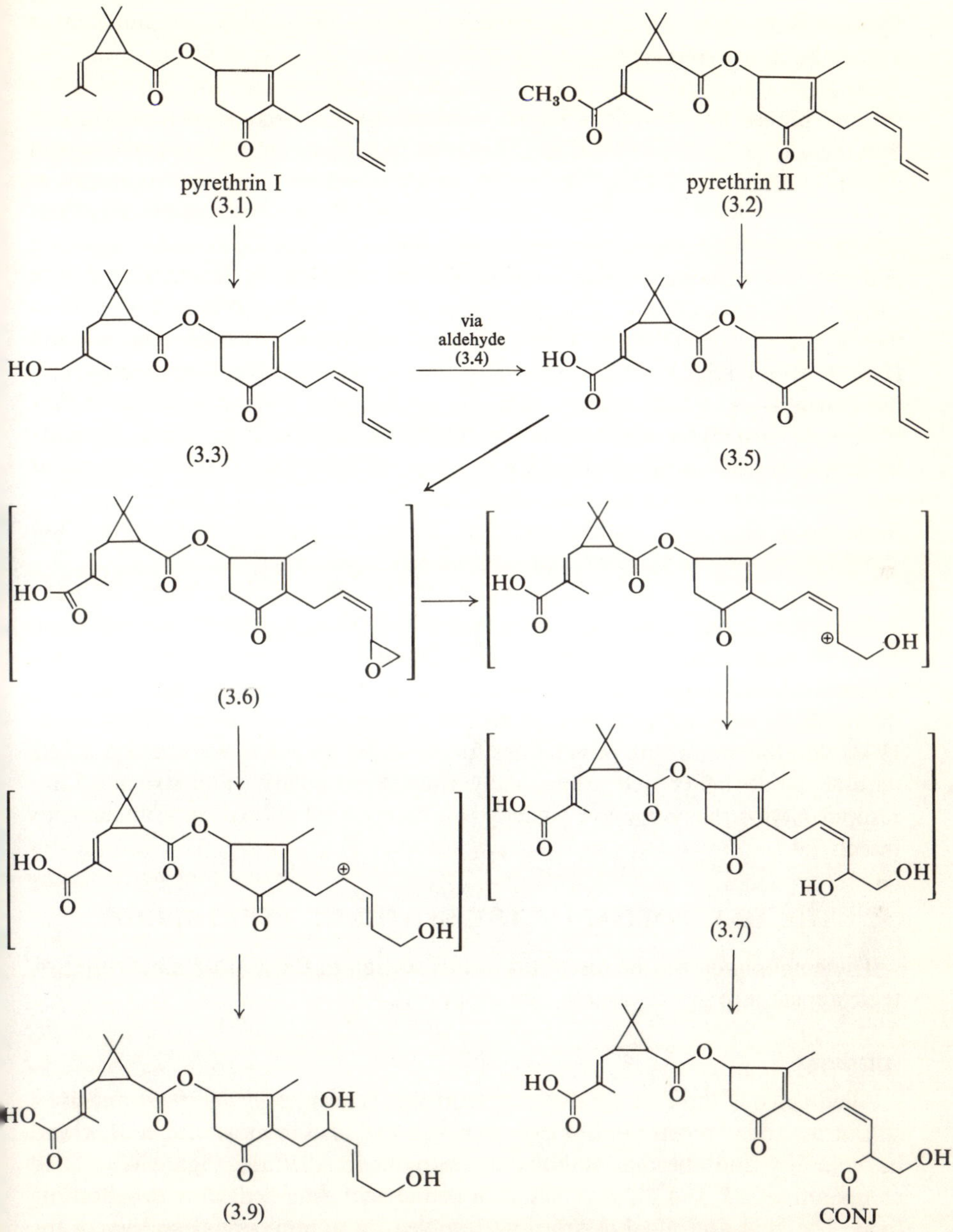

Figure 3 Partial metabolic pathways for pyrethrins I and II in rats

not be obtained in sufficient quantity for firm identification. This possibly new type of conjugate has not since been found or confirmed in foreign compound metabolism. Another interesting metabolite, postulated to arise via the epoxide (3.6), was the 2,5-*trans*-diol (3.9), an isomer of (3.7). The metabolites shown in figure 3 were found in urine and faeces, but the faeces also contained some unmetabolized pyrethrin.

Studies in mice revealed similar elimination data and *in vitro* studies using rat and mouse liver fractions largely confirmed the scheme shown in figure 3. Pyrethrin II (3.2) afforded a similar array of metabolites and a little unchanged pyrethrin II in the faeces. The most readily observed reaction, especially *in vitro*, was the hydrolysis of the methoxycarbonyl bond to afford the acid (3.5) which lies on the pathway of pyrethrin I metabolism. The microsomal location, and the lack of cofactor requirements for the reaction, indicated that it was catalysed by microsomal carboxylesterase. The location and cofactor requirements of the oxygenation reactions, together with the fact that pyrethrins I and II both afford type I substrate binding spectra with hepatic liver microsomes (Kulkarni *et al*, 1975), suggest that the cytochrome P-450-dependent monooxygenase system is responsible for these oxidations. Presumably epoxide hydratase is responsible for the ring opening of (3.6) to (3.7); the formation of the 2,5-diol (3.9) may also be a consequence of the action of this enzyme. Its mechanism is poorly understood; the biotransformation of (3.6) to (3.9) supports the intermediacy of a carbonium ion in the reaction.

The metabolism of the cinnerins and the jasmolins (figure 1) has not been studied but it has been reasonably suggested (Casida, 1973) that the same reactions will occur at the acid moiety as those found in pyrethrin metabolism (figure 3). Analogous reactions at the alcohol moiety, together with terminal methyl hydroxylation, may be expected. It is thought (Elliott *et al*, 1972; Casida, 1973) that the multiroute possibilities for the rapid oxidative metabolism of the natural pyrethrins (which dramatically alters their polarity and structure) are responsible for their very low toxicity to experimental animals as compared to insects.

THE METABOLISM OF THE SYNTHETIC PYRETHROIDS

The compounds will be discussed in this section in the approximate order of their appearance in use or active development.

Allethrins

Allethrin was the first synthetic pyrethroid (Schechter *et al*, 1949) and it is still in use today mostly in domestic aerosols and also in mosquito coils where its volatility and thermal stability are exploited. Allethrin (figure 4, 4.1) is composed of 1*R* and 1*S trans*-chrysanthemic acid esterified with *RS*-allethrolone. The acid and alcohol are now resolved on a commercial scale and are used to make bioallethrin (1*R trans* acid/4′*RS* alcohol). The allethrins, like the pyrethrins, have low mammalian toxicity. The acute oral toxicity (LD_{50}) of the allethrins to rats ranges from 430 to 2,430 mg/kg depending on sex and isomer. *S*-Bioallethrin (1) (from the 4′*S* alcohol), ^{14}C-acid labelled and ^{3}H-alcohol labelled, and bioallethrin (^{14}C-alcohol labelled) were included in the study of the pyrethrins cited above (Elliott *et al*, 1972). Compounds were administered orally

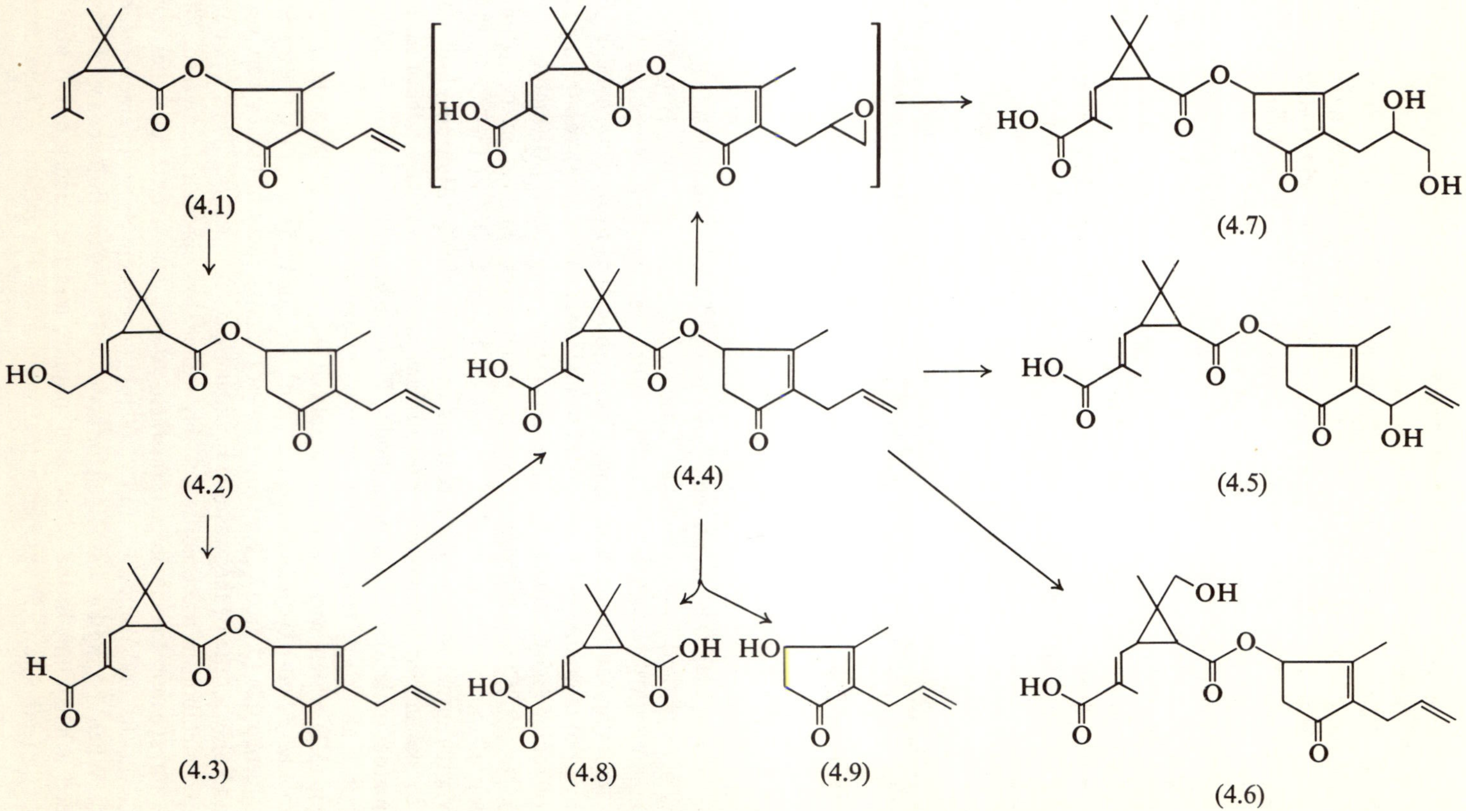

Figure 4 Partial metabolic pathway for allethrin in rats

to rats at doses of 1–5 mg/kg. Large doses (8×450 mg/kg) were used for the isolation of specific urinary metabolites. Radioactivity was eliminated in urine and faeces. Tissues were not examined. The urinary radioactivity (up to 51% after 48 hours) was contained mostly in esters (i.e. common to both labelling patterns). However, small amounts of chrysanthemum dicarboxylic acid (figure 4, 4.8) and allethrolone (4.9) were detected, indicating that some hydrolysis occurred. The three major metabolites were isolated, and identified by chromatographic and spectroscopic techniques as the diol (4.7), the monohydroxyallethrin acid (4.5), and allethrin acid hydroxylated at one of the *geminal* dimethyl groups (*trans* to the original isobutenyl group) (4.6). It is interesting that allethrin acid itself (4.4) was not observed as a metabolite *in vivo*; however, it could be detected *in vitro* (rat liver microsomes) as could allethrin alcohol (4.2) and aldehyde (4.3). Faecal metabolites, about 30% of the dose after 48 hours, were not investigated. A tentative scheme for allethrin metabolism is shown in figure 4. This study was the first to reveal hydroxylation of one of the *geminal* dimethyl groups—a phenomenon that is now found with increasing frequency. Like the pyrethrins, the allethrins are metabolized mainly by peripheral hydroxylation probably catalysed by hepatic microsomal monooxygenase.

Tetramethrin

Tetramethrin, 3,4,5,6-tetrahydrophthalimidomethyl *trans*-chrysanthemate (figure 5, 5.1) (also known as neopynamin and phthalthrin), was the second synthetic pyrethroid to be produced commercially. It was first reported in 1964 (Kato *et al*, 1964). The compound possesses good knock-down activity, fair killing activity, and low mammalian toxicity. Its acute oral toxicity to rats is 8,300 mg/kg (Miyamoto *et al*, 1968). When tetramethrin, prepared from 1*RS* *trans*-chrysanthemic acid and [^{14}C-carbonyl]-N-hydroxymethyl-3,4,5,6-tetrahydrophthalimide (5.2), was dosed to male rats (500 mg/kg), rapid elimination of radioactivity, equally in urine and faeces, was found (Miyamoto *et al*, 1968). No [^{14}C]CO_2 was liberated. Similar results were obtained on the administration of the labelled alcohol (5.2), but in this case 80% of the elimination was via the urine. Most of the faecal radioactivity from [^{14}C]tetramethrin was due to unchanged compound. The urinary metabolites were identified by chromatographic and physical methods. Their structures (figure 5) indicated that, once absorbed, tetramethrin was rapidly hydrolysed to its alcohol component (5.2) which was further metabolized via (5.3) and (5.4) to the major metabolite, 3-hydroxycyclohexane-1,2-dicarboximide (5.5), which was excreted as a glucuronide (5.6). The concentrations of radioactivity in tissues were very low and only a little of this was due to unchanged tetramethrin. Thus a pattern of rapid metabolism preceded by possibly rather slow absorption emerged. The acute intravenous toxicity of tetramethrin to rats was over 2,000 times that found via the oral route (3·5 and 8,300 mg/kg respectively) (Miyamoto *et al*, 1968). When 1·5 mg/kg was given intravenously, tetramethrin concentration reached a maximum in the blood at 1 minute, and the concentration of the primary metabolite (5.2) reached a maximum after 4–5 minutes. These data, together with the presence of unchanged (unabsorbed) compound in the faeces, suggest that the low toxicity of orally ingested tetramethrin is due to both limited absorption and rapid metabolism. In a study directed mainly at the mechanism of degradation of tetramethrin in houseflies (Suzuki and Miyamoto, 1974) some preliminary results with rat liver microsomes indicated that the

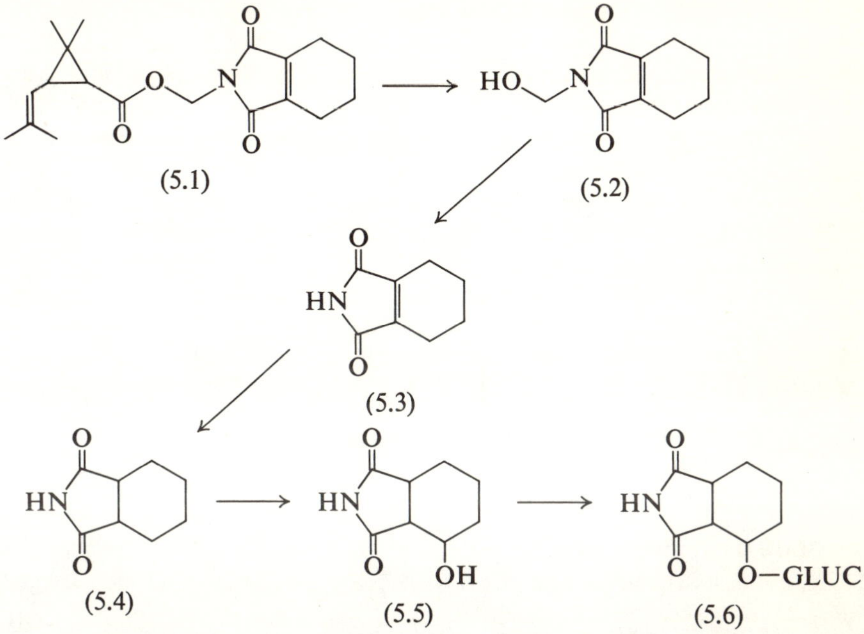

(5.1)   (5.2)   (5.3)   (5.4)   (5.5)   (5.6)

Figure 5   Partial metabolic pathway for tetramethrin in rats

hydrolysis was catalysed by a carboxylesterase. It was independent of NADPH and was inhibited by pretreatment with paraoxon. In the presence of NADPH, tetramethrin underwent oxidation to unidentified metabolites. Mouse liver acetone powder (a crude preparation containing microsomal carboxylesterase and other esterases, but with the monooxygenase denatured) hydrolysed $1R$ *trans*-tetramethrin about 3 times faster than the $1R$ *cis*-isomer (Abernathy *et al*, 1973). This is a general phenomenon which will emerge clearly as more pyrethroids are discussed. The *cis*-isomer of tetramethrin is about twice as acutely toxic to mice compared with the *trans*-isomer.

Resmethrin, Bioresmethrin, and Cismethrin

Resmethrin, 5-benzyl-3-furylmethyl chrysanthemate (figure 6, 6.1), is the most important member of a series of substituted furan-containing pyrethroids. It was synthesized in 1966 (Elliott *et al*, 1967). It is a mixture of isomers; bioresmethrin (6.1 *trans*) is the ester of $1R$ *trans*-chrysanthemic acid. The latter possesses the very favourable insect/mammalian toxicity ratio of about 32,000 (Elliott, 1971). Its acute oral LD_{50} (rat) is 8,000 mg/kg (Verschoyle and Barnes, 1972). In the first metabolic study with this series of compounds (Miyamoto

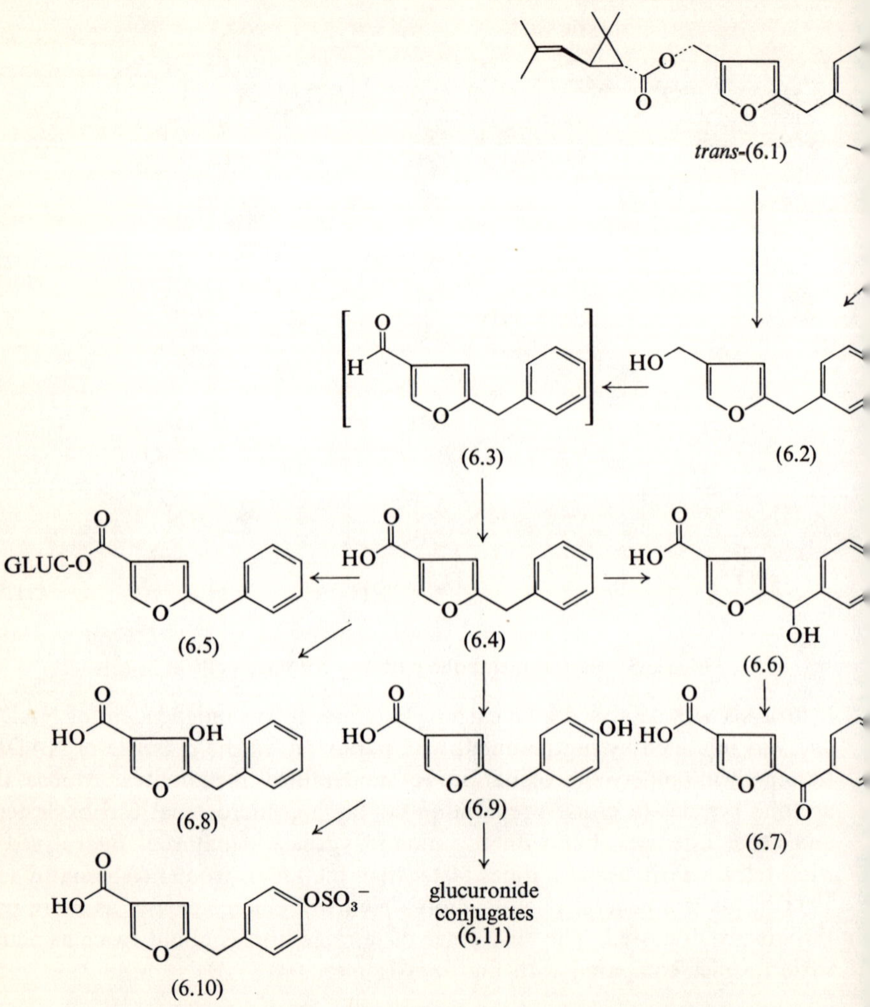

Figure 6 Partial metabolic pathways of resmethrin in rats

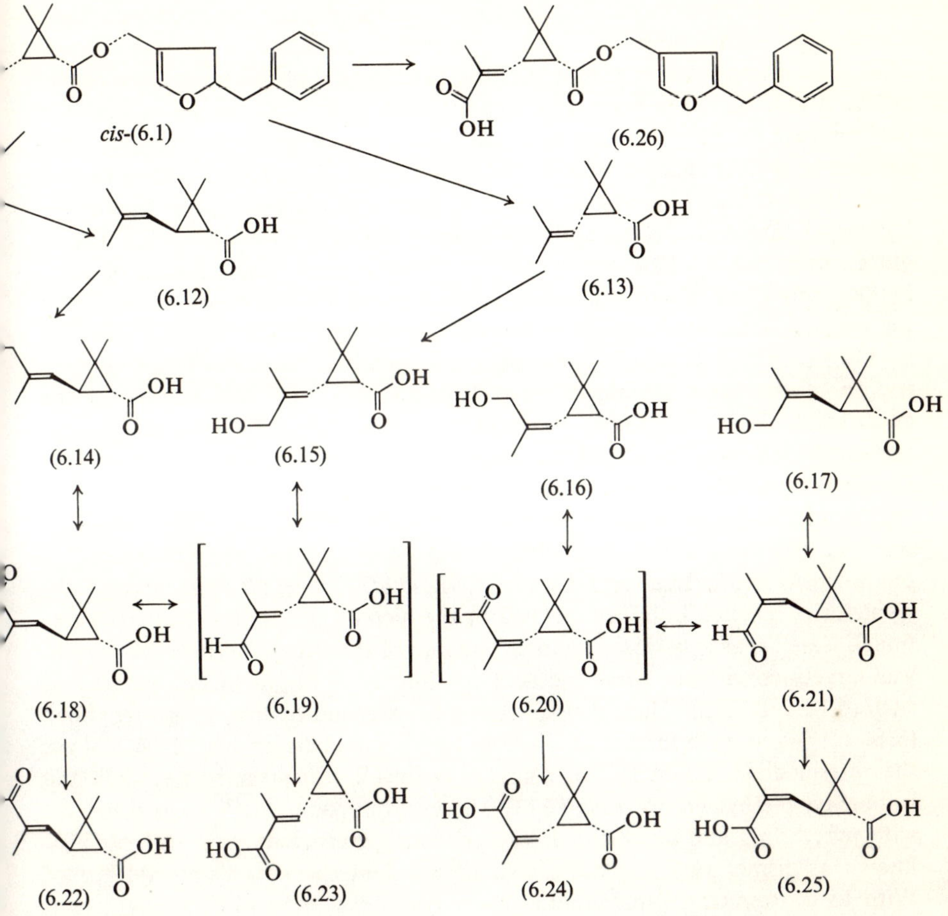

cis-(6.1)

(6.26)

(6.12)

(6.13)

(6.14)

(6.15)

(6.16)

(6.17)

(6.18)

(6.19)

(6.20)

(6.21)

(6.22)

(6.23)

(6.24)

(6.25)

et al, 1971), [^{14}C-furan]resmethrin was given orally to rats (500 mg/kg). The initial elimination of radioactivity in urine and faeces was rapid and 80% of the administered radioactivity was excreted in 5 days; however, a further 15 days elapsed before the excretion approximated to 100% (faeces, 60%; urine, 35%). A study of biliary elimination indicated that much of this delay was probably due to enterohepatic circulation. Intravenously administered resmethrin (50 mg/kg) resulted in radioactivity elimination data similar to those found after oral administration except that the faeces/urine proportions were nearer 50/50. Much of the urinary radioactivity was accounted for as metabolites derived from the benzylfurylmethyl moiety. The major metabolite was 5-benzyl-3-furoic acid (6.4) and the ester glucuronide thereof (6.5). Hydroxylated derivatives of (6.4) such as α-(4-carboxy-2-furyl)benzyl alcohol (6.6), 5-benzyl-4-hydroxy-3-furoic acid (6.8), and 5-(4-hydroxybenzyl)-3-furoic acid (6.9) (as its glucuronide and sulphate conjugates) were also present. Examination of liver, kidney, and blood after intravenous administration of resmethrin showed that the original compound rapidly disappeared and that the alcohol (6.2) and the acid (6.4) could be detected. The former was rapidly eliminated but the concentration of the latter remained relatively stable over the 120 minutes of the experiment. The concentration of resmethrin in the brain at 2·5 minutes (24 μg/g) remained constant for about an hour (22·7 μg/g). This concentration was associated with toxicological symptoms (but not with death). Faecal metabolites were not investigated in this study and the biliary metabolites, while containing some of the compounds described above, contained mostly metabolites of unknown structure. In a second study (Ueda *et al*, 1975a), 1*R trans*- and 1*R cis*-resmethrin, labelled in either the acid or the alcohol moiety (i.e. four preparations), were separately dosed to rats. The fate of the benzylfurylmethyl portion was largely confirmed, while the acid portions were found to be liberated as such (6.12 and 6.13). They also suffered methyl group hydroxylation to afford (6.14–6.17) and were further oxidized to the dicarboxylic acids (6.22–6.25), via the intermediate aldehydes (6.18–6.21). With 1*R trans*-resmethrin, only the isobutenyl methyl group *trans* (*E*) to the cyclopropane ring was oxidized (as with pyrethrin I and allethrin). However, with 1*R cis*-resmethrin (6.1 *cis*, also known as cismethrin), oxidation also occurred at the *cis* (*Z*) methyl group. With 1*S cis*-resmethrin, preferential hydroxylation at the *cis* (*Z*) methyl group occurred. A complicating feature of this work was that these products epimerized (probably at the aldehyde stage). The biotransformations of resmethrin are summarized in figure 6.

Rat liver microsomes oxidize the *cis*-isomers of 1*R* and 1*S* resmethrin more rapidly than the *trans*-isomers (Abernathy *et al*, 1973; Casida *et al*, 1976). The microsomal esterases hydrolyse the isomers in the reverse order. An extensive product analysis (Ueda *et al*, 1975b) confirmed the reactions found *in vivo* and also allowed the detection of side-chain hydroxylation of the intact 1*R cis*-ester observed as a carboxylic acid (6.26). Very little such hydroxylation was observed from the 1*S cis*-isomer. Rat and mouse liver microsomes were compared in this study. As *in vivo*, side-chain hydroxylation by rat microsomes occurred *trans* to the cyclopropane ring; with mouse liver microsomes, hydroxylation *cis* to the cyclopropane ring was preferred. Mouse liver microsomal esterases hydrolyse $1R$ *trans*-resmethrin 8- to 15-fold more rapidly than $1R$ *cis*-resmethrin. Rates of microsomal oxidation are of the same order for both isomers (Abernathy *et al*, 1973; Jao and Casida, 1974a; Casida *et al*, 1976). This difference may account in part for the differences in acute toxicity between the $1R$ *trans*- and the $1R$ *cis*-isomers to mice (i.p. LD_{50} values $> 1,500$ and 320 mg/kg respectively). The *trans*-isomer is so non-toxic that it may exert its lethal action via a metabolite. Verschoyle and Barnes (1972) noted a delay in symptoms when a lethal dose was given intravenously. This is in accord with the observation that three of the resmethrin metabolites ($1R$ *trans*-chrysanthemic acid (6.12), 5-benzyl-3-furylmethanol (6.2), and 5-benzyl-3-furoic acid (6.4)) were more toxic than the parent compound (Ueda *et al*, 1975a). However, a later report (White *et al*, 1976) that the time-course of symptoms compared closely with the time-course of the concentration of pyrethroid in the brains of rats (20–25 μg/g at death) does not support the toxic metabolite theory. Oral doses of $1R$ *trans*-resmethrin to rats (300 mg/kg) gave rise to very low brain concentrations up to 2 hours (0.45 μg/g). It would appear therefore that absorption and metabolism protect rats from the effects of orally ingested *trans*-resmethrin. There is also some evidence for an intrinsic difference in toxicity between the isomers. Death from the *cis*-isomer occurred at a brain concentration of 3.9–5.1 μg/g (female rats); the corresponding value for the *trans*-isomer was 30.5 ± 4.5 μg/g.

An esterase in blood plasma has been reported by White *et al* (1976). It is of interest in that it did not exhibit the stereoselectivity towards the *cis*- and *trans*-isomers that is characteristic of the hepatic esterase. Activity towards resmethrin was low, and comparable with that of the hepatic enzyme to the *cis*-isomer:

Enzyme	Hydrolysis (nmol/min/g liver or per ml plasma) of	
	Cismethrin	Bioresmethrin
Liver	3.1 ± 0.36	40.8 ± 5.50
Plasma	3.4 ± 0.21	3.15 ± 0.43

Its role in the detoxication of resmethrin and other pyrethroids is unknown. If it is identical with the serum carboxylesterase of rats, the finding will probably not be relevant to many other common species, including man, which do not contain measurable amounts of serum carboxylesterase.

The distinction between hydrolysis and oxidation is potentially important. The (hepatic) hydrolytic enzyme can be inhibited *in vitro* by tetraethylpyrophosphate (TEPP) and *in vivo* by prior administration of S,S,S-tributyl phosphorothioate (DEF) (Abernathy *et al*, 1973). The oxidative reactions can be inhibited *in vitro* simply by leaving out the cofactors necessary for microsomal monooxygenation. An interesting possibility emerged from the study of *cis*-resmethrin *in vitro*, that of the oxidative deesterification of carboxylic esters.

Microsomal esterase action on the *cis*-isomer was very slow but, in the presence of NADPH, both 1*R* and (particularly) 1*S cis*-resmethrin afforded chrysanthemic acid (6.13) and its oxidized metabolites. Similar results were obtained with the *trans*-isomer when TEPP-inhibited microsomes were used as the enzyme source. The mechanism and significance of this reaction will be discussed further below.

Ethanomethrins

The ethanochrysanthemates are derivatives of the chrysanthemates in which the butenyl methyl groups are incorporated into a 5-membered ring. The most successful ester is that of the *trans*-acid with 5-benzyl-3-furylmethanol (**8**). It is also known as K-othrin and RU (Roussel-Uclaf, France) 11679 (Lhoste and Rauch, 1969). This is a very effective insecticide, but it has a somewhat higher mammalian toxicity than have those discussed so far (Elliott, 1971). Its acute toxicity i.p. to mice is > 1,500 mg/kg but some mortality was observed at 500–1,500 mg/kg; the acute toxicity of the *cis*-isomer is 10 mg/kg (Abernathy *et al*, 1973). Studies on the metabolism of these compounds *in vivo* have not been

(**8**)

published but the results of *in vitro* work suggest pathways and mechanisms of metabolism. The esterase inhibitor DEF, when predosed to mice, had a > 188-fold synergizing action on the acute toxicity of the *trans*-isomer. It even synergized the *cis*-isomer by a factor of four, lowering the LD_{50} to 2·4 mg/kg (Abernathy *et al*, 1973). This suggests that the esteratic breakdown of the *trans*-isomer *in vivo* is very important in its detoxication. Fresh mouse liver microsomes in the presence and absence of NADPH and paraoxon (esterase inhibitor) hydrolyse and oxidize the 1*R trans*-isomer at 0·21 and 0·11 nmol/min/mg protein respectively. Sites of oxidation in the molecule could be the cyclopentylidene ring, a (cyclopropyl) methyl group, and, by analogy with resmethrin (figure 6), the 4-position of the phenyl ring in the alcohol moiety. The esterase is inhibited 86% in DEF-treated animals. Inhibitors of microsomal monooxygenation do not increase the toxicity of this pyrethroid so it would appear that its detoxication is almost completely dependent on hydrolysis.

Kadethrin (RU 15525)

Kadethrin, also developed by Roussel-Uclaf, is a derivative of ethanoresmethrin (Lhoste and Rauch, 1976). It has very high knock-down activity. No *in vivo* metabolism studies have been reported. It is the 5-benzyl-3-furylmethyl ester of a 1*R cis*-acid (**9**) and therefore should be rather slowly hydrolysed.

Soderlund and Casida (1977a), in a comparative study that will be discussed in more detail below, found that indeed hydrolysis of (9) was very slow but that its oxidation was the fastest of the 44 pyrethroids studied. It is likely that the sulphur atom in the thiolactone ring is the major site of oxidation in this molecule. *S*-Oxygenation would lead to ring opening and to a dramatic change in

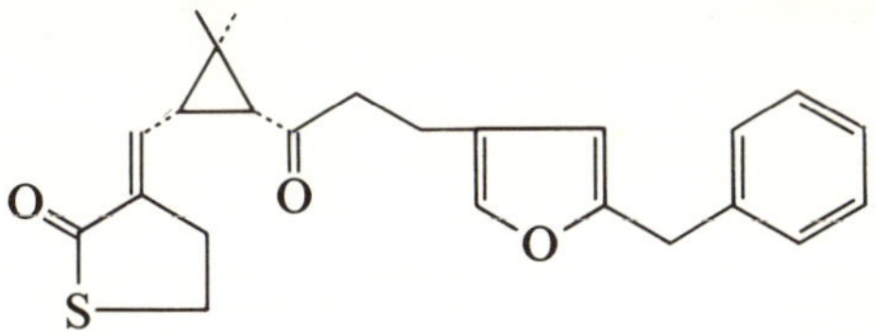

(9)

polarity and probably also in toxicity. Analogy with resmethrin (figure 6) would suggest that 4-(phenyl)-hydroxylation should also occur.

Proparthrin (Kikuthrin)

Proparthrin (figure 7, 7.1) is the 2-methyl-5-(2-propynyl)-3-furylmethyl ester of *trans*-chrysanthemic acid (Nakanishi *et al*, 1970). Its volatility makes it useful in some aerosol preparations. When [³H-alcohol]proparthrin was orally administered to rats (100 mg/kg), the tritium label was eliminated in the urine (40%) and faeces (35%) during 4 days. Biliary elimination (in a separate study)

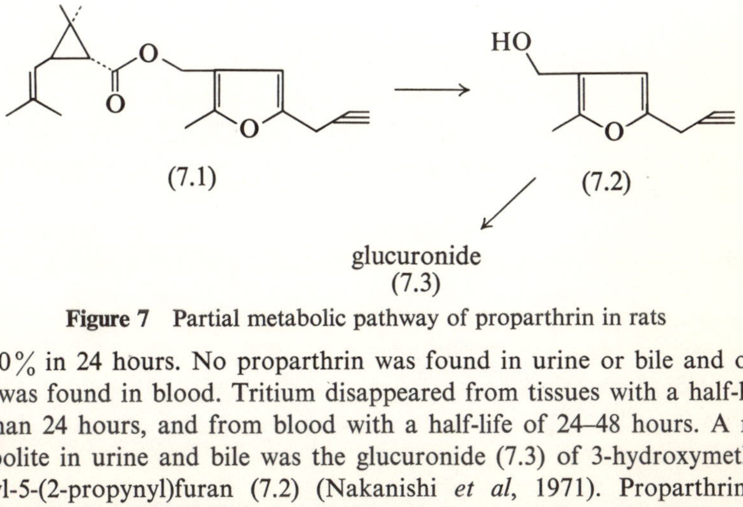

(7.1)   (7.2)

glucuronide
(7.3)

Figure 7   Partial metabolic pathway of proparthrin in rats

was 40% in 24 hours. No proparthrin was found in urine or bile and only a trace was found in blood. Tritium disappeared from tissues with a half-life of less than 24 hours, and from blood with a half-life of 24–48 hours. A major metabolite in urine and bile was the glucuronide (7.3) of 3-hydroxymethyl-2-methyl-5-(2-propynyl)furan (7.2) (Nakanishi *et al*, 1971). Proparthrin was very rapidly hydrolysed (more than twice as fast as *trans*-resmethrin) *in vitro* (Soderlund and Casida, 1977a). Oxidation, to unspecified products, occurred at about one-third of the rate of hydrolysis.

Prothrin (Furamethrin)

Prothrin (**10**, Ogami *et al*, 1970) is similar in structure, properties, and uses to proparthrin (figure 7). Its acute toxicity (intraperitoneal) to mice is

232

>1,500 mg/kg and 400 mg/kg for the *trans*- and *cis*-esters respectively (Abernathy *et al*, 1973). Studies *in vivo* have not been reported but *in vitro* studies (Abernathy *et al*, 1973) revealed a typical 50-fold difference in the rates of hydrolysis of the *trans*- and *cis*-isomers (*trans*>*cis*). Oxidation plays a minor role in the metabolism of *trans*-isomer *in vitro* (*c*. 10%), but plays a major role in the metabolism of the *cis*-isomer.

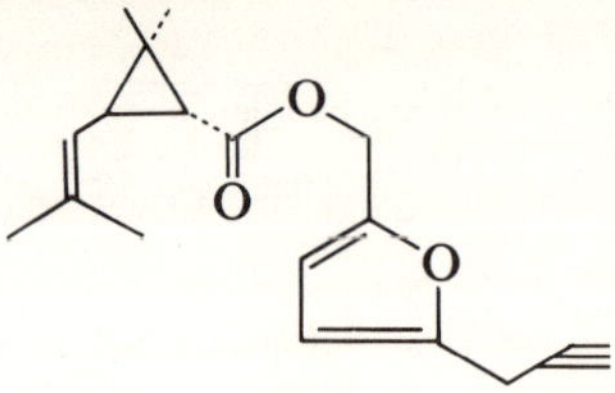

(10)

Benzyl Esters

Dimethrin

2,4-Dimethylbenzyl 1*R*,1*S trans*-chrysanthemate (figure 8) is a relatively early example of a benzyl ester (Barthel, 1958). Its acute toxicity to rats and rabbits is >15,000 mg/kg (Ambrose, 1964). Rabbits given 5 ml of dimethrin per kilogram excreted more glucuronic acid (total) than controls. Masri *et al*

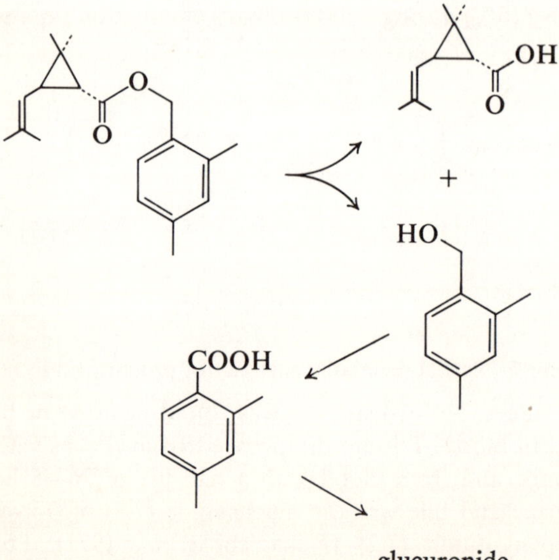

glucuronide

Figure 8   Partial metabolic pathway for dimethrin in rabbits

(1964) fed dimethrin to rabbits (2% in synthetic diet) and isolated crystalline *trans*-chrysanthemic acid from the urine. Dimethylbenzoic acid was tentatively identified via its equivalent weight. The fate of the chrysanthemic acid moiety was similar, in terms of ^{14}C-elimination data, to that of other chrysanthemate esters (Elliott *et al*, 1972).

Barthrin

Barthrin (figure 9, 9.1) was developed at the same time as dimethrin (figure 8) (Barthel and Alexander, 1958). Its acute toxicity to rats is 15,000–20,000 mg/kg (Ambrose, 1963). Masri and coworkers (1964) isolated 1·2 g of crystalline potassium chrysanthemate from 2·5 litres of urine from rabbits receiving barthrin at a rate of 2% in the diet for 3 days. 6-Chloropiperonylic acid (9.4)

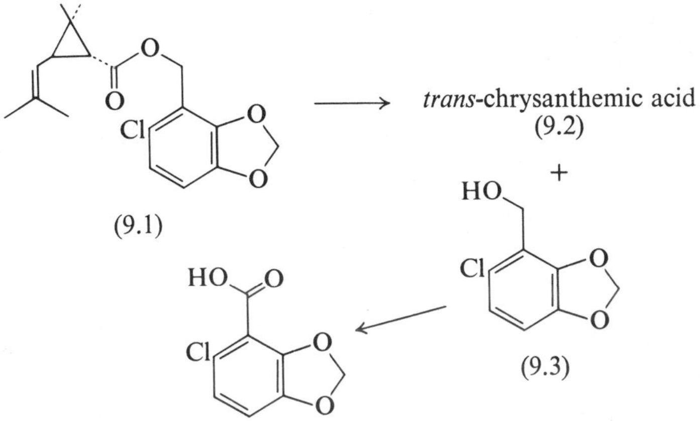

trans-chrysanthemic acid
(9.2)

(9.1)

(9.3)

(conjugate) (9.4)

Figure 9 Partial metabolic pathway for barthrin in rabbits

was also obtained and its structure proved by m.p., analytical data, and n.m.r. spectroscopy. A partial metabolic pathway for barthrin may therefore be constructed (figure 9). In the light of current knowledge it would be interesting to reinvestigate this compound, and particularly the *cis*-isomer (presumably resistant to hydrolysis), for an inhibitory effect of the methylenedioxy group on its oxidative metabolism.

Phenothrin

The discovery that *meta*-substituted benzyl groups served as stereoanalogues of the furylmethyl moiety was an important advance in pyrethroid chemistry and led to the 3-phenoxybenzyl esters (Elliott, 1971; Fujimoto *et al*, 1973). The first of these, the chrysanthemate, is not as active as resmethrin (figure 6) but this was thought at one time to be offset by the ready availability, cheapness, and stability of 3-phenoxybenzyl alcohol. Phenothrin (Sumitomo 2539) is 3-phenoxybenzyl 1*R trans*-chrysanthemate (figure 10, 10.1). Its acute oral toxicity to rats and mice is >5,000 mg/kg (Miyamoto, 1976). Its metabolism has been studied by Miyamoto *et al* (1974) using ^{14}C-label in the methylene group. The absorption and distribution of an oral dose to rats (200 mg/kg) were rapid and the radioactivity was virtually all eliminated within 3 days (57% in urine and 44% in faeces). None was eliminated via the lungs. The distribution of radioactivity in the tissues at 0·5, 1, 3, 6, 12, and 24 hours was followed by whole-body autoradiography. Nothing unusual was observed. After

234

24 hours, only the intestines contained detectable radioactivity. Radioactivity in the blood, brain, liver, and kidneys reached a maximum at 3 hours after dosing. At this time phenothrin was a minor component (2·9%) of the 161 µg equivalents per gram of liver and also constituted only 7·1% of the 167 µg equivalents per millilitre of blood. The major metabolite in both tissues was 3-phenoxybenzoic acid (10.3, 3PBA). About half of the intestinal radioactivity

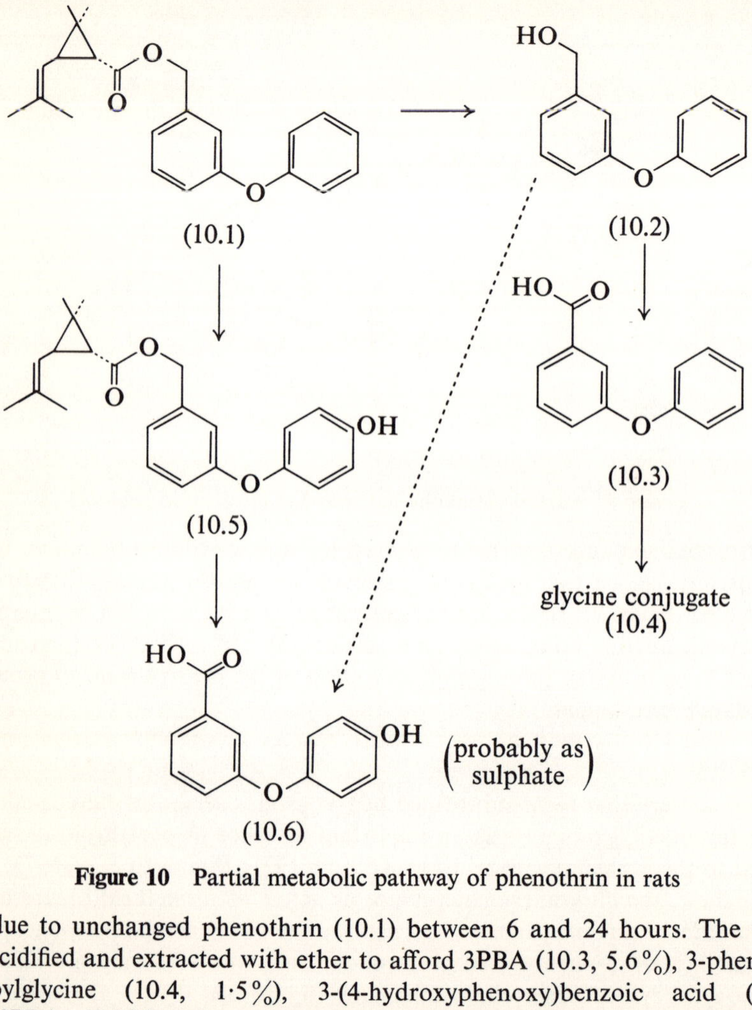

Figure 10   Partial metabolic pathway of phenothrin in rats

was due to unchanged phenothrin (10.1) between 6 and 24 hours. The urine was acidified and extracted with ether to afford 3PBA (10.3, 5.6%), 3-phenoxy-benzoylglycine (10.4, 1·5%), 3-(4-hydroxyphenoxy)benzoic acid (10.6, 4′HO3PBA, 42·3%), other ether-soluble metabolites (7%), and water-soluble metabolites (0.6%). Faeces afforded phenothrin (10.1, 9%), 3PBA (10.3, 3·8%), glycine conjugate (10.4, 1·2%), 4′HO3PBA (10.6, 11·9%), other ether-extractable metabolites (11·6%), water-soluble metabolites (0·4%), and residue (5·5%). More recent work with other 3-phenoxybenzyl esters would suggest that 4′HO3PBA (10.6) would have been present in the urine, mainly as its sulphate conjugate which was hydrolysed during the extraction procedure and that the faeces contained hydroxylated phenothrins. 3-Phenoxybenzyl alcohol (10.2; 3PBAlc) was not detected. Most of the above metabolites, including 3PBAlc (10.2), were detected when phenothrin (10.1) (1 mM) was incubated with rat liver 8,000 **g** supernatant. The *cis*-isomer was also tested in this system and found to be only slowly hydrolysed; however, it is noteworthy that when NADPH was added to the system, the overall rate of metabolism of both isomers was very similar, the *cis*-isomer affording 'other ether-soluble metabolites'. This report contains some of the few kinetic measurements made in pyrethroid metabolism to date. 1*R* *trans*-, 1*S* *trans*-, 1*R* *cis*-, and 1*S* *cis*-phenothrins were incubated with liver microsomes (no cofactors) and the released 3PBAlc (10.2) was measured by gas–liquid chromatography.

The resulting values are tabulated below.

	K_m (mM)	V_{max} (nmol/h/mg protein)
1*R trans*	0·17	60
1*S trans*	0·17	50
1*R cis*	0·11	2·0
1*S cis*	0·16	2·8

They demonstrate once again the *trans/cis* rate difference, reveal that the difference is due to V_{max}, and also show that the configuration at cyclopropyl C-1 (very important in insecticidal activity) has little effect on hydrolytic metabolism). In the mouse liver system of Soderlund and Casida (1977a) (substrate concentration 0·1 mM), the esterase contribution was twice that of oxidation for the *trans*-isomer. For the *cis*-isomer the esterase contribution was not detectable and oxidative metabolism was 1·4 times that for the *trans*-isomer. Three metabolites retaining the ester bond were recently found in the faeces of rats dosed with 1*R cis*-phenothrin (200 mg/kg) (Suzuki *et al*, 1976). These were 4′-hydroxy-1*R cis*-phenothrin (the *cis*-isomer of 10.5, 1·4% of dose), the derivative of phenothrin in which the *E* methyl group was oxidized to carboxyl (10·4%) and finally the compound in which both of these biotransformations had occurred together with hydroxylation of one of the (cyclopropyl) *gem*-dimethyl groups (2·1%), i.e. a metabolite formed via oxidation of the parent compound at three positions.

Permethrin

Permethrin (figure 11, 11.1) is the phenothrin analogue in which chlorine atoms replace the methyl groups of the isobutenyl side-chain of chrysanthemic acid (Elliott, 1973). It is about as active as bioresmethrin (**2**), but it represents an exciting step forward because the last site of photoinstability (see figure 2) has now been removed and the resultant molecule (11.1) is stable enough to control insects in the field and therefore it represents a new generation of pyrethroid insecticides.

Racemic permethrin (3-phenoxybenzyl 2-(2,2-dichlorovinyl)-3,3-dimethyl-cyclopropanecarboxylate) has an acute oral LD_{50} of 490 mg/kg to male and

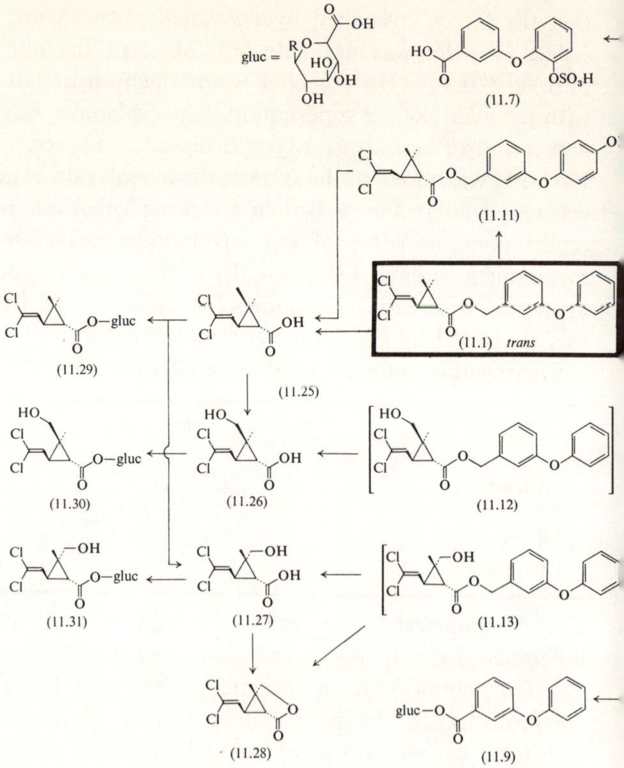

236

Figure 11   Metabolic pathways of permethrin in rats (from Gaughan, 1977a)

female mice and > 5,000 mg/kg to male and female rats (Miyamoto, 1976).
The individual isomers have the following oral LD_{50} values to mice: 1R *trans*,
3,150; 1R *cis*, *c*. 96; 1S *trans*, and 1S *cis*, > 5,000 mg/kg (Miyamoto, 1976). It
should be noted that only 1R isomers exhibit acute toxicity. The toxicity of
isomer mixtures approximates to that expected of their components and no
synergism is found.

A brief report of the radiosynthesis and metabolism of the 1R isomers
(Elliott *et al*, 1976) has now been superseded by perhaps the most comprehensive
paper on pyrethroid metabolism published to date. In this study (Gaughan *et al*,
1977a), the 1R *trans*-, 1RS *trans*-, 1R *cis*-, and 1RS *cis*-isomers, separately
labelled in the acid and in the alcohol moieties, were dosed orally to rats (1·6–
4·8 mg/kg) and the metabolites in urine and faeces were identified. Twelve days
after administration, 97–100% of the radioactivity was recovered in urine and
faeces. Virtually no $^{14}CO_2$ was expired. The concentrations of radioactivity in all
tissues, with the exception of fat, were low at 4 and 12 days. Radioactivity from
the *cis*-isomers tended to be retained longer than that from the *trans*-isomers,
and that from the alcohol label, longer than that from the acid label. The most

striking difference was that only 45–54% of the radiocarbon from the *cis*-isomer appeared in the urine whereas 81–90% of that from the *trans*-isomer was excreted thus. This was due to the fact that the more (hydrolytically) stable *cis*-isomer afforded metabolites that retained the ester bond and these were excreted in the faeces, presumably via the bile. The major metabolites from both isomers were the sulphate of 4′HO3PBA (11.5) and the glucuronides of the cyclopropanecarboxylic acids (11.23 and 11.29). 3PBA-glucuronide (11.9) from the *trans*-isomer was the next most abundant metabolite. All of the other metabolites shown in figure 11 were present in quantities between 0·5% and 5% of the dose. Six metabolites from each label remain unidentified (three of these from each source may be identical). Some of the metabolites were difficult to handle; for example, hydroxylation at a methyl *cis* to carboxyl led to metabolites that lactonized very readily (e.g. 11.27). [^{14}C]-3-Phenoxybenzyl alcohol, when dosed to rats, afforded a very similar picture to that from the ^{14}C-3PBAlc moiety of *trans*-permethrin; likewise the *trans*-cyclopropanecarboxylic acid afforded the same metabolites as those from acid-labelled *trans*-permethrin. These features are included in figure 11.

The relative contributions of the esterase and oxidase in the *in vitro* hepatic metabolism of permethrin (0·1 mM) have been estimated (rates relative to 1*R trans*-resmethrin) by Soderlund and Casida (1977a) as follows:

	Oxidase	Esterase
1*R trans*	30	77
1*S trans*	17	109
1*RS trans*	18	78
1*R cis*	26	<2
1*S cis*	22	<4
1*RS cis*	16	<2

These values confirm that, as with other pyrethroids, *trans*-isomer metabolism is dominated by hydrolysis and that of *cis*-isomers by oxidation. The products and mechanism of ester cleavage of the *cis*-isomer remain an intriguing problem. The major metabolite *in vivo* is the *cis*-acid (11.19) (as glucuronide). This may arise from esterase action which, though slow, probably operates to some extent *in vivo*, or it may arise from oxidative ester cleavage of the type postulated above for resmethrin (figure 6). An artefactual mechanism of oxidative ester

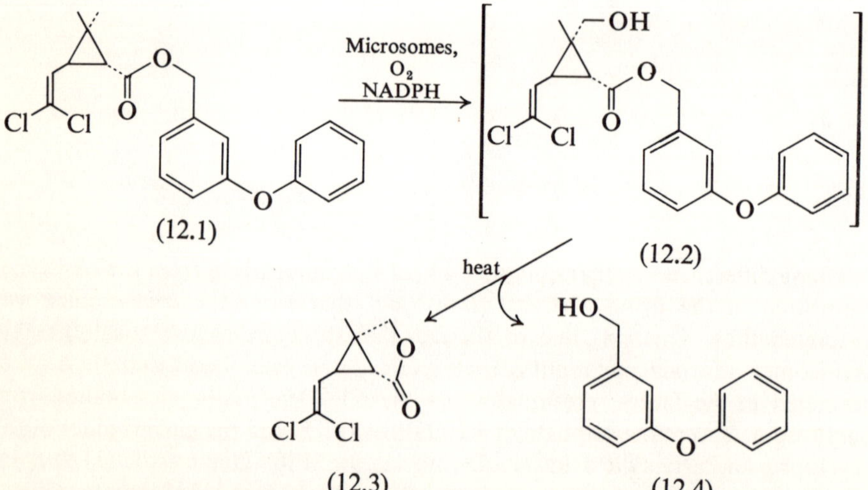

Figure 12 Ester cleavage of permethrin *in vitro* via oxidation

cleavage has been elucidated using deuteropermethrin and mouse liver microsomes (Soderlund and Casida, 1977b). It involves hydroxylation at the *gem*-dimethyl group of the acid moiety. Hydroxylation of 1*R trans*-permethrin *trans* to the carboxyl group afforded a stable product (11.12). However, hydroxylation *cis* to the carboxyl group affords the analogous ester (figure 12, 12.2). Under the analytical conditions used to detect hydrolysis *in vitro* (g.l.c.), this ester cleaved in an intramolecular reaction to afford 3PBAlc (12.4) and the *cis*-hydroxy acid lactone (12.3). This artefactual sequence was avoided by trimethylsilylation before g.l.c. It is not known if this mechanism operates to any extent *in vivo*. The fact remains that the major metabolite *in vivo* is the *unhydroxylated* acid and this must arise via esterase action or oxidation at the benzyl methylene group (such a reaction is illustrated in figure 14).

The NADPH-dependent metabolism of permethrin by esterase-inhibited (TEPP-treated) mouse liver microsomes has been briefly described (Unai and Casida, 1977). The products were approximately quantitated as follows:

Product	*trans*-Permethrin	*cis*-Permethrin
trans-HO-Permethrin (12, 16)	−	−
cis-HO-Permethrin (13, 17)	+ + + +	+ + + +
cis-CHO-Permethrin*	+ +	(+)
2′-HO-Permethrin (15)	−	+
4′-HO-Permethrin (11, 14)	+	+ + + +
6-HO-Permethrin	+ +	+ +
trans-,4′Di-OH permethrin	−	+ +

* Metabolite in which a *cis*-hydroxymethyl group has been oxidized to an aldehyde group. Numbers in parentheses refer to structure numbers in figure 11.

Hydroxylation in the alcohol moiety differed qualitatively and quantitatively from that found with rat; the isomers also varied in their reactivity. Thus the extent of hydroxylation for the *trans*-isomer lay in the order $6 > 4' > 2'$ and, for the *cis*-isomer, $4' > 6 > 2'$. The preferred site of hydroxylation for both of the $1R$ isomers was the *cis*-methyl group on cyclopropyl. There was less apparent specificity in the $1RS$ series but this was because of the stereoselectivity for *trans*-methyl hydroxylation with $1S$ *trans*-permethrin (Soderlund and Casida, 1977b).

Unai and Casida (1977) have described the chemical synthesis of 44 possible metabolites of permethrin, 29 of which have actually been detected as metabolites in rats, cows, or insects. A preliminary account of the fate of permethrin (3 daily oral doses of 1 mg/kg) in lactating cows (Gaughan *et al*, 1977b) indicates that the metabolism is similar to that in rats. However, more hydroxylated esters were excreted (in the faeces) by cows, suggesting that ester cleavage, even of the *trans*-isomer, was less efficient than in the rat. The conjugation pattern was somewhat different from that in the rat in that the dichlorovinyl acid (11.25) was excreted in the urine as a glutamic acid conjugate and an unknown conjugate as well as the glucuronide. The major metabolite of the 3PBAlc moiety was N-(3-phenoxybenzoyl)glutamic acid which was not detected in rats. No 2′-hydroxylation was detected in cows. Details of milk and tissue metabolites are not yet available. The elimination of radioactivity from lactating goats dosed orally (0·2–0·28 mg/kg) with ^{14}C-acid and ^{14}C-alcohol-labelled *cis*- and *trans*-permethrin has been reported (Hunt and Gilbert, 1977). Radioactivity from the *cis*-isomer was excreted mostly in the faeces (52–67%); that from the *trans*-isomer was excreted mostly in the urine (72–79%). Milk residues were less than $0.1\ \mu g/g$ and lay in the order $[^{14}C\text{-acid}]trans < [^{14}C\text{-alcohol}]$-$trans < [^{14}C\text{-acid}]$ $cis = [^{14}C\text{-alcohol}]cis$. No respired $^{14}CO_2$ was detected. Tissue residues at 24 hours after the last dose were generally low (0.002–$0.005\ \mu g/g$) except in fat. The *cis*-isomer labels afforded a residue in fat of $0.25\ \mu g/g$ and the *trans*-isomer labels, $0.02\ \mu g/g$. This suggests that the *cis*-isomer was more biostable than the *trans*-isomer in goats as in the few other species so far studied.

Cyanobenzyl esters

Esters derived from 3-phenoxybenzaldehyde cyanohydrin are approximately 3 times more insecticidally active than those from 3-phenoxybenzyl alcohol (Elliott, 1976). The insertion of the cyano-group at the benzyl carbon atom results in a greater than 10-fold decrease in the rate of hydrolysis of *trans*-substituted cyclopropanecarboxylate esters by rat liver microsomal esterase (Miyamoto, 1976). The rate of hydrolysis of *cis*-esters, already low, drops by a similar factor. Rates relative to *trans*-phenothrin for the permethrins and their cyano analogues (cypermethrins) are as follows: *trans*-permethrin, 135; *trans*-cypermethrin, 10.7; *cis*-permethrin, 1.8; *cis*-cypermethrin, 0. The latter value should be regarded as 'undetectable' rather than zero. Slow rates can be measured, particularly at low substrate concentrations, especially if sensitive radiochemical methods are used. Values found in the comparative study of Soderlund and Casida (1977a) also confirm that the cyanopyrethroids are hydrolysed much more slowly than their primary alcohol analogues. They also appear to be somewhat more resistant to oxidation by mouse liver microsomal monooxygenase. The presence of the cyano-group introduces another chiral centre into the pyrethroid molecule, a factor that further complicates the study of efficacy, metabolism, and toxicity and also creates further opportunities for development. Whereas permethrin exists as four isomers (two diastereoisomeric pairs), cypermethrin exists as eight isomers. An exceptional example of optimization of the stereochemistry is that of decamethrin, α-cyano-3-phenoxybenzyl 2-(2,2-dibromovinyl)-3,3-dimethylcyclopropanecarboxylate ($1R$ *trans*-acid–*S*-alcohol) (NRDC 161) (Elliott *et al*, 1974). This compound (see **11**) has an activity more than 1,000 times that of pyrethrin I to houseflies (LD_{50} approximately 0.05 mg/kg). This value is even lower (0.002 mg/kg) when activity is synergized with sesamex. The combination of *cis*-acid and α-cyano-alcohol apparently affords the most biostable pyrethroids known to date. In the *in vitro* studies so far reported, they are apparently not hydrolysed and only slowly oxidized (Miyamoto, 1976; Soderlund and Casida, 1977a). However, it is important to note that metabolism occurs rapidly in whole animals (see below).

α-Cyano-3-phenoxybenzyl tetramethylcyclopropanecarboxylate (WL 41706)

This compound (figure 13, 13.1) has the proposed common name fenpropathrin (also known as Sumitomo compound S3206 and Shell compound WL 41706). The acid (13.4) possesses no asymmetric centre, being fully substituted at C-2 and C-3 with methyl groups. In terms of enzymic hydrolysis, it

(13.1) should be, and in fact is (Soderlund and Casida, 1977a), analogous to a *cis*-pyrethroid. Its acute oral LD_{50} in mice is 18–36 mg/kg and in rats 20–26 mg/kg. It possesses one asymmetric centre (the α-carbon atom) and its metabolism has been studied as the *RS* mixture. Labelled as the 3-phenoxy-[14C]benzyl ester, an oral dose to rats (1·5 mg/kg) was eliminated rapidly in the urine (57 %) and faeces (40 %) in 48 hours, and the mean recovery from four animals after 8 days was 100·4 % (Crawford and Hutson, 1977). No sex differences were observed in rates or routes of elimination or in the structures and

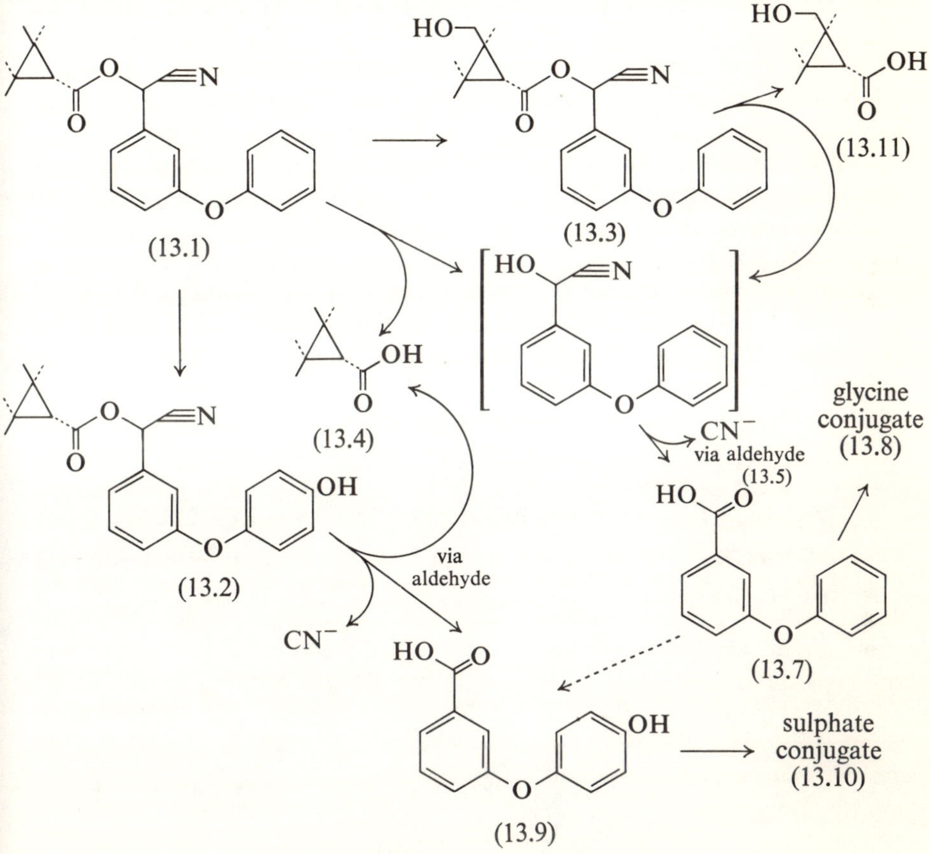

Figure 13 Metabolism of WL 41706 in rats

quantities of excreted metabolites. The highest residue was in fat from which its elimination was slowest. The urinary metabolites (derived from benzyl-labelled WL 41706) were very similar to those afforded by permethrin (see figure 11). The major metabolite was the sulphate conjugate (13.10) of 4′HO3PBA (13.9). Neither 2′HO3PBA nor its sulphate conjugate could be detected. The major metabolite from the 14C-cyclopropyl-labelled pyrethroid was the glucuronide conjugate of tetramethylcyclopropanecarboxylic acid (13.4). Another major metabolite was the *trans*-hydroxy acid (13.11) which was mostly excreted in urine unconjugated. Hydroxylation products retaining the ester bond (e.g. 13.2 and 13.3) were eliminated via the bile (conjugated) and the faeces. No unchanged pyrethroid was eliminated in the bile; such elimination would not be expected in view of the lipophilic character of these compounds. The known metabolic pathways are summarized in figure 13. When benzyl-labelled WL 41706 was fed to cows daily for 21 days in an amount equivalent to 0.1 μg/g of total diet, urinary and faecal elimination of radioactivity attained equilibrium with input after 4 days. The milk residues were below 0.0005 μg/ml throughout the study. Muscle residues were low (< 0.004 μg/g) after 21 days. These data suggest that the compound was rapidly metabolized by the cows (Crayford and Hutson, 1977). This type of experiment is necessary in order to confirm that low residues which may reach an animal via its diet under certain circumstances are disposed of by that animal rather than passed on to humans via milk or meat.

The metabolism of WL 41706 (13.1) by rat liver microsomes followed the typical pattern expected for a *cis*-isomer. Hydrolysis rate was less than 0.2 nmol/min/mg protein at 0.1 mM. However, in the presence of NADPH, metabolism occurred at a rate (of substrate disappearance) of 2.2 nmol/min/mg protein. The major aryl-labelled metabolites were *trans*-hydroxy-WL 41706 (13.3, 73%), 3PBA (9%), and 3PBAlc (6%). Only traces (1%) of 4′HO3PBA (13.9) and 4′HO-WL 41706 (13.2) were detected, i.e. the aryl hydroxylation was difficult to achieve *in vitro* using the usual cofactors (NADPH generators). Microsomes from phenobarbitone-treated rats were twice as effective as normal

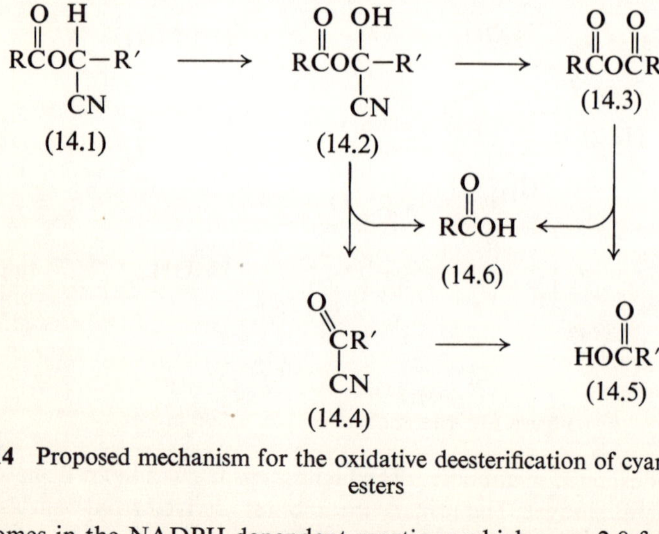

Figure 14 Proposed mechanism for the oxidative deesterification of cyanopyrethroid esters

microsomes in the NADPH-dependent reactions which were 2.8-fold inhibited by carbon monoxide (Crawford and Hutson, 1977). In an attempt to demonstrate the relative importance of oxidative and hydrolytic detoxication *in vivo*, rats were pretreated with phenobarbitone or with the carboxylesterase inhibitor tri-*o*-tolyl phosphate (TOTP) and the LD_{50} of WL 41706 was determined in comparison with appropriate controls. Phenobarbitone protected against the toxicity by a factor of five to six. TOTP had no effect. Although these results were in accord with an oxidative process predominating in detoxication (increased activity of the oxidizing enzymes affording rapid metabolism), they must be viewed with caution because the protection may have been due to a pharmacological action of the barbiturate.

Oxidative deesterification of the cyanopyrethroids via α-carbon hydroxylation would result either in 3-phenoxybenzoyl cyanide (14.4) or the anhydride of 3PBA and the cyclopropanecarboxylic acid (14.3). In either case these acylating reagents would mostly react with water to afford the observed acids (figure 14).

Cypermethrin

The cyano analogue of permethrin (which is cypermethrin (NRDC 149, Shell WL 43467) (figure 15, 15.1)) may prove to be a useful development of permethrin (see figure 11) (Elliott, 1976). Acute oral LD_{50} values in the rat are 160–300 mg/kg (*cis*-isomer) and > 10,000 mg/kg (*trans*-isomer). The relative rates of oxidation and hydrolysis respectively in the *in vitro* test system (Soderlund and Casida, 1977a) are: *trans*-isomer 4 and 17, and *cis*-isomer 5

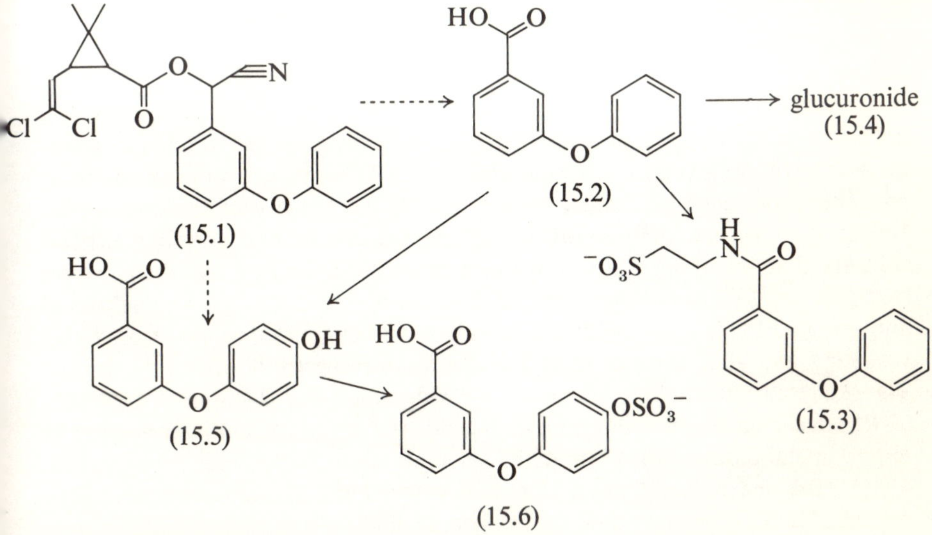

Figure 15 Fate of 3-phenoxybenzyl group of cypermethrin in mice

and < 2, i.e. typically, the *trans*-isomer is hydrolysed and oxidized and the *cis*-isomer is apparently metabolized mainly by oxidation. *In vivo* studies in rats, not yet completed (Crawford *et al*, 1978), using ^{14}C-benzyl- and ^{14}C-cyclopropyl labelling, indicated that the fate of cypermethrin was similar to that of permethrin in terms of rates of excretion, routes of excretion, tissue residues, and the structures of the excreted metabolites. The urinary metabolites of *cis*- and *trans*-^{14}C-benzyl]cypermethrin in the mouse were very different from those in the rat. The major rat metabolite (the sulphate of 4'HO3PBA,

244

15.6) was a minor metabolite in the mouse; the major mouse metabolite was not excreted by the rat (Hutson and Casida, 1978). This major mouse metabolite was N-(3-phenoxybenzoyl)taurine (15.3), the first example of the taurine conjugation of a benzoic acid (cf. arylacetic acids). Free 4′HO3PBA (15.5) was also eliminated in good yield. In this study 3-phenoxy-[^{14}C]benzoic acid was dosed to mice and afforded a profile of metabolites almost identical to that from the parent pyrethroid. It would appear likely therefore that 4′-hydroxylation can occur *after* hydrolysis (or oxidation) of the ester bond.

Decamethrin (NRDC 161)

This compound (Elliott *et al*, 1974) combines many of the features discussed in the introduction, including the selection of the most effective isomers, to afford one of the most active insecticides known. The stereochemistry is a combination of 1R *cis*-acid and S-cyanohydrin and is shown in (**11**). In the *in vitro* test system using mouse liver microsomes (Soderlund and Casida, 1977a)

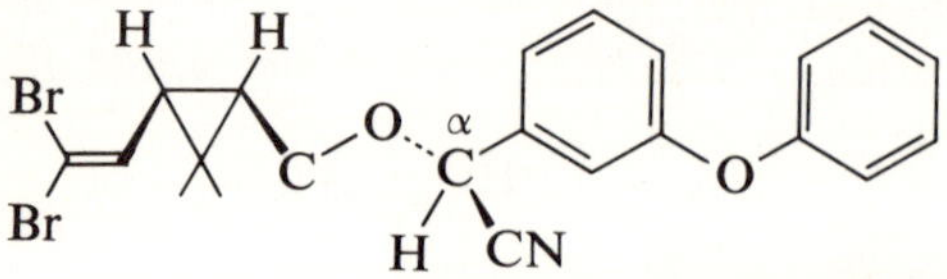

(11)

the esterase, oxidase, and total rates of hydrolysis (relative to 1R *trans*-resmethrin) were given as <4, <3 and $<4\%$. These values represent a rather biostable molecule which must be a factor in the toxicity of the compound. However, its acute toxicity to rats (25–63 mg/kg) (Barnes and Verschoyle, 1974) suggests that metabolism and clearance must occur *in vivo*. A recent report (Ruzo *et al*, 1977) confirmed that decamethrin (0·5–2 mg/kg) is metabolized and excreted by rats as rapidly as the other synthetic pyrethroids. ^{14}C-α-Label was 92% and 98% eliminated at 1 and 8 days respectively after oral dosing. The excreted metabolites included α-RS-decamethrin, 2′- and 4′-hydroxy-(α-RS)-decamethrin, the dibromovinyl acid and its glucuronide conjugate (a major metabolite), 3PBA (and its glycine and glucuronide conjugates), 4′HO3PBA and its sulphate (major) and glucuronide (minor) conjugates. The partial racemization at α-S is an interesting finding and merits confirmation and further investigation. Additional minor metabolites were tentatively identified as 6-hydroxydecamethrin and metabolites hydroxylated at one of the *gem*-dimethyl groups of the acid moiety. Tissue concentrations at 8 days were equivalent to less than 0·02 μg/g except for blood (^{14}C-α-label), liver (^{14}C-α-label), and fat (both labels).

The fate of ^{14}CN-label was interestingly different from that of other labels. Excretion was slower: 42% at 24 hours and 82% at 48 hours, the label being excreted as thiocyanate and 2-iminothiazolidine-4-carboxylic acid (**12**). These are well-known products of the cyanide ion in mammals (Wood and Cooley, 1956; Williams, 1959). The latter is formally a product of the reaction of CN$^-$

with cysteine or cystine but it is most unlikely to occur via such an interaction in the animal. It is more likely to be derived from mercapturic acid biosynthesis initiated through S-cyanoglutathione but terminated by cyclization at the S-substituted cysteine stage (i.e. cylization prevents N-acetylation). Some [14]CN-label was retained in the stomach and the skin. *In vitro* studies indicated that some of the decamethrin (**11**) may have been metabolized in the stomach wall. The fragment from the [14]CN-label that was slowly released from the tissue was

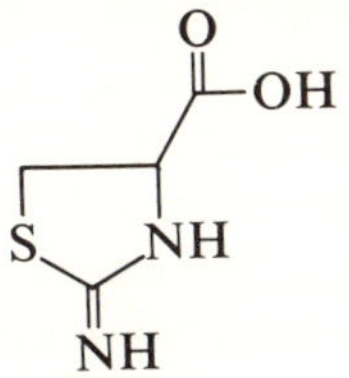

(12)

tentatively characterized as thiocyanate ion. The rather slow elimination of this ion is in accord with the suggestion that it is distributed in the extracellular fluid and is also partially bound to serum albumin (Tolbert and Hughes, 1959).

Fenvalerate

Fenvalerate (**7**) is also known as Sumitomo S5602, Shell WL 43775; it has recently reached field use (on cotton). It is α-cyano-3-phenoxybenzyl 2-(4-chlorophenyl)-3-methylbutyrate. This class of compound was first reported by

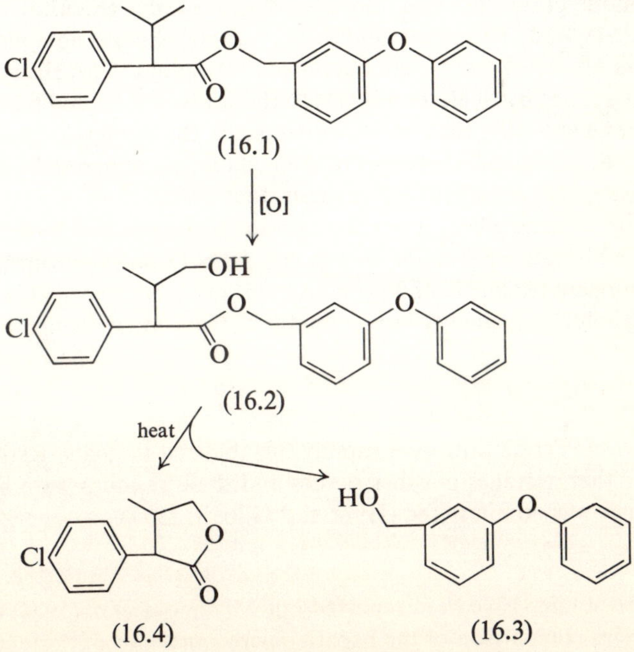

Figure 16 Cleavage of the ester bond of fenvalerate *via* oxygenation and heat

246

Ohno *et al* (1974, 1976). *In vitro* the *SαRS* isomer is oxidized but poorly hydrolysed, and the *RαRS* isomer is oxidized and hydrolysed (Soderlund and Casida, 1977a). This suggests that in terms of metabolism the *R* acid is analogous to the *trans*-dihalovinyl acid series, and the *S* acid to the *cis*-acids. The fate of the 3-phenoxybenzyl group in rats *in vivo* is similar to that in permethrin (figure 11) and cypermethrin (figure 15). *In vitro* studies on the non-cyano analogue (Sumitomo S5439) using rat and mouse liver microsomes (Soderlund and Casida, 1977b) revealed that hydroxylation of a methyl group was the most common reaction (figure 16). The hydroxyderivative (16.2) was unstable when handled unsympathetically. (e.g. gas–liquid chromatography without prior derivatization) and the reaction could be mistakenly observed as a 'hydrolysis' to 3-phenoxybenzyl alcohol (16.3). However, full product analysis, affording the γ-lactone (16.4), or trimethylsilyl-derivatization, revealed the true nature of the reaction.

SPECIES DIFFERENCES

Most of the pyrethroid metabolism studies to date have been carried out using rats. The results from the relatively few studies in other species may be briefly summarized.

Cows

Metabolism/residue studies in this species are a necessary part of the development of a modern agricultural chemical. Such studies are carried out if there is even a remote possibility that the use-pattern of the chemical may afford residues in cow feed. The compound (often radiolabelled) is administered daily and the milk and edible tissues are examined for residues. The urinary and faecal metabolites are not particularly relevant to the study of milk and tissue residues, but the experiments offer the opportunity to study the metabolic fate in a species other than rat. A preliminary report of the metabolism of permethrin (figure 11) in cows (Gaughan *et al*, 1977b) suggests that metabolism is fairly efficient; however, the 3-phenoxybenzyl portion appears to be handled rather differently compared with rat. The major metabolite is N-(3-phenoxybenzoyl)glutamic acid; the sulphate conjugate of 3-(4-hydroxyphenoxy)benzoic acid is a relatively minor metabolite. Apparently less aromatic hydroxylation occurs in cows than in rats.

Goats

cis- and *trans*-Permethrin were rapidly metabolized in goats. Residues in fat were higher than residues in other tissues and these residues were higher after the *cis*-isomer was administered (Hunt and Gilbert, 1977).

Dogs

No *in vivo* studies have been reported but Miyamoto *et al* (1974) carried out an interspecies comparison of the hepatic microsomal carboxylesterase (8,000 **g** supernatant) that hydrolyses *trans*-phenothrin (figure 10). Rat, dog, guinea-pig, rabbit, and mouse were compared. The dog preparation contained 1·3 times the activity of the rat preparation. The rate of metabolism was increased by the addition of NADPH.

Guinea-pigs

In the comparative study reported above (Miyamoto *et al*, 1974) the guinea-pig was shown to possess the highest hydrolase activity of the species studied (1·5 times that of rat).

Rabbits

No *in vivo* studies have been reported. Miyamoto *et al* (1974) reported that rabbit hepatic 8,000 **g** supernatant hydrolysed *trans*-phenothrin 1·3 times faster than that from rat. Rabbit microsomal carboxylesterase may have a much greater activity than that of the rat enzyme to *cis*-pyrethroids. When α-cyano-3-phenoxy-[^{14}C]benzyl tetramethylcyclopropanecarboxylate (figure 13) was incubated with rat or rabbit liver microsomes in the absence of cofactors for monooxygenation, the latter readily hydrolysed the substrate to 3-phenoxy-benzaldehyde at a rate several times greater than did rat microsomes (Crawford *et al*, 1978).

Mice

More than half of an oral intake of *trans*-[^{14}C-benzyl]cypermethrin (1–20 mg/kg) was eliminated in the urine of mice within 24 hours of dosing (Hutson and Casida, 1978). The major metabolite, N-(3-phenoxybenzoyl)-taurine (figure 15, 15.3), was unique to mouse (cf. rat and cow) and an appreciable amount of unconjugated 3-(4-hydroxyphenoxy)benzoic acid (4′HO3PBA) was also excreted. Several *in vitro* studies by Casida and coworkers using mouse liver microsomes have been discussed above under various compound headings. Mouse microsomes exhibit differences from rat liver microsomes in the stereo-specificity of hydroxylation at the *gem*-dimethyl group of permethrin (figure 11) (Soderlund and Casida, 1977b). In addition, aromatic hydroxylation occurs with less specificity than that with rat microsomes, affording some 5- and 6-hydroxylated metabolites (Unai and Casida, 1977).

In summary, scant though the information is, it is enough to indicate that the ester bond of the synthetic pyrethroids is as labile in other mammals as it is in the rat; hydroxylation occurs in all the species studied but with variable chemical and stereochemical specificity; the conjugation reactions of 3-phenoxybenzoic acid vary with respect to species. There is at present no information on any of these reactions in man.

THE ENZYMOLOGY OF PYRETHROID METABOLISM

Hydrolysis

The major pyrethroid-hydrolysing esterase is located in mammalian liver microsomes. The activity is probably a property of 'microsomal carboxyl-esterase' (EC 3.1.1.1). The most dramatic substrate specificity is that exhibited by *cis*- and *trans*-pyrethroid isomers, the latter being hydrolysed up to 50 times faster than the former (Casida *et al*, 1976). Liver cytosol (mouse) contains about one-fifth of the activity of microsomes and this enzyme exhibits less specificity for the two isomer classes (Soderlund, 1976). The microsomal enzyme has been solubilized from mouse liver microsomes using phospholipase A. This soluble form exhibited greater *cis/trans* specificity than the bound form (Soderlund, 1976). An effective purification of the enzyme has just been reported. The extensive studies on the isolation, purification, and properties of beef liver microsomal carboxylesterase by Krisch and coworkers (Heymann *et al*, 1974) could be a reasonable starting point for a thorough study of 'pyrethroid hydrolase'. However, a 45-fold purification of pyrethroid carboxylesterase has been effected in 38% yield from rat liver microsomes by cholic acid solubilization, ammonium sulphate fractionation, heat treatment, and DEAE-Sephadex A-50 column chromatography. The preparation appears to contain only one protein with a molecular weight of 74,000, a pH optimum of 7–9, a K_m (*trans*-phenothrin) of 0·21 mM and V_{max} 12·1. It is inhibited by insecticidal organophosphates and carbamates but it is unaffected by *p*-chloromercuribenzoate, mercuric ion, and cupric ion. It predictably hydrolyses *trans*-isomers about 10 times faster than *cis*-isomers. The protein retained a high activity towards malathion and *p*-nitrophenyl acetate, hydrolysing them both (e.g. for malathion, K_m, 1·54; V_{max}, 1,002) (Suzuki and Miyamoto, 1978).

Pyrethroid hydrolysis is inhibited by dialkyl phosphorylating agents of the type used as insecticides (organophosphorus pesticides) both *in vitro* and *in vivo*. The acute toxicity of some pyrethroids is increased by pretreatment of animals with these compounds (Abernathy *et al*, 1973; Abernathy and Casida, 1973; Casida, 1973). This interaction raises the possibility of a utilizable synergistic action of organophosphates on pyrethroids in the field (Jao and Casida, 1974b). It also raises the question of hazard to pesticide formulators and users who may be exposed simultaneously or sequentially to the two types of pesticide. This situation is by no means unlikely and therefore the possibility will be taken into account in toxicological studies on the pyrethroids.

Oxidation

The importance of oxidation in pyrethroid metabolism must not be underrated. It is certain that hydrolysis plays a major part in the detoxication of *trans*-pyrethroids but oxidation may be of paramount importance with the *cis*-isomers. Oxidative reactions occur at the cyclopropanecarboxylic acid moiety (or its equivalent), at the alcohol moiety (e.g. 3-phenoxybenzyl), and also probably in the proximity of the ester bond such that its cleavage is catalysed. The latter process may be very important with *cis*-isomers (Ueda *et et al*, 1975b; Crawford and Hutson, 1977). Oxidation at peripheral sites, while leaving the ester bond intact, affords points at which conjugation reactions occur, leading to biliary and faecal elimination of the esters. The various C-hydroxylations are probably catalysed by cytochrome P-450 but this has not been confirmed unequivocally.

The enzymology of pyrethroid metabolism is complicated by the stereo-chemistry of the substrates and the diversity of reactions occurring on the same substrate. Analysis of the various products as a function of time and protein concentrations is difficult, time-consuming, and tedious. Thus, with the exception of the hydrolysis of *trans*-phenothrin, we have no data on the K_m values, and it is difficult to assess the relative importance of the various reactions *in vivo*. Very little is known about enzyme activity, specificity, and distribution in non-hepatic tissues.

THE RELATIONSHIP BETWEEN METABOLISM AND TOXICITY

It is clear that the rate of metabolism of a pyrethroid is profoundly important to its acute toxicity (Casida *et al*, 1976). The *trans*-isomers (rapidly hydrolysed) are more rapidly eliminated and much less toxic than their *cis*-analogues. Intro-duction of the α-cyano group reduces the rate of hydrolysis and increases toxicity to some extent. The inhibition of hydrolytic reactions enhances toxicity (Aber-nathy *et al*, 1973; Miyamoto, 1976). The inhibition of oxidative metabolism also increases toxicity (Soderlund and Casida, 1977c). Pretreatment of animals with phenobarbitone to induce the hepatic microsomal monooxygenase lowers the acute toxicity of the tetramethylcyclopropanecarboxylate (13.1) (Crawford and Hutson, 1977). These facts suggest that both hydrolysis and oxidation are important in limiting acute toxicity. It should be stressed, however, that the rate of metabolism is by no means the only factor controlling acute toxicity. Both the insecticidal activity and the acute toxicity to mammals are largely features of the 1*R* acid esters as opposed to the 1*S* acid esters, yet the former are generally metabolized as rapidly as the latter (Soderlund and Casida, 1977a).

A chronic low intake of a synthetic pyrethroid is unlikely to affect the enzymes that metabolize these compounds. Pyrethrum itself is an inducer of hepatic microsomal monooxygenase in rats when given daily at 200 mg/kg, but the effect is reversible and the enzyme activities and protein concentrations return to normal within 7 days of ceasing the treatment (Springfield *et al*, 1973). Increases in liver weight have been reported in feeding studies with very high dietary levels (about 5,000 μg/g) of permethrin, resmethrin, phenothrin, fura-methrin, and allethrin (Kadota *et al*, 1976; Miyamoto, 1976). This may be of the hypertrophic type usually accompanied by microsomal enzyme induction. The response is not accepted as a toxic reaction (Hunter and Chasseaud, 1976).

Several classes of biotransformation reaction may result in the formation of reactive intermediates that may cause toxic reactions. Ruzo and Casida (1977) have considered the known biotransformations of the pyrethroids in relation to mutagenicity, a phenomenon that is often initiated by electrophilic intermediary metabolites. Vinyl group oxygenation (epoxidation) is one such biotransforma-tion. This can occur at the unsaturated side-chains of the natural pyrethrins (figure 1) and allethrin (1). It is theoretically possible at the dimethylvinyl side-chain in the acid moiety of many pyrethroids but it has not been reported. Perhaps of more concern is the dihalovinyl side-chain as in permethrin (figure

11), cypermethrin (figure 15), and decamethrin (**11**). Since the vinyl chloride issue has been widely publicized, molecules bearing even a remote resemblance to this chemical have been under scrutiny. However, in the metabolism studies so far reported, there has been no evidence of oxygenation at the dihalovinyl group. In addition, it is encouraging to note that conventional mutagenicity screening and the use of bacterial test systems (Miyamoto, 1976) have failed to reveal mutagenicity with several pyrethroids including permethrin (figure 11) (Ruzo and Casida, 1977).

CONCLUSIONS

Some general principles have emerged from the metabolic studies so far carried out on these rather complex molecules. The dominant effect of stereochemistry on metabolism is that resulting from the relative orientations of the vinyl and carboxyl groups on the cyclopropane ring (i.e. '*cis-*' and '*trans-*' isomerism). The difference is seen in rate, route, and even possibly mechanisms of metabolism. The synthetic pyrethroids are in a phase of rapid development at the moment. Increased regulation of the use of pesticides and an increased level of environmental/ecological awareness will combine to ensure that this class of pesticides will be very extensively studied. As metabolic fate plays a central role in these considerations, we can expect studies of biotransformation to be very thorough. Increasing use and extensive toxicological research will undoubtedly throw up unexpected phenomena which will require further research. The field promises to be a very active one for some years.

REFERENCES

Abernathy, C. O. and Casida, J. E. (1973), *Science*, **179**, 1235.

Abernathy, C. O., Ueda, K., Engel, J. L., Gaughan, L. C. and Casida, J. E. (1973), *Pestic. Biochem. Physiol.*, **3**, 300.

Ambrose, A. M. (1963), *Toxicol. Appl. Pharmacol.*, **5**, 414.

Ambrose, A. M. (1964), *Toxicol. Appl. Pharmacol.*, **6**, 112.

Barnes, J. M. and Verschoyle, R. D. (1974), *Nature*, **248**, 711.

Barthel, W. F. (1958), U.S. Pat. 2,857,309.

Barthel, W. F. and Alexander, B. H. (1958), *J. Org. Chem.*, **23**, 1012.

Brooks, G. T. (1973), *Chlorinated insecticides*, CRC, Cleveland, Ohio.

Casida, J. E. (1973), in Casida, J. E. (ed.), *Pyrethrum, the natural insecticide*, p. 101, Academic, New York.

Casida, J. E., Kimmel, E. C., Elliott, M. and Janes, N. F. (1971), *Nature*, **230**, 326.

Casida, J. E., Ueda, K., Gaughan, L. C., Jao, L. T. and Soderlund, D. M. (1976), *Arch. Environ. Contam. Tox.*, **3**, 491.

Crawford, M. J., Crayford, J. V., Croucher, A. and Hutson, D. H. (1978), Unpublished work.

Crawford, M. J. and Hutson, D. H. (1977), *Pestic. Sci.*, **8**, 579.

Crayford, J. V. and Hutson, D. H. (1977), Unpublished work.

Elliott, M. (1971), *Bull. W.H.O.*, **44**, 315.

Elliott, M. (1973), *Proc. of the 7th British Insecticide and Fungicide Conf.*, p. 721, Brit. Crop Prot. Council, London.

Elliott, M. (1976), *Environ. Hlth. Perspect.*, **14**, 3.

Elliott, M. (1977), in *Synthetic pyrethroids*, ACS Symposia Series No. 42, p. 1.

Elliott, M., Farnham, A. W., Janes, N. F., Needham, P. H. and Pearson, B. C. (1967), *Nature*, **213**, 493.

Elliott, M., Farnham, A. W. Janes, N. F., Needham, P. H., Pulman, D. A. and Stevenson, J. H. (1973), *Nature*, **246**, 169.

Elliott, M., Farnham, A. W., Janes, N. F., Needham, P. H. and Pulman, D. A. (1974), *Nature*, **248**, 710.

Elliott, M. and Janes, N. F. (1973), in Casida, J. E. (ed.), *Pyrethrum, the natural insecticide*, p. 56, Academic, New York.

Elliott, M., Janes, N. F., Kimmel, E. C. and Casida, J. E. (1972), *J. Agr. Food Chem.*, **20**, 300.

Elliott, M., Janes, N. F., Pulman, D. A., Gaughan, L. C., Unai, T. and Casida, J. E. (1976), *J. Agr. Food Chem.*, **24**, 270.

Eto, M. (1974), *Organophosphorus pesticides: Organic and biological chemistry*, CRC, Cleveland, Ohio.

Fujimoto, K., Itaya, N., Okuno, Y., Kadota, T. and Yamaguchi, T. (1973), *Agr. Biol. Chem.*, **37**, 2681.

Gaughan, L. C., Unai, T. and Casida, J. E. (1977a), *J. Agr. Food Chem.*, **25**, 9.

Gaughan, L. C., Unai, T. and Casida, J. E. (1977b), in *Synthetic pyrethroids*, ACS Symposia Series No. 42, p. 186.

Heymann, E., Junge, W., Krisch, K. and Marcussen-Wulf, G. (1974), *Z. Physiol. Chem.*, **355**, 155.

Hunt, L. M. and Gilbert, B. N. (1977), *J. Agr. Food Chem.*, **25**, 673.

Hunter, J. and Chasseaud, L. F. (1976), in Bridges, J. W. and Chasseaud, L. F. (eds), *Progress in drug metabolism*, vol. 1, p. 129, Wiley, London.

Hutson, D. H. and Casida, J. E. (1978), *Xenobiotica*, **8**, 565.

Jao, L. T. and Casida, J. E. (1974a), *Pestic. Biochem. Physiol.*, **4**, 456.

Jao, L. T. and Casida, J. E. (1974b), *Pestic. Biochem. Physiol.*, **4**, 465.

Kadota, T., Okuna, Y., Kohda, H. and Miyamoto, J. (1976), *Botyu-Kagaku*, **41**, 143.

Kato, T., Ueda, K. and Fujimoto, K. (1964), *Agr. Biol. Chem.*, **28**, 914.

Kuhr, R. J. and Dorough, H. W. (1976), *Carbamate insecticides: chemistry, biochemistry and toxicology*, CRC, Cleveland, Ohio.

Kulkarni, A. P., Mailman, R. B. and Hodgson, E. (1975), *J. Agr. Food Chem.*, **23**, 177.

Lhoste, J. and Rauch, F. (1969), *C. R. Acad. Sci. (Paris)*, **268**, 3218.

Lhoste, J. and Rauch, F. (1976), *Pestic. Sci.*, **7**, 247.

Masri, M. S., Jones, F. T., Lundin, R. E., Bailey, G. F. and DeEds, F. (1964), *Toxicol. Appl. Pharmacol.*, **6**, 711.

Matsuo, T., Itaya, N., Mizutani, T., Ohno, N., Fujimoto, K., Okuno, Y. and Yoshioka, H. (1976), *Agr. Biol. Chem.*, **40**, 247.

Miyamoto, J. (1976), *Environ. Hlth. Perspect.*, **14**, 15.

Miyamoto, J., Nishida, T. and Ueda, K. (1971), *Pestic. Biochem. Physiol.*, **1**, 293.

Miyamoto, J., Sato, Y., Yamamoto, K., Endo, M. and Suzuki, S. (1968), *Agr. Biol. Chem.*, **32**, 628.

Miyamoto, J., Suzuki, T. and Nakae, C. (1974), *Pestic. Biochem. Physiol.*, **4**, 438.

Nakanishi, M., Kato, Y., Furuta, T. and Miura, S. (1971), *Botyu-Kagaku*, **36**, 116.

Nakanishi, M., Mukai, T., Inamasu, S., Yamanaka, T., Matsuo, H., Taira, S. and Tsuruda, M. (1970), *Botyu-Kagaku*, **35**, 87.

Ogami, H., Yoshida, Y., Katsuda, Y., Miyamoto, J. and Kadota, T. (1970), *Botyu-Kagaku*, **35**, 45.

Ohno, N., Fujimoto, K., Okuno, Y., Mizutani, T., Hirano, M., Itaya, N., Honda, T. and Yoshioka, H. (1974), *Agr. Biol. Chem.*, **38**, 881.

Ohno, N., Fujimoto, K., Okuno, Y., Mizutani, T., Hirano, M., Itaya, N., Honda, T. and Yoshioka, H. (1976), *Pestic. Sci.*, **7**, 241.

Ruzo, L. O. and Casida, J. E. (1977), *Environ. Hlth. Perspect.*, **21**, 285.

Ruzo, L. O., Unai, T. and Casida, J. E. (1977), *Abstract of 174th ACS Meeting*, Chicago, Abstr. No. 25.

Schechter, M. S., Green, N. and LaForge, F. B. (1949), *J. Amer. Chem. Soc.*, **71**, 3165.

Soderlund, D. M. (1976), *Ph.D. thesis*, University of California, Berkeley.

Soderlund, D. M. and Casida, J. E. (1977a), *Pestic. Biochem. Physiol.*, **7**, 391.

Soderlund, D. M. and Casida, J. E. (1977b), in *Synthetic pyrethroids*, ACS Symposia Series No. 42, p. 173.

Soderlund, D. M. and Casida, J. E. (1977c), in *Synthetic pyrethroids*, ACS Symposia Series No. 42, p. 162.

Springfield, A. C., Carlson, G. P. and DeFed, J. J. (1973), *Toxicol. Appl. Pharmacol.*, **24**, 298.

Suzuki, T. and Miyamoto, J. (1974), *Pestic. Biochem. Physiol.*, **4**, 86.

Suzuki, T. and Miyamoto, J. (1978), *Pestic. Biochem. Physiol.*, **8**, 186.

Suzuki, T., Ohno, N. and Miyamoto, J. (1976), *J. Pestic. Sci. (Nippon Noyaku Gakkaishi)*, **1**, 151.

Tolbert, B. M. and Hughes, A. M. (1959), *Metabolism*, **8**, 73.

Ueda, K., Gaughan, L. C. and Casida, J. E. (1975a), *J. Agr. Food Chem.*, **23**, 106.

Ueda, K., Gaughan, L. C. and Casida, J. E. (1975b), *Pestic. Biochem. Physiol.*, **5**, 280.

Unai, T. and Casida, J. E. (1977), *J. Agr. Food Chem.*, **25**, 979.

Verschoyle, R. D. and Barnes, J. M. (1972), *Pestic. Biochem. Physiol.*, **2**, 308.

White, I. N. H., Verschoyle, R. D., Moradian, M. H. and Barnes, J. M. (1976), *Pestic. Biochem. Physiol.*, **6**, 491.

Williams, R. T. (1959), in *Detoxication mechanisms*, p. 390, Chapman and Hall, London.

Wood, J. L. and Cooley, S. L. (1956), *J. Biol. Chem.*, **218**, 449.

Yamamoto, I., Elliott, M. and Casida, J. E. (1971), *Bull. W.H.O.*, **44**, 347.

CHAPTER 5

Epoxide hydratase

F. Oesch

INTRODUCTION

The first pure chemical compounds recognized to induce cancer were synthetic dibenz[*a,h*]anthracene (Kennaway, 1930) and benzo[*a*]pyrene isolated from coal tar (Cook *et al*, 1933), both compounds being polycyclic aromatic hydrocarbons possessing no other structural features but aromatic rings. Due to the lack of chemical reactivity of these compounds, their physical interactions with cellular constituents were initially suspected to be the critical events in chemical carcinogenesis. Since these compounds were planar and of an 'appropriate' size, intercalation between base-pairs of the double-stranded DNA was the favoured mechanism, but adsorption to the exterior of the DNA helix was also suggested. However, it was soon shown that isomers of these potent carcinogens, also planar, similar in size, and consisting exclusively of aromatic rings were non-carcinogenic or much less so (for a review, see Sims and Grover, 1974).

Research of the last two decades has shed considerable light on this enigma. It was realized that many chemical carcinogens, including polycyclic aromatic hydrocarbons, need biotransformation to chemically reactive metabolites before they can exert their biological effects (for a review see Miller and Miller, 1974). The same is true for the mutagenic (Ames *et al*, 1973) and cytotoxic (Brodie *et al*, 1971) activity of many compounds.

Compounds possessing carbon–carbon double bonds, that is compounds with olefinic or aromatic structural features, are widely distributed both in our natural as well as in our man-made environment. Such compounds can be metabolized by microsomal monooxygenases to epoxides. For olefinic compounds, which are metabolized to usually fairly stable alkene oxides, this has been known for quite some time (for references see Ocsch, 1973). The first rigorous demonstration of the metabolic transformation of an aromatic compound to an arene oxide was for naphthalene (Jerina *et al*, 1968, 1970). Soon it was also shown that many carcinogenic polycyclic aromatic hydrocarbons are metabolized to epoxides (for reviews see Daly *et al*, 1972; Oesch 1973; Jerina and Daly, 1974; Sims and Grover, 1974; Heidelberger, 1975).

Due to ring tension and electronic polarization, epoxides are chemically reactive (for a review on the chemistry of epoxides see Jerina *et al*, 1973). Thus they can chemically react with and thereby irreversibly bind to many tissue constituents, including macromolecules of prime importance for the normal functioning of a cell such as DNA, RNA, and proteins. Thus, enzymes which control the concentrations of such epoxides in the tissue are very important.

Further biotransformation of such epoxides can be catalysed by epoxide hydratase (epoxide hydrase) (Oesch, 1973; Jerina and Daly, 1974; Sims and Grover, 1974) or glutathione S-transferases (Booth *et al*, 1960; Jerina *et al*, 1970; Nemoto *et al*, 1975; Arias and Jakoby, 1976). As epoxide hydratase is localized (Oesch *et al*, 1971a) in the microsomal fraction where epoxides are formed, it may be especially important for their further bioalteration and thus for the control of the tissue levels of such epoxides. On the other hand, some of the dihydrodiols formed, if derived from large polycyclic hydrocarbons, retain sufficient lipophilic character to serve again as substrates for microsomal monooxygenases. Thus dihydrodiol-epoxides may be produced, which are also capable of irreversible binding to cellular macromolecules (Sims *et al*, 1974). Epoxide hydratase may therefore play a dual role: inactivating monofunctional epoxides and providing precursor molecules for dihydrodiol-epoxide biosynthesis. This enzyme is the subject of this review.

A review on epoxide hydratase has already appeared (Oesch, 1973). Several reviews on mammalian metabolism of aromatic compounds also include epoxide hydratase (Daly *et al*, 1972; Jerina and Daly, 1974; Sims and Grover, 1974; Heidelberger, 1975; Nebert *et al*, 1975). Material already treated extensively in one of these reviews, without substantial progress in the topic since then, has been omitted (e.g. stereochemistry of epoxide hydratase reaction) or only briefly mentioned (e.g. structure–activity relationships of epoxide hydratase substrates and inhibitors with respect to substituents around the oxirane ring) in the present review.

ISOLATION OF EPOXIDE HYDRATASE IN APPARENTLY HOMOGENEOUS FORM

The major difficulties encountered in the isolation of epoxide hydratase, are all due to the fact that epoxide hydratase is a hydrophobic membrane-bound enzyme:

1. Solubilization from the membrane in an active form.
2. Separation of the mixture (obtained after precipitation and ion-exchange chromatography) which consists of many very hydrophobic components adhering tightly together.
3. Removal of the detergent used for solubilization as well as for elution during hydrophobic chromatography.

The following procedure (Bentley and Oesch, 1975), which is summarized in Table 1, led to a preparation which proved homogeneous according to four independent criteria (Bentley and Oesch, 1975; Bentley *et al*, 1975). Solubilization of epoxide hydratase from male Sprague–Dawley rat (200–250 g) liver

Table 1 Purification of rat liver epoxide hydratase

Purification step	Total protein (mg)	Specific activity*	Yield (%)	Relative purifi- cation
10,000 g supernatant fraction	49,800	1·67	100	1
Solubilized microsomes	11,454	8·91	124	5·3
Ammonium sulphate precipitate	5,184	19·15	120	11·5
DEAE–cellulose effluent	740	93·8	84	56
Cellulose phosphate effluent	80	300	29	179
n-Butyl–Sepharose effluent	21	690	17·7	415
Final preparation	15·7	516	9·8	310

* Specific activity nmoles styrene glycol per milligram protein per minute.

microsomes was effected by their resuspension in 10 mM sodium phosphate buffer, pH 7·0, containing 1% Cutscum, a non-ionic detergent. This agent had previously been found effective in solubilizing epoxide hydratase from guinea-pig (Oesch and Daly, 1971) and human (Oesch, 1974) liver microsomes. Ammonium sulphate was then added to a final concentration of 140 g/litre, and the precipitate dissolved in 5 mM sodium phosphate buffer, pH 7·0, which was dialysed against the same buffer and then applied to a DEAE–cellulose column that had been equilibrated with the same buffer. In contrast to much of the contaminating material, epoxide hydratase was not retained on the column, and the eluate therefore contained a highly purified epoxide hydratase in a relatively high yield. The fractions incorporating the active enzyme were then applied to a cellulose phosphate column which had been equilibrated with the same buffer. The detergent, containing a minor proportion of epoxide hydratase, was not retarded on the column, and the subsequent fractions which were eluted with 5 mM and 50 mM sodium phosphate buffer, pH, 7·0, contained no detectable epoxide hydratase. Epoxide hydratase was then eluted with 50 mM sodium phosphate buffer, pH 7·0, containing 0·5 M NaCl. The fact that a portion of epoxide hydratase was not retarded by this column was not due to overloading since the same portion was not retarded when reapplied to another phosphocellulose column. The observation that the ratio of specific epoxide hydratase activity towards two different substrates, styrene 7,8-oxide and benzo[*a*]pyrene 4,5-oxide, was the same in both fractions did not support the assumption that two different epoxide hydratases were present in these two fractions. Indeed, two peaks of enzyme activity eluting from an ion-exchange column do not necessarily imply the presence of two different enzyme proteins, since the charged groups of the same enzyme molecule could be masked by non-specific association with other proteins or lipids thereby causing different chromatographic properties. On the other hand, the possibility that two different epoxide hydratases are present in the two fractions is not excluded by the observation of identical ratios of specific activities in these two fractions for only two investigated substrates.

The hydrophobic character of the enzyme rendered the removal of contaminating hydrophobic proteins difficult. Therefore, an attempt was made to exploit the relative hydrophobic properties of the components of the impure preparation. Hydrophobic arms of different size and geometry were coupled to Sepharose 4B using the method of Er-el *et al* (1972) with some modifications. Selective adsorption of epoxide hydratase followed by its elution with low concentrations of detergent (0·05% Cutscum in 5 mM sodium phosphate buffer, pH 7·0) proved most satisfactory when using *n*-butyl-residues as hydrophobic arms. The detergent was then removed by chromatography on a small phosphocellulose column. This removal of the detergent at two different stages during purification was necessary since epoxide hydratase was not amenable to hydrophobic chromatography in the presence of the detergent. The final preparation was, prior to use or storage, dialysed at 0–5 °C against 50 mM sodium phosphate buffer, pH 7·0.

Figure 1 Criteria for the homogeneity of the purified epoxide hydratase. Upper part: SDS–gel electrophoresis of purified epoxide hydratase and cellulose phosphate effluent. Electrophoresis was performed in 2 mm thick slab gels containing 10% acrylamide and 0·1% SDS. The fractions shown are, from left to right, cellulose phosphate effluent 20 μg, and 0·5 μg, 1 μg, 2 μg, and 5 μg of pure epoxide hydratase. Lower part: Ouchterlony double diffusion analysis of purified epoxide hydratase. The centre well contained 7·5 μg purified epoxide hydratase. The outer wells from upper left to lower middle each contained 10 μl of (1) control serum, (2) ⅛ dilution of antiserum, (3) ¼ dilution of antiserum, (4) ½ dilution of antiserum, (5) undiluted antiserum. From Bentley *et al* (1975), reprinted by permission of North-Holland Publishing Company, Amsterdam

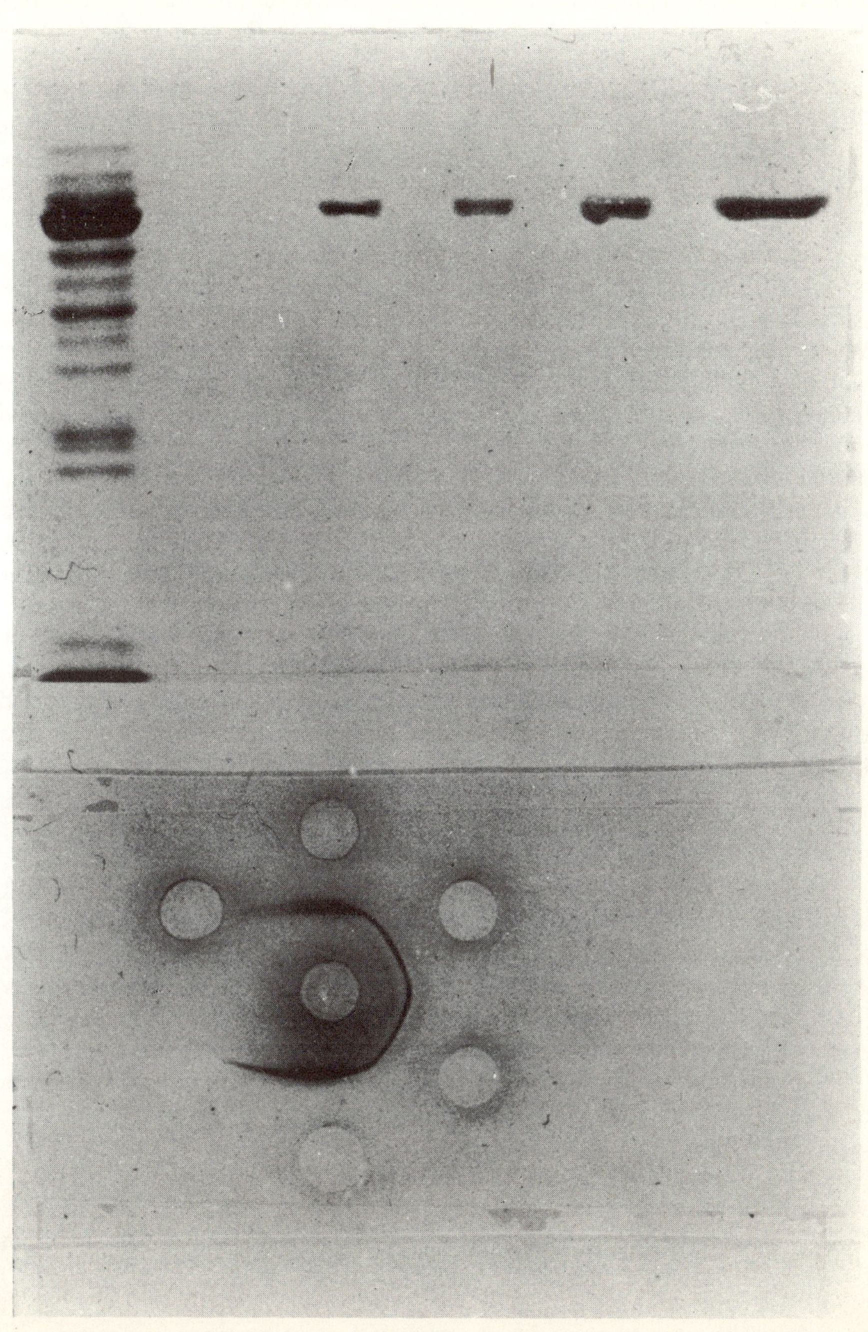

Typically, the final preparations had 510–600 units per milligram protein while the overall yield of epoxide hydratase activity was around 10% (a unit is defined as that amount of epoxide hydratase catalysing the formation of 1 nmol of styrene glycol from styrene oxide under the assay conditions described (Oesch, 1974)). During gel electrophoresis in 10% polyacrylamide gels the enzyme did not migrate into the separating gel in the absence of SDS, while in the presence of SDS one single band was observed (figure 1). Similarly, in the analytical ultracentrifuge a single band was observed in the absence of SDS with a high S_{20w} value of 14·5 while in the presence of 0·2% SDS a single symmetrical peak with a S_{20w} value of 3 was observed (protein concentration 2·5 mg/ml). Double-diffusion tests of various concentrations of the final preparation and antiserum raised against the same preparation in New Zealand White rabbits showed one single precipitation line both before (data not shown) and after staining with Coomasie blue (figure 1). Thus, the preparation appears homogeneous by SDS–electrophoretical, analytical, ultracentrifugal, and immunological criteria as well as according to the analysis of the C-terminal and N-terminal amino acid (see below).

A purification procedure by Lu and associates also led to a preparation which was characterized as homogeneous by one criterion, SDS–gel electrophoresis (Lu *et al*, 1975). Their procedure takes advantage of the fact that during purification of cytochrome P-450, there is a step where the cytochrome and epoxide hydratase separate quite clearly. Thus if pure cytochrome P-450 and pure epoxide hydratase are required, this procedure is particularly suitable.

A third method of purification of epoxide hydratase has recently been reported by Knowles and Burchell (1977). This procedure is quite rapid, but suffers from the disadvantage that the detergent remains in the final preparation.

CHARACTERIZATION OF THE PURE EPOXIDE HYDRATASE

The pure epoxide hydratase (Bentley and Oesch, 1975) has been characterized with respect to physicochemical properties, amino acid composition, and kinetics of enzyme action (Bentley *et al*, 1975) as well as substrate specificity (Bentley *et al*, 1976). Several properties of the epoxide hydratase purified by Lu *et al* (1975) were investigated by these authors, with essentially similar results (Lu *et al*, 1975, 1977).

The molecular weight of the smallest subunit of epoxide hydratase was estimated by SDS–gel electrophoresis on polyacrylamide gels. In separate experiments using two entirely different enzyme preparations, values for the molecular weight of 49,500 and 48,500 were obtained (Bentley *et al*, 1975). This indicates that the minimum molecular weight of the epoxide hydratase is 49,000, which is of the order of magnitude suggested by the sedimentation coefficient measured in the presence of 0·2% SDS of $S_{20w} = 3$. Lu *et al* (1975) reported a molecular weight of 53,000–54,000, Knowles and Burchell (1977) of 49,500. The molecular weight was estimated in the presence of standards of known molecular weight, by Lu *et al* (1975) according to the method of Neville

(1971), by Bentley and Oesch (1975), and by Knowles and Burchell (1977) according to the method of Weber and Osborn (1969). The three epoxide hydratase preparations were all from the livers of male rats, albeit from different strains: Sprague–Dawley, untreated (Bentley and Oesch, 1975); Long–Evans, phenobarbitone-pretreated (Lu *et al*, 1975); and Wistar, untreated (Knowles and Burchell, 1977). In the absence of detergent the enzyme aggregated to a very high molecular weight oligomer which sedimented with a sedimentation coefficient of $S_{20w} \sim 14.5$ and did not migrate into the separating gel during polyacrylamide gel electrophoresis (Bentley *et al*, 1975).

The absorption spectrum of pure enzyme is shown in figure 2. The extinction maximum at 280 nm and the A_{280}/A_{260} ratio of 1·46 suggest that the preparation is largely free of Cutscum, the detergent used for solubilizing the enzyme from the microsomal membrane, which has a very strong absorption with λ_{max} at 277 nm. The shoulder in the spectrum at 290 nm is indicative of the high

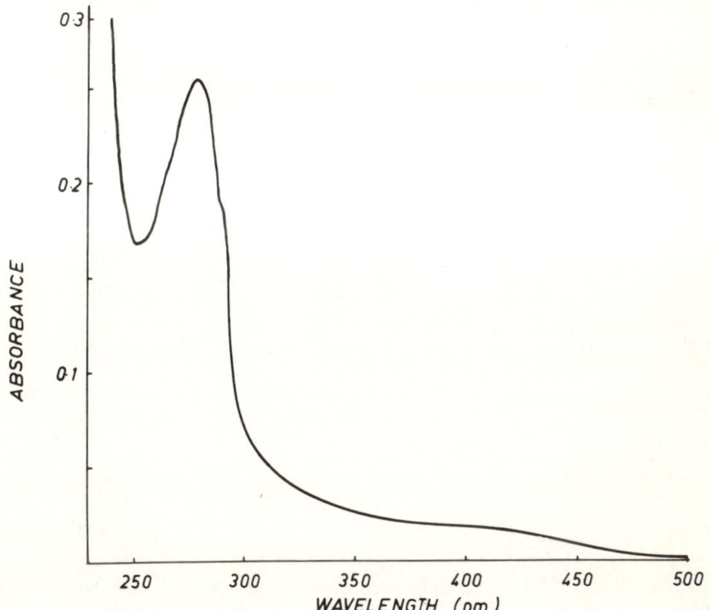

Figure 2 The absorption spectrum of epoxide hydratase. The enzyme was dissolved in filtered 5 mM sodium phosphate buffer, pH 7·0, at a protein concentration of 0·14 mg/ml and measured at 25 °C. From Bentley *et al* (1975), reprinted by permission of North-Holland Publishing Company, Amsterdam

tryptophan content as demonstrated by the amino acid analysis shown in Table 2. The amounts of tryptophan and tyrosine estimated from the enzyme spectrum were slightly lower than those estimated chemically, which confirms the detergent-free character of the preparation. The small but significant absorption between 500 nm and 300 nm accounts for the fact that enzyme solutions with a protein concentration of 2–3 mg/ml are a faint yellow colour (Bentley *et al*, 1975; see also Lu *et al*, 1975).

Table 2 summarizes the results of the amino acid analysis of pure epoxide hydratase. The residues per monomer were calculated from the % contribution of the single amino acids to the entire protein by assuming 43 glutamate (Glx) residues. Based on this assumption, in the range of molecular weights from 10,000 to 100,000, the sum of total deviations from integral numbers of the single residues was a minimum for a molecular weight of 48,300–49,000

Table 2 Amino acid analysis of epoxide hydratase*

| | Residues per monomer† | | | |
Residue	Hydrolysis time (hours) 24	144	Values from extrapolation or from other methods	Integral values
Lysine	32·1	32·1		32
Histidine	13·5	13·3		13–14
NH₃	36·2	44·3	34·8‡	(<35)
Arginine	19·1	18·5		19
Aspartate (Asx)	28·7	28·9		29
Threonine	19·3	18·8	19·4‡	19
Serine	31·8	29·5	32·1‡	32
Glutamate (Glx)	43·0	43·0		43
Proline	25·7	24·3		24–26
Glycine	33·5	33·6		33–34
Alanine	18·1	18·2		18
Half-cystine	3·3	2·0	3·6‡ 4·8§	4–5
Valine	20·3	23·0		23‖
Methionine	12·0	10·5	8·6** 12·2§	12
Isoleucine	19·6	21·8		22‖
Leucine	41·7	41·8		42
Tyrosine	22·4	22·6	22·0¶	23
Phenylalanine	25·5	26·1		26
Tryptophan			8·3* 7·1¶	7–8
			Total	421–427

* From Bentley *et al* (1975), reprinted by permission of North-Holland Publishing Company, Amsterdam.

† Analysis involves ±5% error.

‡ Subject to time-dependent deviation from true value. Value obtained by extrapolation to zero hydrolysis time.

§ Determined by performic acid oxidation.

‖ Acid-resistant residues, results based on the value after 144 hours hydrolysis time.

¶ Determined spectrophotometrically.

** Determined with 5% thioglycolic acid.

which is in agreement with the minimum molecular weight of 49,000 as determined by SDS–gel electrophoresis. The integer values are based on extrapolation to zero hydrolysis time for acid-labile amino acid residues (threonine, serine, cysteine, tyrosine), on values after 144 hours hydrolysis for acid resistant residues (valine, isoleucine), and on average values for the rest of the residues.

As shown in Table 2, there is a relatively high content of aromatic amino acids and hydrophobic amino acids. The hydrophilic amino acids lysine, histidine, arginine, aspartic acid, asparagine, threonine, serine, glutamic acid, and glutamine account for only 44% of the sum of amino acid residues of the protein. This hydrophobic character could account for the aggregation of the protein in the absence of detergents. The partial specific volume of the protein calculated from the amino acid analysis is 0·740–0·742 ml/g at 25 °C (Bentley *et al*, 1975). The amino acid composition was also analysed by Lu *et al* (1975). After correction for the approximately 10% higher molecular weight estimated by Lu *et al* (1975) compared to Bentley and Oesch (1975), the number of individual amino acid residues estimated by the two groups agree fairly well. Deviations from the average are not larger than ±5% for most of the amino acids and not larger that ±10% for the remainder (tryptophan, threonine, serine, alanine, methionine).

No N-terminal amino acid could be detected as [^{14}C]-dinitrofluorobenzene or phenylthiohydantoin derivatives implying that the terminal residue at the end of the monomer opposite to the C-terminal does not have a free α-amino group. Free C-terminal amino acids were detected by some but not all methods, indicating the presence of a free C-terminal amino acid and allowing some conclusions with respect to its chemical nature. Digestion with carboxypeptidases A and B and hydrazinolysis did not result in detectable amounts of free amino acids. Carboxypeptidase Y digestion, however, resulted in the liberation of a considerable number of amino acids. Carboxypeptidase P digestion liberated only threonine and asparagine or glutamine. Since hydrazinolysis would be expected to detect C-terminal threonine it may be concluded that the C-terminal amino acid of epoxide hydratase is either asparagine or glutamine (Bentley *et al*, 1975).

The pure epoxide hydratase preparation is exceedingly stable. There was no detectable loss of activity (measured with styrene oxide and benzo[*a*]pyrene 4,5-oxide as substrates) throughout 2 months' storage at 0 °C (in an ice bath) in 50 mM sodium phosphate buffer, pH 7·0. Similarly an enzyme solution at a concentration of 0·23 mg/ml in 10 mM sodium phosphate buffer, pH 7·0 was completely stable for 5 hours at 37 °C and showed less than 10% inactivation when maintained at room temperature (25 °C) for 24 hours (Bentley *et al*, 1975).

The pH optimum of the purified enzyme was estimated in 0·125 M Tris buffer over a pH range from 8·0 to 10·0, in 0·1 M sodium phosphate buffer between pH 7·0 and pH 10·0 and in 0·05 M glycine buffers between pH 9·0 and pH 10·0 with 2 mM styrene oxide as substrate (Bentley *et al*, 1975). Non-enzymic hydration rates were less than 10% over the entire pH range studied. The pH optimum in Tris buffer was at pH 8·9 and that in sodium phosphate buffer at pH 9·0. In glycine buffer the optimum pH appeared to be somewhat higher, at pH 9·4.

Epoxide hydratase activity did not appear to depend on the ionic strength of the medium. Thus, the activity of the enzyme was not affected by variations in the Tris buffer concentrations at pH 8·9 from 0·025 M to 0·375 M. Lu *et al* (1977) determined the pH optimum of their purified preparation with a range of substrates. Optima as different as pH 7·4 for benzo[a]pyrene 4,5-oxide and pH 8·9 for benzo[a]pyrene 7,8-oxide and benzo[a]pyrene 9,10-oxide were observed.

A double reciprocal plot of the variation of the initial specific rate with substrate (styrene oxide) concentration was linear throughout the range of substrate concentrations used (0·2–6 mM) at protein concentrations between 8 and 31 μg/ml. An apparent K_m of 0·67 nM with a maximum specific rate of 800 nmol styrene glycol formed per minute per milligram protein was obtained (pure enzyme, no lipid added). The maximum specific rate suggests a turnover number of 40 molecules of styrene glycol produced per minute per molecule of epoxide hydratase using a molecular weight of 49,000 (Bentley *et al*, 1975). Lu *et al* (1977) investigated the effect of dilauroyl phosphatidyl choline on the apparent K_m value of the purified enzyme for benzo[a]pyrene 11,12-oxide as substrate. In the absence of added lipid or in its presence at a concentration below the critical micelle concentration, the observed K_m remained constant at various enzyme concentrations. However, when the lipid concentration exceeded the critical micelle concentration, the apparent K_m increased with increasing lipid concentrations, consistent with partition of the lipid-soluble substrate between the lipid micelle and the aqueous environment.

The pure epoxide hydratase was active with a wide variety of substrates including arene and alkene oxides (Bentley *et al*, 1976; Lu *et al*, 1977). However, the possibility remained that some other possibly more important epoxide hydratase enzyme(s) were removed during the purification. Antibodies were therefore raised in rabbits against the pure epoxide hydratase isolated from rat liver (Oesch and Bentley, 1976). These antibodies precipitated epoxide hydratase activity towards both styrene oxide and benzo[a]pyrene 4,5-oxide. This precipitation, which was dose-dependent, occurred when antiserum was incubated with either the pure enzyme or the crudest soluble preparation (solubilized microsomes). At the higher concentrations of antiserum, the immunoprecipitation was complete (Oesch and Bentley, 1976). This could be taken to indicate the presence of one single enzyme responsible for the hydration of the two substrates. On the other hand, some alternative explanations cannot be excluded, such as the presence of several epoxide hydratases with immunological cross-reactivity or differential but complete inactivation of some epoxide hydratase species during solubilization of the microsomes. However, although the extent of inhibition of epoxide hydratase activity by antiserum was different in microsomes (20–30%) as compared to soluble preparations (70–80%), the inhibition was always similar ($\pm$ less than 10% of the mean) towards the two substrates. Moreover, the relative potency of low molecular weight epoxide hydratase inhibitors remained essentially the same throughout purification. This was true for either of the two substrates. Finally, only one single side-fraction during purification had detectable epoxide hydratase activity towards either of the two substrates. The ratio of the specific activities towards the two substrates was the same in this single side-fraction as in the fraction containing the bulk of epoxide hydratase activity (Bentley and Oesch, 1975). Taken together these findings very strongly suggest that rat liver microsomal fractions contain a single epoxide hydratase which catalyses the hydration of substrates with structures as different as benzo[*a*]pyrene 4,5-oxide and styrene oxide, and that this is the enzyme purified to homogeneity. This does not exclude the existence of other epoxide hydratases for classes of epoxides which were not investigated.

ROLE OF EPOXIDE HYDRATASE IN THE CONTROL OF MUTAGENIC METABOLITES DERIVED FROM POLYCYCLIC AROMATIC HYDROCARBONS AND TOXICOLOGICAL CONSEQUENCES OF DIFFERENT EPOXIDE HYDRATASE ACTIVITIES IN DIFFERENT ANIMAL SPECIES

Role

The epoxide hydratase purified to homogeneity according to four independent criteria (see p. 258) was used as a tool to investigate the role of the enzyme in the control of mutagenic metabolites derived from polycyclic aromatic hydrocarbons.

To study this role several model compounds were used. As a typical example the results obtained with benzo[*a*]pyrene will be discussed here. Benzo[*a*]pyrene was activated by liver microsomes from C3H mice to mutagens reverting *his Salmonella typhimurium*. Inhibitors, homogeneous epoxide hydratase, different *his Salmonella typhimurium* strains, the mutagenicity assessment of benzo[*a*]-pyrene metabolites in the absence of microsomes, and the activation of benzo-[*a*]pyrene and benzo[*a*]pyrene metabolites by microsomes possessing different forms of monooxygenase were used as tools (Glatt, 1976; Oesch and Glatt, 1976; Oesch *et al*, 1976; Oesch *et al*, 1977a).

Benzo[*a*]pyrene as such is not mutagenic for *Salmonella typhimurium* but is transformed to mutagenically active metabolites by liver microsomes in the presence of a NADPH generating system (figure 3).

When microsomes from *non-treated* mice were used, the number of revertant colonies from *Salmonella typhimurium* strain TA 1537 could be increased 3-fold by addition of epoxide hydratase inhibitors such as cyclohexene oxide or 1,1,1-trichloropropene oxide (Oesch *et al*, 1971b) to the activating system (figure 3). In contrast to the situation discussed below (microsomes from 3-methylchol-anthrene-pretreated animals), this increase was observed at all benzo[*a*]pyrene concentrations used. Addition of pure epoxide hydratase to the activating system reduced the mutagenicity of benzo[*a*]pyrene towards TA 1537 and TA 98 (figure 4). The extent of this reduction depended upon the amount of epoxide hydratase added. At high epoxide hydratase concentrations, the mutagenicity towards TA 1537 was reduced by more than 95% while about 25% of the mutagenicity towards TA 98 was resistant to epoxide hydratase.

When benzo[*a*]pyrene was incubated with microsomes from *phenobarbitone-induced* mice, the results obtained were similar to those obtained with microsomes from non-treated animals. The mutagenicity of benzo[*a*]pyrene towards both TA 1537 and TA 98 was increased by addition of trichloropropene oxide (data not shown) and decreased by addition of epoxide hydratase (figure 4).

However, in this case epoxide hydratase was unable to lower completely the number of revertant colonies from TA 1537 or from TA 98 to the number arising spontaneously. Under conditions where further addition of epoxide hydratase no longer reduced the number of revertant colonies, at least 10% of the benzo[a]pyrene-induced TA 1537 revertant colonies persisted.

A completely different situation was observed when microsomes from 3-*methylcholanthrene-treated* mice were used in the activating system. The

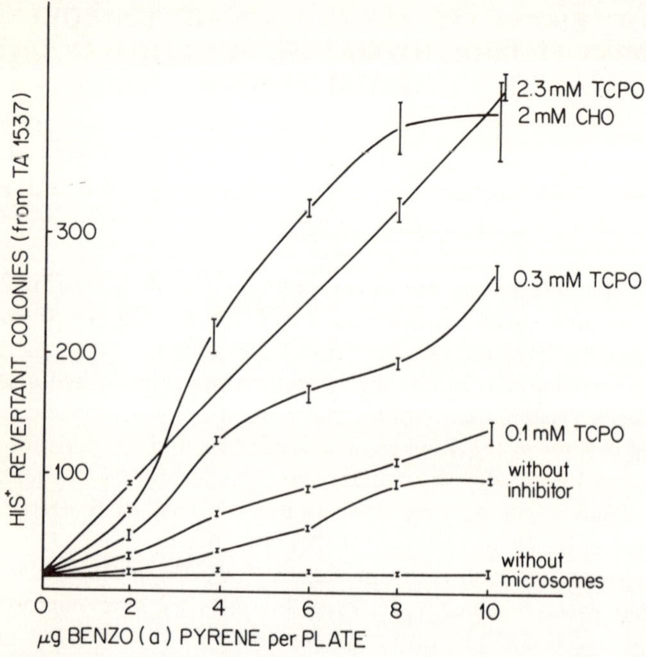

Figure 3 Activation of benzo[a]pyrene to a mutagen: potentiation by epoxide hydratase inhibitors. Number of *his⁺* revertant colonies from *Salmonella typhimurium* Ta 1537 as a function of benzo[a]pyrene concentration in the presence or absence of a microsomal preparation from female C3H mouse liver, and epoxide hydratase inhibitors: 1,1,1-trichloropropene 2,3-oxide (TCPO) or cyclohexene oxide (CHO). The concentrations indicated are calculated with respect to the top agar. Bars represent the standard error of the mean. From Oesch and Glatt (1976), reprinted by permission of IARC, Lyon

dependence of the reversion of TA 1537 on the benzo[a]pyrene concentration was unlike that observed when control microsomes were used in the activating system (compare figures 5 with figures 3). The initial slope was much steeper and the maximum was reached at much lower benzo[a]pyrene concentrations. These differences cannot be explained simply by quantitative differences in the monooxygenase activity of the activating systems because the optimal benzo-[a]pyrene concentration was independent of the amount of microsomal protein (0·1–1·5 mg protein per plate). Thus they must reflect qualitative differences in benzo[a]pyrene metabolism which occur upon induction of the monooxygenases by 3-methylcholanthrene. With 3-methylcholanthrene-induced microsomes, the epoxide hydrase inhibitor 1,1,1-trichloropropene oxide had a complex effect upon the mutagenicity: the number of revertant colonies was reduced at low benzo[a]pyrene concentrations and increased at high benzo[a]pyrene concentrations (figure 5). The addition of pure epoxide hydratase had less marked effects upon the number of revertant colonies when microsomes from 3-methylcholanthrene-treated mice were used than when microsomes from phenobarbitone-treated or untreated mice were used (figure 4). Both increases and decreases in the mutagenic effect were observed depending upon the amount of

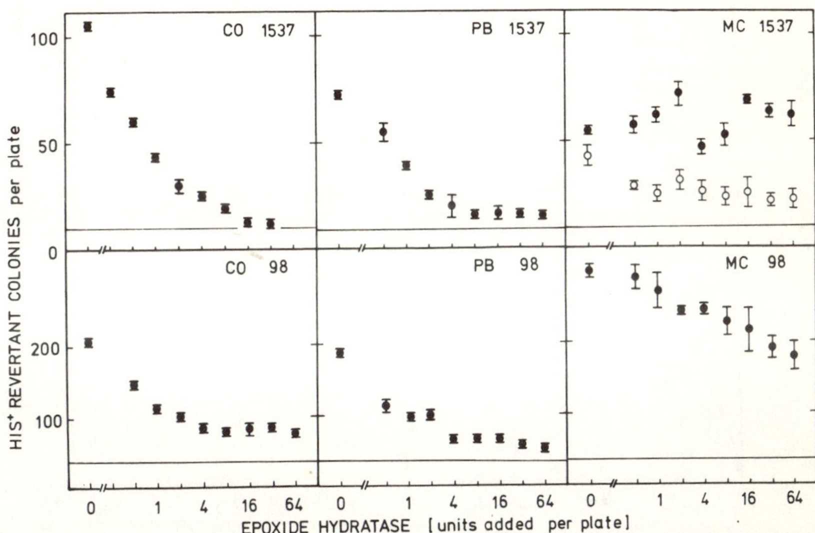

Figure 4 Effect of homogeneous epoxide hydratase on the number of *Salmonella typhimurium* revertant colonies induced by metabolically activated benzo[a]pyrene. 'CO' = control, liver microsomes from untreated C3H mice; 'PB', same after pretreatment with 80 mg/kg phenobarbitone; 'MC', same after pretreatment with 40 mg/kg 3-methylcholanthrene; 1537 = *S. typhimurium* strain TA 1537; 98 = TA 98. Horizontal lines represent the mean of the number of revertant colonies arising spontaneously. Units of epoxide hydratase defined as that amount which catalyses formation of 1 nmol styrene glycol per minute. From Oesch (1977), reprinted by permission of Editio Cantor, Aulendorf

microsomal protein added, the benzo[a]pyrene concentration, and the amount of epoxide hydratase added. Decreases in the mutagenic effect were seen at high benzo[a]pyrene concentrations or with low levels of microsomal protein while increases in the mutagenic effect were seen when low concentrations of benzo[a]pyrene or high concentrations of microsomal protein were used (figure 5). If a constant benzo[a]pyrene concentration was used, increasing amounts of epoxide hydratase had a multiphasic effect upon the mutagenicity (figure 4). Even at very high epoxide hydratase concentrations a considerable proportion of the mutagenicity remained.

Wood *et al* (1976a) tested the effect of their purified epoxide hydratase preparation on the mutagenicity of benzo[*a*]pyrene metabolites generated by a reconstituted system consisting of highly purified cytochrome P-448, NADPH cytochrome c reductase, and phosphatidyl choline. 3-Methylcholanthrene is known to induce cytochrome P-448 (Conney *et al*, 1973; Nebert *et al*, 1975). As observed during metabolic activation of benzo[*a*]pyrene with liver microsomes from 3-methylcholanthrene-pretreated animals (see above), this system containing purified cytochrome P-448 led to a high proportion of mutagenically

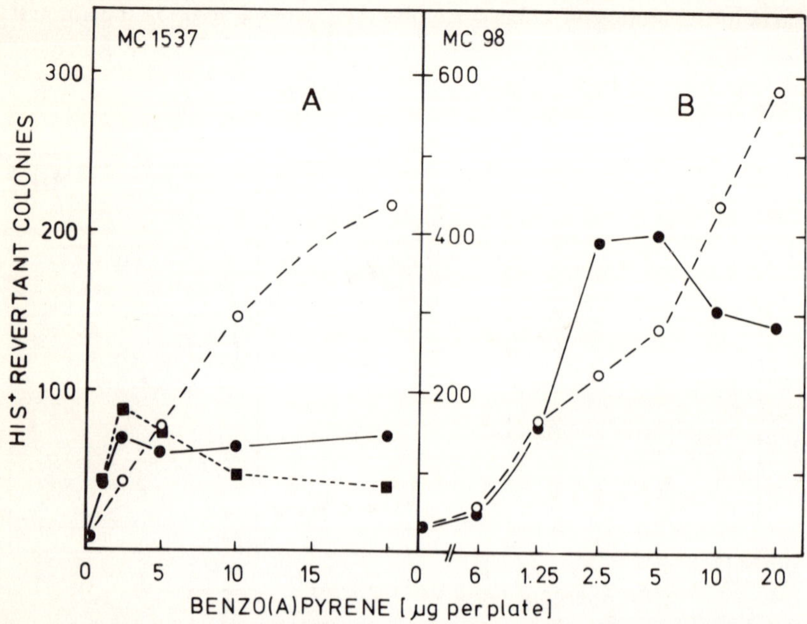

Figure 5 Activation of benzo[*a*]pyrene by microsomes from methylcholanthrene-treated mice: effect of benzo[*a*]pyrene concentration. The number of *his*+ revertant colonies from *his Salmonella typhimurium* TA 1537 (A) and TA 98 (B) is shown as a function of benzo[*a*]pyrene concentration (— ● —). The same incubations were performed in the presence of the epoxide hydratase inhibitor 1,1,1-trichloropropene 2,3-oxide (2·3 µmol/plate) (— ○ —) and pure epoxide hydratase (32 units/plate) (— ■ —). Values represent means of 2 incubations. Deviations from the means were always less than 10%. From Bentley *et al* (1977), reprinted by permission of Springer-Verlag, Heidelberg

active benzo[*a*]pyrene metabolites which were resistant to epoxide hydratase, presumably 7,8-dihydrodiol-9,10-epoxides, since the mutagenicity of these diol-epoxides was virtually unaffected by epoxide hydratase, while that of the preimmediate precursor of 7,8-dihydrodiol-9,10-epoxides, the 7,8-oxide, was potently increased by epoxide hydratase. Moreover, the immediate precursor, the *trans*-7,8-dihydrodiol, but not its analogue in which the 9,10-double bond is reduced (Levin *et al*, 1977), is converted by this reconstituted system containing cytochrome P-448 to metabolite(s) which efficiently revert the *Salmonella* mutants.

From these results two conclusions may be drawn:

1. The pattern of mutagenic metabolites produced from benzo[*a*]pyrene by an activating system containing microsomes from 3-methylcholanthrene-treated mice or by a reconstituted system containing purified cytochrome P-448 was very different from that produced by activating systems containing microsomes from control or phenobarbitone-treated mice.

2. In each different situation at least two different metabolites contributed to the mutagenicity.

When liver microsomes from *untreated* mice were used in the activating system, most of the mutagenicity was prevented by addition of pure epoxide hydratase. This epoxide hydratase-sensitive mutagenicity must be caused by monofunctional arene oxides or their non-enzymic reaction products (e.g. phenols). The only potent mutagen among all the monofunctional arene oxides, phenols, and dihydrodiols formed from benzo[*a*]pyrene is benzo[*a*]pyrene 4,5-oxide (Wood *et al*, 1975; Glatt and Oesch, 1976; Oesch and Glatt, 1976). In this situation (microsomes from untreated animals), the parent hydrocarbon was much more efficiently activated to mutagens detected by TA 1537 than were the known phenols and dihydrodiols (Oesch and Glatt, 1976). Moreover, the ratio of the number of revertant colonies from TA 98 to those from TA 1537 (R 98/1537) was very similar to that obtained using benzo[*a*]pyrene-4,5-oxide (1·5 compared to 1·6) (Bentley *et al*, 1977). These results therefore strongly suggest that benzo[*a*]pyrene 4,5-oxide was the main contributor to the epoxide hydratase-sensitive mutagenicity. Benzo[*a*]pyrene 4,5-oxide is also a relatively good substrate for epoxide hydratase with a low apparent K_m value (Bentley *et al*, 1976; Lu *et al*, 1977). The mutagenic metabolites which were not removed by epoxide hydratase were detected much more readily by TA 98 than by TA 1537 (R 98/1537 > 10). This mutagenicity could be caused by phenols which are weakly mutagenic towards TA 98 (Glatt and Oesch, 1976; Wislocki *et al*, 1976a) and by dihydrodiol-epoxides, but was not pronounced enough to allow further investigation.

When liver microsomes from *phenobarbitone-induced* mice were used in the activating system, the results were similar to those obtained using control microsomes. The number of revertant colonies of both strains was markedly reduced by addition of epoxide hydratase. However, the ratio R 98/1537 in the presence of epoxide hydratase was less when phenobarbitone-induced microsomes were used, indicating that the pattern of mutagenic metabolites was not identical under both conditions (Bentley *et al*, 1977).

Marked changes in the metabolic activation of benzo[*a*]pyrene to mutagens were obtained when liver microsomes from *3-methylcholanthrene-treated* rats were used in the activating system. The optimum benzo[*a*]pyrene concentration was decreased, the effect of epoxide hydratase and epoxide hydratase inhibitors was more complex, and the ratio R 98/1537 was increased.

The low optimal benzo[*a*]pyrene concentration could be explained by either production of toxic metabolites killing the bacteria or two steps in the activation, whereby benzo[*a*]pyrene inhibited the second step. The former explanation is unlikely since the optimum did not shift towards higher benzo[a]pyrene concentrations when the amount of microsomal protein was reduced, a situation which would be expected to produce fewer toxic metabolites. Moreover, the production of dihydrodiol-epoxides from benzo[a]pyrene does require two oxidation steps. Since dihydrodiol-epoxides are known to be strong mutagens (Huberman *et al*, 1976; Newbold and Brookes, 1976; Thakker *et al*, 1976; Wislocki *et al*, 1976b; Wood *et al*, 1976b), the latter explanation is more probable. In the presence of the epoxide hydratase inhibitor 1,1,1-trichloropropene oxide, when dihydrodiol formation was practically zero, the dependence of the mutagenicity upon the benzo[a]pyrene concentration was similar to that obtained using control microsomes. This supports the assumption that the low optimum benzo[a]pyrene concentration obtained using microsomes from 3-methylcholanthrene-treated mice is the result of activation of metabolically produced dihydrodiols.

A significant contribution of dihydrodiol-epoxides towards the mutagenicity when benzo[a]pyrene was activated by microsomes from 3-methylcholanthrene-treated mice would account for the effects of epoxide hydratase and epoxide hydratase inhibitors. Epoxide hydratase is required to produce the dihydrodiols from benzo[a]pyrene. Consequently inhibition of the hydratase would reduce the amount of dihydrodiol available for further oxidation. Similarly, addition of hydratase to the activating system would increase the amount of dihydrodiol available. Wood *et al* (1976a) have shown that addition of epoxide hydratase to an activating system containing highly purified cytochrome P-448 greatly increased the mutagenicity of benzo[a]pyrene 7,8-oxide towards TA 98, indicating that benzo[a]pyrene 7,8-dihydrodiol-9,10-oxide is more mutagenic than benzo[a]pyrene 7,8-oxide. The results of Bentley *et al* (1977) showed that at low benzo[a]pyrene concentrations with an activating system containing microsomes from 3-methylcholanthrene-treated mice, the addition of epoxide hydratase increases the mutagenic effect of benzo[a]pyrene and inhibition of epoxide hydratase decreases the mutagenic effect. Furthermore, the ratio R 98/1537 when benzo[a]pyrene was activated by 3-methylcholanthrene-induced microsomes was similar to that obtained when benzo[a]pyrene 7,8-dihydrodiol was activated by liver microsomes. Addition of epoxide hydratase had no effect upon the mutagenicity of the metabolically activated 7,8-dihydrodiol. These results, therefore, strongly suggest that the further oxidation of metabolically formed dihydrodiols contributed predominantly to the overall mutagenicity when microsomes from 3-methylcholanthrene-treated mice were used to activate benzo[a]pyrene. 3-Methylcholanthrene induced the benzo[a]pyrene monooxygenase activity strongly. The induced enzyme oxidizes benzo[a]pyrene more in the 7,8- and 9,10-positions than the constitutive enzymes which preferentially oxidize the 3- and 4,5-positions (Holder *et al*, 1974; Rasmussen and Wang, 1974; Wiebel *et al*, 1975). Pretreatment of animals with 3-methylcholanthrene also enhanced the activation of benzo[a]pyrene 7,8-dihydrodiol (Bentley *et al*, 1977) and a reconstituted system containing purified cytochrome P-448 was much more efficient in this activation than purified cytochrome P-450 (Levin *et al*, 1977). This induction of two sequential reactions in the activation pathway may explain the potent effect of 3-methylcholanthrene pretreatment upon the metabolic activation of benzo[*a*]pyrene.

Dihydrodiol-epoxides cannot, however, be the sole contributors to the mutagenicity of benzo[*a*]pyrene activated by microsomes from 3-methylcholanthrene-treated mice because at high benzo[*a*]pyrene concentrations the mutagenicity is partially sensitive to epoxide hydratase. Under these conditions the further oxidation of the primary metabolites would be inhibited by high concentrations of the first substrate, benzo[*a*]pyrene. The mutagenicity is probably caused by a mixture of K-region and non-K-region epoxides since the ratio R 98/1537 was larger than expected for the K-region oxide (benzo[*a*]pyrene 4,5-oxide) alone.

Thus the activation of benzo[*a*]pyrene to mutagens is very complex, and great differences are found when different activating systems are used. Fundamentally different effects of epoxide hydratase were observed in the presence of different forms and amounts of monooxygenase and different benzo[*a*]pyrene concentrations. Several activating pathways contribute to the mutagenicity. These pathways are not independent but interconnected by a limited number of enzymes, primarily monooxygenase and epoxide hydratase.

Interestingly, benzo[*a*]pyrene 7,8-oxide was the most active of the three benzo[*a*]pyrene-derived arene oxides tested (the 4,5-, 7,8-, and 9,10-oxide) for carcinogenicity in mice by topical application to the skin, although much less active than benzo[*a*]pyrene itself (Levin *et al*, 1976a), and the *trans*-7, 8-dihydrodiol was much more active, inducing a 100% tumour incidence at the dose level used; the same dose of benzo[*a*]pyrene also induced a 100% tumour incidence (Levin *et al*, 1976b).

Consequences

Epoxide hydratase activity varies quite remarkably between different organs (Oesch *et al*, 1977b) and animal species (Walker *et al*, 1978). In the light of the results discussed above, it would seem probable that such differences in epoxide hydratase activity are very important contributing factors in controlling tissue concentrations of epoxides which are substrates of this enzyme, and that this factor should be taken into account when attempting to relate experimental data to human risk.

Accumulation of mutagenically reactive benzo[*a*]pyrene metabolites by liver microsomes from animal species possessing different epoxide hydratase activities proved very different (Oesch and Glatt, 1976). Other factors such as differences in monooxygenase were, of course also contributing.

In the presence of a system generating NADPH (the cofactor necessary for monooxygenase activity), benzo[*a*]pyrene was activated by liver preparations from all mammalian species and strains investigated, to metabolites mutagenic for *Salmonella typhimurium* TA 1537 and TA 98, but the extent of increase in the number of revertant colonies differed drastically for the various species and strains. As an example, it can be seen in figure 6 that the maximal increase in

the number of revertant colonies is 1·7-fold with respect to spontaneous muta-
tions when benzo[*a*]pyrene is activated by liver microsomes from untreated
Sprague–Dawley rats, but more than 20-fold by liver microsomes from untreated
C3H mice. The 1·7-fold increase using Sprague–Dawley rat microsomes was
statistically highly significant ($P < 0.01$), but would, according to widespread
practice, not be considered 'biologically' significant—a positive assignment of
'mutagenic' generally only being attributed to substances increasing the number
of revertant colonies by at least 2-fold. Increasing the amount of benzo[*a*]pyrene
above the maximum shown in figure 6 did not lead to a further increase in

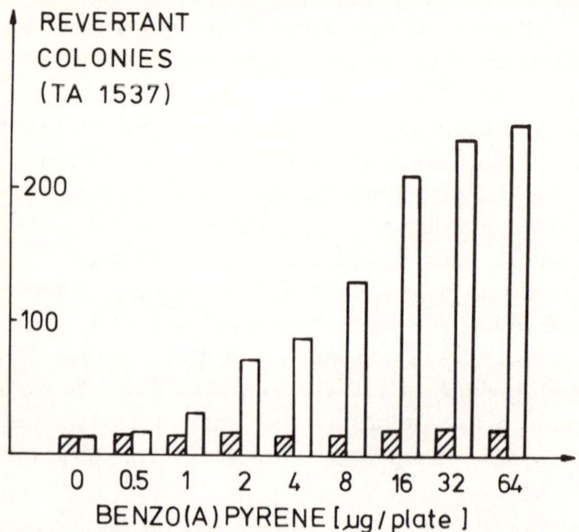

Figure 6 Activation of benzo[*a*]pyrene to mutagenic metabolites by rat and mouse
liver microsomes. The number of *his*+ revertant colonies from *Salmonella typhimurium*
TA 1537 is shown. Hatched bars represent activation by Sprague–Dawley rat microsomes, open bars by C3H mouse microsomes. Values are means of 2–4 incubations.
From Oesch *et al* (1977c), reprinted by permission of Springer-Verlag, Heidelberg

mutagenicity (data not shown). Thus one of the most powerful carcinogens
known, benzo[*a*]pyrene, might have been dismissed as non-mutagenic when
tested as an unknown using as activating system liver microsomes from untreated male Sprague–Dawley rats which possess high epoxide hydratase and
rather modest monooxygenase activity (Table 3) (Oesch and Glatt, 1976).

However, when using liver microsomes from Sprague–Dawley rats which
had been pretreated with Arochlor 1254 the situation was very different. Arochlor
1254 induces a wider spectrum of monooxygenase forms (Alvares *et al*, 1973;
Ryan *et al*, 1977) than the more classical types of monooxygenase inducers
whose prototypes are phenobarbitone, 3-methylcholanthrene, and pregnenolone
16α-carbonitrile (Conney *et al*, 1973). Therefore one of the schedules recommended by Ames *et al* (1975) for routine mutagenicity screening uses liver
microsomes from rats pretreated with Arochlor 1254. Arochlor 1254 induction
may indeed be expected to lead to a liver preparation which increases the

sensitivity of the liver enzyme mediated bacterial mutagenicity test towards many compounds, but the opposite may occur in cases where the control monooxygenases form more potent mutagens than the induced monooxygenases. Moreover, it is important to realize that Arochlor 1254 also induces epoxide hydratase (Oesch *et al*, 1977b). When liver microsomes from Arochlor 1254-pretreated Sprague–Dawley rats were used for metabolic activation of benzo-[*a*]pyrene, the increase in mutation rate was very high (Oesch *et al*, 1977c). The same was observed after 3-methylcholanthrene pretreatment (see below). Thus metabolically activating systems possessing different patterns of activating and inactivating enzymes may lead to very drastically different accumulations of mutagenically active metabolites. This may occur to the extent that an obviously extremely powerful mutagen when activated by a liver preparation from a particular species or strain may be apparently a non-mutagen when using an activating system from a different species or strain.

Epoxide hydratase activity (with styrene oxide as substrate) is lower in liver microsomes from untreated C3H mice compared to Sprague–Dawley rats by a factor of about 7, monooxygenase activity (with benzo[*a*]pyrene as substrate) is higher by a factor of about 2 (Table 3). Both factors would be expected to lead to a higher accumulation of intermediate epoxides in the former species. Thus, the much higher number of revertant colonies during metabolic activation of benzo[*a*]pyrene by liver microsomes from C3H mice as compared to Sprague–Dawley rats appears quite logical. However, very many other parameters will also be different between microsomal preparations from two different species. If the difference in mutagenic potential were in fact causally linked to these differences in enzyme patterns, it should be possible to compensate for them by enzyme modulations. Inhibition of epoxide hydratase in Sprague–Dawley rat liver microsomes indeed led to a large potentiation of the mutagenic effect (figure 7 and Table 3). This was true for two quite different types of epoxide hydratase inhibitors: cyclohexene oxide, a moderately potent inhibitor of the non-competitive type, and 1,1,1-trichloropropene 2,3-oxide, an extremely potent inhibitor of the uncompetitive type (Oesch *et al*, 1971b). Both inhibitors were used at concentrations where no influence on monooxygenase activity (with benzo[*a*]pyrene as substrate) was observed.

From the data in figure 8 and Table 3, it can be seen that an increase in monooxygenase activity in the liver microsomes from Sprague–Dawley rats due to pretreatment of the animals with the inducer 3-methylcholanthrene also leads to a very substantial potentiation of the mutagenic effect. However, the situation with respect to monooxygenases is complex. While inhibitor and antibody studies indicated the existence of only a single epoxide hydratase catalysing the hydration of both styrene oxide and benzo[*a*]pyrene 4,5-oxide (Oesch and Bentley, 1976) (and quite likely of many other epoxides), several different monooxygenase forms exist. They possess overlapping but quantitatively quite different specificities for attack of large molecules at different positions (Lu *et al*, 1972; Nebert *et al*, 1973; Holder *et al*, 1974; Rasmussen and Wang, 1974; Haugen *et al*, 1975; Wiebel *et al*, 1975). Thus modulation of monooxygenase

Table 3 Enzyme activities in the liver microsomes used for the mutagenicity experiments shown in figure 6–8*

Activity data corresponding to experiment of figure number indicated	Species and strain	Modulator	Epoxide hydratase†	Monooxygenase‡
6	Rat (Sprague–Dawley)	none	7·2 ± 0·2	410 ± 32
	Mouse (C3H)	none	1·0 ± 0·1	850 ± 54
7	Rat (Sprague–Dawley)	none	9·8 ± 0·7	364 ± 41
	Rat (Sprague–Dawley)	2·4 mM cyclohexene oxide (*in vitro*)	1·2 ± 0·6	390 ± 66
	Rat (Sprague–Dawley)	0·36 mM 1,1,1-trichloropropene oxide (*in vitro*)	0·8 ± 0·5	421 ± 24
8	Rat (Sprague–Dawley)	none	7·5 ± 0·4	429 ± 36
	Rat (Sprague–Dawley)	3-methylcholanthrene (*in vivo* pretreatment)§	7·6 ± 0·5	1780 ± 60

* Values represent means ± SEM of 4–6 incubations (duplicate determinations at 2–3 protein concentrations).
† nmoles Styrene glycol formed per minute per milligram protein.
‡ pmoles 3-Hydroxybenzo[*a*]pyrene fluorescence equivalents per minute per milligram protein.
§ Treated rats received a single intraperitoneal injection of 3-methylcholanthrene (10 mg/kg) in sunflower oil 3 days before sacrifice.

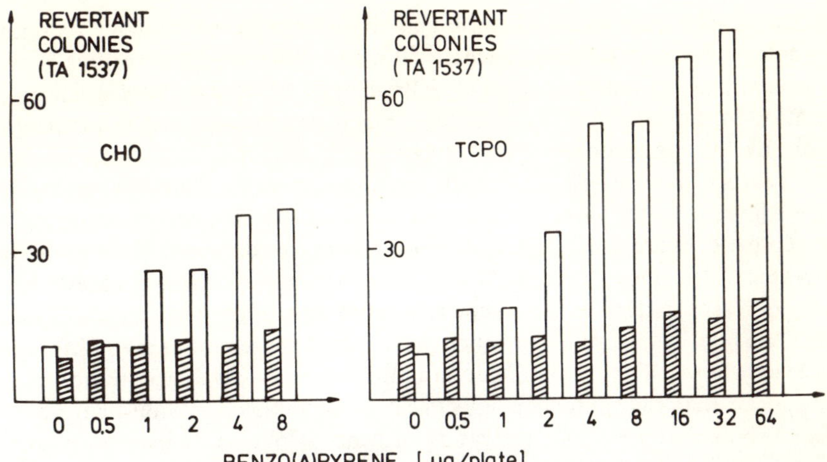

Figure 7 Activation of benzo[a]pyrene by Sprague–Dawley rat liver microsomes to mutagenic metabolites: effect of epoxide hydratase inhibitors. The open bars show the effect of the epoxide hydratase inhibitors cyclohexene oxide (2·4 mM in the top agar, CHO) and 1,1,1-trichloropropene 2,3-oxide (0·36 mM, TCPO). The hatched bars represent the number of revertant colonies in the absence of the inhibitors. Values are means of 2–4 incubations. From Oesch *et al* (1977c), reprinted by permission of Springer-Verlag, Heidelberg

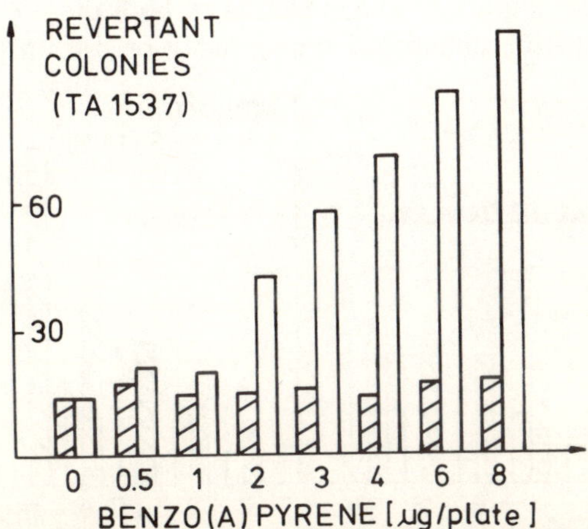

Figure 8 Activation of benzo[a]pyrene to mutagenic metabolites: effect of enzyme induction by 3-methylcholanthrene. Benzo[a]pyrene was activated to mutagenic metabolites by liver microsomes from untreated male Sprague–Dawley rats (hatched bars) or from rats that had been pretreated intraperitoneally with 10 mg/kg of 3-methylcholanthrene in sunflower oil and killed 3 days later (open bars). Values represent means of 2–4 incubations. From Oesch *et al* (1977c), reprinted by permission of Springer-Verlag, Heidelberg

will not simply lead to an alteration in the rate of production of oxidative metabolites, because different agents will affect differently the various monooxygenase forms (Conney *et al*, 1973; Ullrich *et al*, 1975) and thereby lead to an alteration of the pattern of metabolites. Thus metabolic activation of benzo[*a*]pyrene by liver microsomes from untreated or phenobarbitone-induced C3H mice ('cytochrome P-450-dependent monooxygenases') leads to mutagenic benzo[*a*]pyrene metabolites the majority of which are efficiently inactivated by pure epoxide hydratase while liver microsomes from 3-methylcholanthrene-pretreated C3H mice ('cytochrome P-448-dependent monooxygenases') form a very different pattern of mutagenically active benzo[*a*]pyrene metabolites on which epoxide hydratase has a much weaker and more complex (multiphasic) effect (see above). Thus, an increase in monooxygenase activity does not necessarily mean that the mutagenic effect will be potentiated. While figure 8 and Table 3 show that metabolic activation of benzo[*a*]pyrene by liver microsomes from 3-methylcholanthrene-treated rats leads to a potentiation of the mutagenic effect as compared to control microsomes, figure 9 and Table 4 show that pretreatment with a dose of phenobarbitone leading to a similar increase in 'overall' monooxygenase activity (in this experiment determined with 7-ethoxycoumarin as substrate) caused a decrease, rather than an increase in mutagenicity. This underlines the importance of keeping the complexity of such systems in mind. Phenobarbitone induces a pattern of monooxygenase forms which differ greatly from the forms induced by 3-methylcholanthrene. Moreover, the dose of 3-methylcholanthrene used in this study did not bring about any change in epoxide hydratase activity, but that of phenobarbitone led to a considerable increase in epoxide hydratase. The induction of both those enzymes would be expected to lead to the diminished mutagenicity of benzo[*a*]pyrene activated

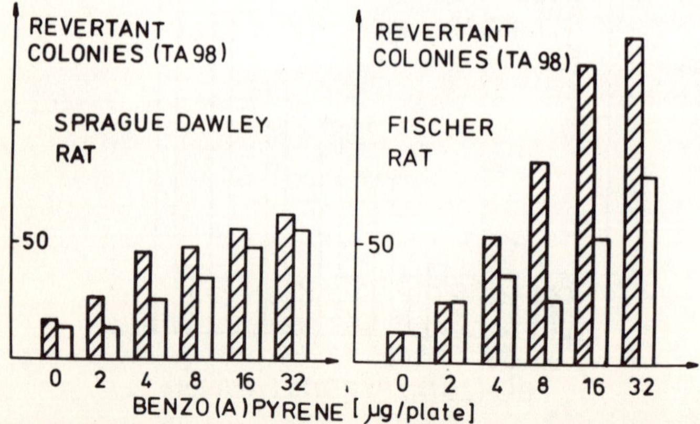

Figure 9 Activation of benzo[*a*]pyrene to mutagenic metabolites by rat liver postmitochondrial supernatant fraction: effect of enzyme induction by phenobarbitone. Hatched bars represent the mutagenicity in the presence of the postmitochondrial supernatant fraction from untreated male rats, open bars from rats that had been pretreated intraperitoneally with 80 mg/kg phenobarbitone in 0·9% NaCl on the 4th, 3rd, and 2nd day before sacrifice. Values represent means of 2 incubations. From Oesch *et al* (1977c), reprinted by permission of Springer-Verlag, Heidelberg

Table 4 Microsomal enzyme activities of the livers used for the mutagenicity experiments shown in figures 9 and 10*

Activity data corresponding to experiment of figure number indicated	Species and strain	Pretreatment†	Epoxide hydratase‡	Monooxygenase§ in presence of modifier			
				None	Metyrapone 10^{-5} M	7,8-Benzo-flavone 2×10^{-5} M	Tetrahydrofuran 10^{-2}
9	Sprague–Dawley rat	none	7.4 ± 0.3	372 ± 40 (100%)	344 ± 41 (93%)	451 ± 62 (122%)	104 ± 11 (28%)
9 and 10	Sprague–Dawley rat	phenobarbitone	13.3 ± 0.7	1210 ± 66 (100%)	593 ± 52 (49%)	1310 ± 110 (108%)	448 ± 36 (37%)
9	Fischer rat	none	3.2 ± 0.2	414 ± 12 (100%)	369 ± 50 (90%)	504 ± 65 (123%)	123 ± 16 (30%)
9 and 10	Fischer rat	phenobarbitone	10.7 ± 0.5	1640 ± 200 (100%)	623 ± 41 (38%)	1870 ± 210 (114%)	1017 ± 82 (62%)
10	CF-1 mouse	none	2.7 ± 0.3	900 ± 40 (100%)	693 ± 44 (77%)	855 ± 62 (95%)	423 ± 21 (47%)
10	CF-1 mouse	phenobarbitone	2.3 ± 0.1	2410 ± 110 (100%)	988 ± 58 (41%)	2220 ± 160 (92%)	1010 ± 88 (42%)

* Values represent means $\pm$ SEM of four incubations (duplicate determinations at two different protein concentrations).
† Phenobarbitone-treated animals received intraperitoneal injections of phenobarbitone (80 mg/kg body weight in 0.9% NaCl on the 4th, 3rd, and 2nd days before sacrifice.
‡ nmoles 4,5-Dihydroxy-4,5-dihydrobenzo[a]pyrene formed per milligram protein per minute.
§ pmoles 7-Hydroxycoumarin formed per milligram protein per minute.

by microsomes from the phenobarbitone-treated (figure 9) as compared to 3-methylcholanthrene-treated rats (figure 8), and this was observed to be true.

The influence of these enzyme activities on the relative accumulation of mutagenically reactive benzo[a]pyrene metabolites was also observed using other *Salmonella* mutants as detector strains, liver postmitochondrial supernatant instead of microsomes as the metabolically activating system, other rat and mouse strains as sources of the liver preparations, and other substrates for epoxide hydratase and monooxygenase (Oesch *et al*, 1977c). Thus the importance of these enzyme activities for the dramatic differences in the relative accumulation of mutagenically active benzo[a]pyrene metabolite appears to be general. Moreover, three diagnostic inhibitors (metyrapone, 7,8-benzoflavone, and tetrahydrofuran) (Ullrich *et al*, 1975) were used as a crude measure of the different monooxygenase forms present. *Salmonella typhimurium* TA 98 was reverted 3-fold but TA 1537 only 1·7-fold, by benzo[a]pyrene metabolically activated by liver postmitochondrial supernatant from untreated Sprague–Dawley rats (compare figure 9 and figure 6). When the same metabolic activation was performed with liver postmitochondrial supernatant from Fischer rats, the mutation rate in TA 98 was considerably higher (9-fold as compared to 3-fold with respect to the spontaneous rate) (figure 9). Table 4 shows that the 'overall' monooxygenase activity (with 7-ethoxycoumarin as substrate) as well as the contributions of the various monooxygenase forms are similar for the two strains. Only the epoxide hydratase is markedly lower in Fischer rats than in Sprague–Dawley rats. The higher accumulation of mutagenically active metabolites from benzo[a]pyrene by the liver preparation from Fischer rats is in line with their lower epoxide hydratase activity. Phenobarbitone pretreatment leads to a similar induction of 'overall' monooxygenase activity in the two strains and the contribution of the various monooxygenase forms is not drastically different between the two strains after phenobarbitone induction. However, epoxide hydratase is increased more in the strain with the lower constitutive activity than in the other strain, leading to similar epoxide hydratase activities in the two strains after phenobarbitone pretreatment. Accordingly, the differences in mutagenicity also virtually disappear (figure 9).

The differences in enzyme activities are much less between Fischer rats and CF-1 mice after phenobarbitone induction than was the case between untreated Sprague–Dawley rats and C3H mice (compare Tables 3 and 4). Accordingly, the differences in mutagenicity are also much less (compare figure 10 with figure 6). If, in addition, epoxide hydratase activity is inhibited by 1,1,1-trichloropropene oxide, the rather small difference in monooxygenase activity which persists is now accompanied by an accordingly smaller difference in mutagenicity (figure 10).

Thus the differences between species and strains in enzymes activating compounds to electrophilically reactive metabolites and in enzymes inactivating such metabolites invariably lead to differences in the potential of tissue preparations from such species or strains to mediate mutagenic effects of compounds which are substrates of these enzymes. For lipophilic compounds whose active forms are metabolically produced epoxides which are substrates for epoxide hydratase, liver preparations of several mouse strains (e.g. C3H, CF-1) will lead to an accumulation of such epoxides to an extent much higher than many other mammalian species because those strains have high monooxygenase and very low epoxide hydratase activities. In some cases where dihydrodiol-epoxides of an especially high reactivity due to location of the epoxide ring at a bay region

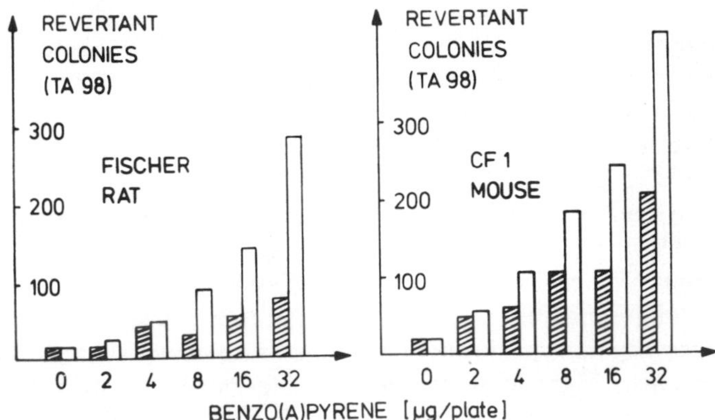

Figure 10 Activation of benzo[*a*]pyrene by liver postmitochondrial fraction of phenobarbitone-treated rats and mice. The open bars represent the mutagenicity when the epoxide hydratase inhibitor 1,1,1-trichloropropene 2,3-oxide was added to the top agar at a concentration of 1 mM. The hatched bars show the mutagenicity in the absence of the inhibitor. Values represent means of 2 incubations. From Oesch *et al* (1977c), reprinted by permission of Springer-Verlag, Heidelberg

can be formed (Jerina and Daly, 1977), epoxide hydratase will have both activating and inactivating properties (Bentley *et al*, 1977). However, with the majority of aromatic and olefinic compounds of pharmaceutical and industrial interest, it is to be expected that epoxide hydratase plays a simple inactivating role. Since man has a much higher epoxide hydratase activity (Oesch *et al*, 1974) than any of the many investigated mice strains (Oesch *et al*, 1973a), it is to be expected that mice are much more susceptible to toxic effects which are mediated by metabolically produced epoxides which are substrates for epoxide hydratase than man, at least for compounds large and lipophilic enough to preclude efficient inactivation by glutathione (Glatt *et al*, 1977). Whether a metabolically produced epoxide will be a substrate for epoxide hydratase can also be predicted for several structural features, since structure–activity relationships have been studied for rodent and human hepatic epoxide hydratase (Oesch, 1974), which may allow more rational design of such drugs which essentially need for their intended properties structural moieties which are metabolically epoxidized.

SELECTIVE INDUCTION OF EPOXIDE HYDRATASE

Rationale

From the results discussed in the preceding section it becomes evident that in mammalian enzyme-mediated bacterial *in vitro* mutagenicity test systems, epoxide hydratase plays a crucial role in the control of the relative concentrations of mutagenically active epoxides which are substrates of the enzyme. Enormous variations in mutagenicity of the same compound from negligible to very potent can frequently be explained by differences in epoxide hydratase activities in the animal species used as source for the *in vitro* metabolizing system.

Do these *in vitro* mutagenicity results have implications with respect to *in vivo* differences in susceptibility of these different animal species to the carcinogenic effect of compounds metabolized via epoxides? To assess this, animals similar in all respects except for epoxide hydratase activity would be helpful. We therefore set out to develop a selective inducer of epoxide hydratase. This task appeared to be very difficult because of the ease with which the monooxygenase system is induced by such different compounds as barbiturates, hormones, insecticides, or carcinogens (Conney, 1967; Remmer, 1972) and by a great number of environmental factors (Vesell *et al*, 1976). Moreover, all epoxide hydratase inducers discovered thus far also induce the monooxygenase system, suggesting that epoxide hydratase and a rate-limiting entity of the monooxygenase system might be under common biosynthetic control. However, in a recent study on transplacental induction of epoxide hydratase and benzo[*a*]-pyrene monooxygenase activities, the latter could be selectively induced in the foetal liver (Oesch, 1976). This finding gave rise to the hope that a selective induction of epoxide hydratase should also be possible. The most likely class of compounds were speculated to be epoxides for which, because they are monooxygenase products or product mimics, little or no affinity to the monooxygenase system, or to the receptor(s) responsible for its induction would be anticipated. However, the receptor(s) responsible for epoxide hydratase induction might be expected to possess a high affinity for them. Therefore in order to find a selective epoxide hydratase inducer a series of structurally varying epoxides was tested.

Effects of Epoxides with varying Structures on Epoxide Hydratase and Monooxygenase Activities

Epoxides which were good substrates of epoxide hydratase turned out not to be epoxide hydratase inducers (Schmassmann *et al*, 1978). This lack of epoxide hydratase induction may be due to their fast hydration by the enzyme. A receptor responsible for epoxide hydratase induction may on the one hand share with the enzyme active site a specificity for epoxides, but on the other hand the affinity and intrinsic activity of such a receptor towards an epoxide may depend on structural features different to those required for a good substrate of the enzyme. Therefore epoxides similar to non-competitive epoxide hydratase inhibitors as well as poor substrates were tested (Schmassmann *et al*, 1978). When rats were treated with the two cyclohexene oxide derivatives 4-vinyl-cyclohexene dioxide and exo-2,3-epoxynorbornane as well as after treatment with 16α,17α-epoxypregnenolone, the liver epoxide hydratase activities were never significantly different from controls. On the other hand, after treatment with these compounds the benzo[*a*]pyrene monooxygenase activity was decreased to 40–70% of the control values.

However, treatment with a low dose (20 mg/kg) of the poor epoxide hydratase substrate dieldrin caused an induction of liver epoxide hydratase to about 170% of control activity without a significant increase of the benzo[*a*]pyrene monooxygenase activity. But twice the dose (40 mg dieldrin/kg) induced also the benzo[*a*]pyrene monooxygenase activity to 170% of control activity (after 3 days). These results indicate that epoxide hydratase can be preferentially induced by dieldrin compared to benzo[*a*]pyrene monooxygenase but only in a narrow range of low doses (see also Vainio and Parkki, 1976).

After treatment with another poor epoxide hydratase substrate, *trans*-stilbene oxide, the epoxide hydratase activities in liver microsomes increased dose-dependently up to 350% of controls, whereas none of the given doses had a significant effect on the benzo[*a*]pyrene monooxygenase activity. Treatment with *trans*-stilbene oxide up to the dose required for maximal epoxide hydratase induction (400 mg/kg per day for 3 days) had no apparent harmful effects on the rats, but after a single intraperitoneal injection of 1,000 mg *trans*-stilbene oxide/kg, the animals showed signs of convulsions.

The effect of treatment with all these epoxy compounds was also followed in rat kidney and lung (Schmassmann *et al*, 1978), because the biosynthetic control of epoxide hydratase in these organs, which are important target organs for certain toxins, may be different from that in the liver. However, as in the liver, most of the epoxides tested had no effect on epoxide hydratase activities in kidney and lung. The exceptions were 4-vinylcyclohexene dioxide, which caused a 30% decrease of epoxide hydratase activities in both organs, and *trans*-stilbene oxide, which was most striking in that it induced epoxide hydratase activities in kidney up to 300% of controls whereas in the lung no induction was observed. In fact in the lung a slight decrease of epoxide hydratase activity (70–90% of controls) was apparent.

Effects of *Trans*-Stilbene Oxide Derivatives on Epoxide Hydratase and Monooxygenase Activities

Various *trans*-stilbene oxide derivatives were synthesized in order to find an even more potent selective epoxide hydratase inducer. However, all these derivatives were less effective epoxide hydratase inducers than the parent compound (Table 5). Moreover, most of them induced also the benzo[*a*]pyrene monooxygenase activity when determined either fluorimetrically ('3-OH-BP') or radiometrically 'overall'). The chlorinated derivatives were most potent in this respect. The more chlorine atoms the *trans*-stilbene oxide derivatives contained, the lower were the epoxide hydratase activities and the higher the benzo[*a*]pyrene monooxygenase activities compared to the enzyme activities after treatment with *trans*-stilbene oxide itself (Schmassmann *et al*, 1978).

Treatment with 2,2′,4,4′-tetrachloro-*trans*-stilbene oxide caused a decrease of epoxide hydratase activity in the liver to 25% of control activity within 3

Table 5 Effect of *trans*-stilbene oxide derivatives on rat liver epoxide hydratase and benzo[a]pyrene monooxygenase activities*

Compound (mmoles/kg body weight)		Epoxide hydratase†		BP monooxygenase†	
		Styrene oxide	BP-4,5-oxide	'Overall'	'3-OH-BP'
trans-Stilbene oxide (TSO)	(0·2)	153	147	114	111
trans-Stilbene oxide (TSO)	(0·5)	173	170	97	90
trans-Stilbene oxide (TSO)	(2·0)	321	295	112	100
4-Methoxy-TSO	(0·5)	145	128	185	132
4-Chloro-TSO	(0·5)	171	150	195	146
4,4′-Dichloro-TSO	(0·5)	n.d.‡	122	220	140
2,2′,4,4′-Tetrachloro-TSO	(0·5)	n.d.	25	370	340
4-Nitro-TSO	(1·5)	133	129	150	128
Diethylstilboestrol α,β-oxide	(0·3)	153	133	32	34
Diethylstilboestrol diacetate					
αβ-oxide	(0·3)	150	141	27	33
trans-Stilbene	(0·2)	120	110	100	90
trans-Stilbene	(2·0)	154	144	57	31

* Male Sprague–Dawley rats (180–240 g) were treated by a daily intraperitoneal injection of the indicated dose in 0·5 ml sunflower oil for 3 days and were killed at 24 hours after the last treatment. Control animals received sunflower oil alone.

† Enzyme activities are expressed as a percentage of the control activities which were (in nmoles product per milligram protein per minute) $7·21 \pm 1·02$ for epoxide hydratase with styrene oxide and $6·65 \pm 0·76$ with benzo[a]pyrene 4,5-oxide as substrate and $0·287 \pm 0·04$ for benzo[a]pyrene monooxygenase as 3-hydroxybenzo[a]pyrene fluorescence equivalents and $5,260 \pm 1,230$ cpm per milligram protein per minute as overall tritium release.

‡ n.d. = not determined.

days when determined with benzo[*a*]pyrene 4,5-oxide as substrate. This decrease was most probably not due to the presence of 2,2′,4,4′-tetrachloro-*trans*-stilbene oxide or metabolites of it in the microsomes, since mixtures of liver microsomes from 2,2′,4,4′-tetrachloro-*trans*-stilbene oxide-pretreated animals always gave—after preincubation for 10 minutes with control microsomes—additive enzyme activities. Moreover, addition of 2,2′,4,4′-tetrachloro-*trans*-stilbene oxide to the incubation mixture up to 5-fold the substrate concentration caused no significant inhibition of epoxide hydratase activity. These observations indicate a repression of the enzyme by this compound. On the other hand, 2,2′,4,4′-tetrachloro-*trans*-stilbene oxide induced the benzo[*a*]pyrene monooxygenase activities more than 3-fold. Because of this lack of selectivity, the repressing effect of this compound on epoxide hydratase activity cannot be utilized in studies on the mechanism of tumour formation caused by compounds which are activated via epoxides.

In order to investigate whether for the induction of epoxide hydratase by *trans*-stilbene oxide, the overall *trans*-stilbene structure or the epoxide moiety or both were critical, animals were treated with *trans*-stilbene. A comparison of the augmentations of the epoxide hydratase activities after pretreatment with equimolar amounts showed that *trans*-stilbene oxide was at least 4-fold more potent than *trans*-stilbene. This higher potency may be due to a higher affinity of the receptor responsible for the induction of epoxide hydratase, for *trans*-stilbene oxide or to the need for *trans*-stilbene to be oxidized to *trans*-stilbene oxide before it can exert its inducing effect, or to pharmacokinetic differences between the two molecules with respect to the availability of the ultimate inducer at the receptor. A marked difference between *trans*-stilbene oxide and *trans*-stilbene was also observed with respect to the benzo[*a*]pyrene mono-oxygenase activities. At a dose where *trans*-stilbene oxide showed no effect (Table 5), *trans*-stilbene treatment caused a decrease of the benzo[*a*]pyrene monooxygenase activities to 31% controls (Schmassmann *et al*, 1978).

It was also interesting to test the oxide of the structurally related clinically used oestrogenic compound diethylstilboestrol. Diethylstilboestrol α,β-oxide and diethylstilboestrol diacetate α,β-oxide showed about the same potency—but not selectivity—as epoxide hydratase inducers as *trans*-stilbene oxide. Treatment with relatively low doses (0·3 mmol diethylstilboestrol α,β-oxide or diethylstilboestrol diacetate α,β-oxide/kg per day for 3 days) caused an induction of epoxide hydratase activity in the liver to about 140–150% of controls, but at the same time these compounds decreased the benzo[*a*]pyrene monooxygenase activities to about 30% of controls. This very marked reduction of the mono-oxygenase activities is most probably due to an *in vitro* effect of diethylstilboestrol α,β-oxide present in the liver microsomes, since this compound proved to be a potent inhibitor of benzo[*a*]pyrene monooxygenase activities *in vitro* (Schmass-mann *et al*, 1978).

Thus, all modifications of the *trans*-stilbene oxide molecule led to compounds which, firstly, were less potent epoxide hydratase inducers than the parent compound, and, secondly, changed (increased or decreased) the benzo[*a*]pyrene monooxygenase activities.

282

Trans-stilbene oxide induced the epoxide hydratase activities in the kidney but not in the lung. An examination was made of whether the kidney epoxide hydratase activities showed the same differences as the liver epoxide hydratase activities in their response to pretreatment with the various *trans*-stilbene oxide derivatives and whether lung epoxide hydratase activities could possibly be induced by one of these compounds. The kidneys and lungs were taken from the same rats as the livers. The effect of the *trans*-stilbene oxide derivatives on kidney epoxide hydratase activities was considerably different from that in the liver (compare Tables 5 and 6). *Trans*-stilbene and 4,4′-dichloro-*trans*-stilbene oxide were about 3-fold more potent epoxide hydratase inducers in the kidney than in the liver, whereas *trans*-stilbene oxide was less effective. Pretreatment with 2,2′,4,4′-tetrachloro-*trans*-stilbene oxide, which decreased liver epoxide hydratase to 25% of control, slightly induced this enzyme in kidney. Diethyl-stilboestrol α,β-oxide and the corresponding diacetate had no apparent effect on kidney epoxide hydratase activity as determined with benzo[a]pyrene-4,5-oxide as substrate, which is in contrast to their inducing ability in the liver. In the lung all the *trans*-stilbene oxide derivatives tested showed a similar slightly reducing effect on epoxide hydratase activities. The different effect of *trans*-stilbene oxide treatment on epoxide hydratase activities in rat liver, kidney, and lung suggests that there is a different biosynthetic control of the enzyme in these organs, if the exposure of the responsible receptor in these organs to the ultimate inducing species is the same. Moreover, the different ratios of the epoxide hydratase induction in liver to the induction in kidney after treatment with various *trans*-stilbene oxide derivatives can be taken to indicate a direct effect of these compounds or their metabolites in the corresponding organs, rather than an induction mechanism via a central target such as the pituitary gland. However, a combined central and peripheral effect of these *trans*-stilbene derivatives cannot be excluded. Furthermore, the high correlation of epoxide hydratase activities when determined either with benzo[a]pyrene 4,5-oxide or with styrene oxide as substrate after treatment with widely varying compounds suggests that at least those structural elements of the active site of the induced and the control epoxide hydratase which are important for catalysis cannot be very different.

Selectivity of Epoxide Hydratase Induction by *Trans*-Stilbene oxide and its Limitations

From a great variety of different epoxides tested, *trans*-stilbene oxide was the only inducer satisfactory in terms of selective epoxide hydratase induction with no change in benzo[a]pyrene monooxygenase activity. This selectivity was therefore investigated more thoroughly for this compound in the liver by monitoring the preferentially cytochrome P-450-dependent and phenobarbitone-inducible aminopyrine N-demethylase, the predominantly cytochrome P-448 (P_1-450)-dependent and polycyclic hydrocarbon-inducible benzo[a]pyrene monooxygenase, the NADPH-cytochrome c reductase and the cytochrome P-450 content. These parameters were followed over a prolonged period of time

Table 6 Effect of *trans*-stilbene oxide and related compounds on kidney and lung epoxide hydratase activity of male rats*

Compound tested (mmoles/kg body weight)		Kidney		Lung	
		Styrene oxide†	BP-4,5-oxide†	Styrene oxide†	BP-4,5-oxide†
trans-Stilbene oxide (TSO)	0·2	92	108	n.d.‡	n.d.‡
trans-Stilbene oxide (TSO)	2·0	147	161	71	82
4,4′-Dichloro-TSO	0·5	n.d.†	176	n.d.	80
2,2′,4,4′-Tetrachloro-TSO	0·5	n.d.	126	n.d.	51
trans-Stilbene	0·2	127	111	n.d.	n.d.
trans-Stilbene	2·0	249	230	n.d.	n.d.
Diethylstilboestrol α,β-oxide	0·3	n.d.	81	n.d.	85
Diethylstilboestrol-diacetate α,β-oxide	0·3	n.d.	95	n.d.	86

* Male Sprague–Dawley rats (180–240 g) were treated by a daily intraperitoneal injection of the indicated dose in 0·5 ml sunflower oil for 3 days and were killed at 24 hours after the last treatment. Control animals received sunflower oil alone.

† Epoxide hydratase activities are expressed as a percentage of controls which were in lung 0·43 ± 0·07 with styrene oxide and 0·33 ± 0·05 with benzo[a]pyrene oxide and in kidney 0·79 ± 0·12 with styrene oxide and 0·75 ± 0·10 with benzo[a]pyrene oxide as substrate (units as in Table 5).

‡ n.d. = not determined.

to see whether the selectivity was perhaps rather more apparent than real due to different time-courses rather than to the absolute presence and absence of induction. The limits of the selectivity with respect to the doses used were also investigated (Schmassmann and Oesch, 1978).

The epoxide hydratase activity, determined with styrene oxide as substrate, increased dose dependently up to about 300 % of controls after daily treatment with 2·0 mmol (about 400 mg) *trans*-stilbene oxide per kilogram body weight

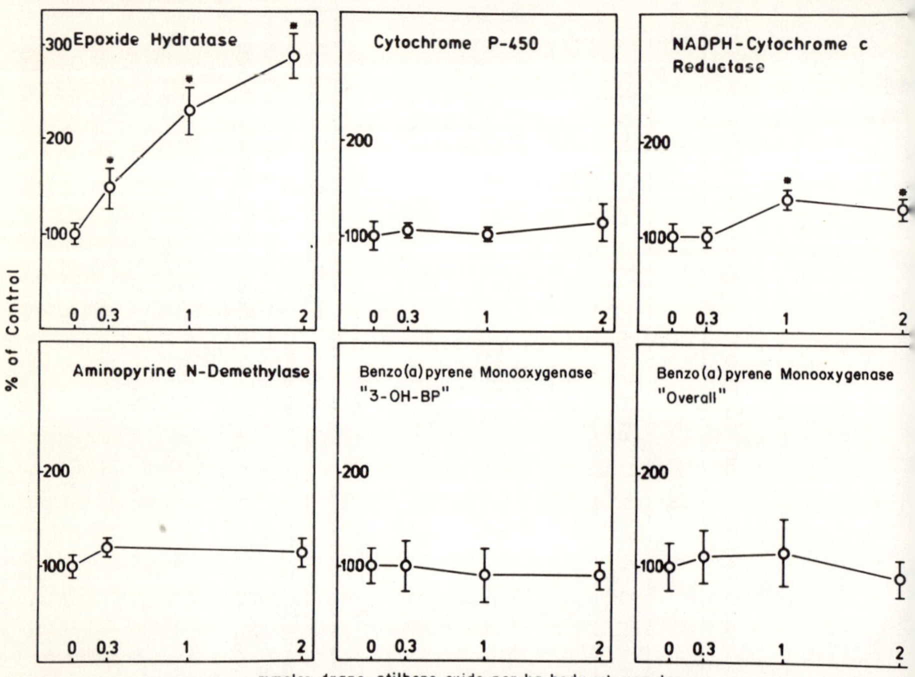

Figure 11 Dose–response curves of rat liver epoxide hydratase activity and monooxygenase parameters after daily intraperitoneal injections of *trans*-stilbene oxide for 3 days. Activities or contents represent the means ± S.D. Control activities expressed as nmol product per mg protein per min ± S.D. were: 6·97 ± 0·88 styrene glycol, 6·96 ± 1·13 benzo[a]pyrene 4,5-dihydrodiol, 324 ± 49 cytochrome c reduced, 4·09 ± 0·52 formaldehyde, and 0·292 ± 0·058 3-hydroxybenzo[a]pyrene. Control activity for the radiometric benzo[a]pyrene monooxygenase was 6,280 ± 1,560 cpm (counts per minute) per mg protein per min and cytochrome P-450 content in controls was 0·852 ± 0·128 nmol per mg protein. $*p < 0.025$ as compared to controls. From Schmassmann and Oesch (1978)

for 3 days (figure 11). The same dose-dependency was seen when epoxide hydratase activity was measured with benzo[a]pyrene 4,5-oxide as substrate. Over the whole range of doses the cytochrome P-450 content, the aminopyrine N-demethylase, and the benzo[a]pyrene monooxygenase activity determined fluorimetrically ('3-OH-BP') and radiometrically ('overall') were never significantly different from controls. Only the NADPH-cytochrome c reductase activity was slightly (but significantly) increased to 140 % and 130 % of controls after doses of 1 and 2 mmol *trans*-stilbene oxide, respectively. An attempt to provoke a higher induction of epoxide hydratase by daily treatment with toxic doses of 4 mmol (about 800 mg) *trans*-stilbene oxide per kilogram body weight. ($LD_{50} \sim 6$ mmol per kilogram body weight) failed in that three of the four treated rats died after the second injection and epoxide hydratase in the liver of the surviving rat was only induced to 225% of controls. Moreover, all measured monooxygenase parameters were now considerably reduced. The cytochrome P-450 content was decreased to 57% of controls.

Trans-stilbene oxide showed no *in vitro* effect on the determination of the cytochrome P-450 content. Thus the decreased cytochrome P-450 content may be taken to indicate a repressing effect of acute toxic doses of *trans*-stilbene oxide on cytochrome P-450 biosynthesis or an enhancement of its breakdown. This loss in cytochrome P-450 content was paralleled by a decrease of the aminopyrine N-demethylase activity to 69% of controls. The benzo[a]pyrene monooxygenase activity was no longer linear with protein concentration—probably due to an inhibition by a relatively high concentration of *trans*-stilbene oxide in the microsomes after this massive treatment—and showed at the lower concentration of microsomal protein (0·13 mg per assay) a decrease to 51%, and at the higher protein concentration (0·26 mg per assay) a reduction to 30% of controls. Moreover, incubations of mixtures of control microsomes with equal amounts (0·15 mg) of microsomes derived from the rat which was treated with daily doses of 4 mmol *trans*-stilbene oxide per kilogram body weight for 3 days resulted (after preincubation for 3 minutes) in a benzo[a]pyrene mono-oxgenase activity which was lower by about 30% than the sum of the two components.

Thus, inhibitors present in one microsomal preparation can obviously diffuse to the monooxygenase of another preparation if the two are incubated together. To investigate whether the monooxygenase activities were also inhibited after the doses of *trans*-stilbene oxide indicated in figure 11, and whether the selectivity of the induction of epoxide hydratase was apparent rather than real being only the result of such an inhibition, liver microsomes from control animals were incubated together with various amounts of liver microsomes from rats which had been treated with daily doses of 2 mmol *trans*-stilbene oxide per kilogram body weight for 3 days. No inhibition of the aminopyrine N-demethylase and the benzo[a]pyrene monooxygenase could be observed when determined at 24 hours after the last application of *trans*-stilbene oxide (instead in some cases a slight activation of these two enzyme activities was noted). Furthermore, it seems rather unlikely that different monooxygenase activities should always be inhibited to the same extent as they are induced after various doses of *trans*-stilbene oxide, the more so as no changes in the cytochrome P-450 content and no spectral shift in the Soret peak of the reduced cytochrome–CO complex could be observed. Nevertheless, a change in the pattern of the multitude of cytochrome P-450 species present in liver microsomes possessing a similar overall ability to metabolize aminopyrine and benzo[a]pyrene as control liver microsomes cannot be excluded.

286

The question remained, whether one or more of the measured parameters of the monooxygenase system may possibly be induced at a later time point. A time-course study (figure 12) showed that at 12 hours after application of *trans*-stilbene oxide, the epoxide hydratase activity increased very rapidly and reached its maximum induction after 2 days. The enzyme activity then declined almost linearly to reach control levels at 12 days after treatment. Epoxide hydratase activity at each time point was very similar when determined with benzo[*a*]pyrene 4,5-oxide or styrene oxide as substrate. Over the whole time-course, the cytochrome P-450 content, the aminopyrine N-demethylase, and the benzo[*a*]pyrene monooxygenase activities when determined fluorimetrically ('3-OH-BP') and radiometrically ('overall') were never significantly increased. Only NADPH-cytochrome c reductase activity was at one time point slightly (and just significantly) increased to 130% of controls. At the earliest time point investigated (at 12 hours after application) the aminopyrine N-demethylase and benzo[*a*]pyrene monooxygenase activities were reduced to about 60% of controls (Schmassmann and Oesch, 1978). This effect is most likely due to the relatively high concentrations of *trans*-stilbene oxide in the microsomes at this time point. Thus, with the possible exception of a small increase of the NADPH-cytochrome c reductase activity, the induction of liver epoxide hydratase by *trans*-stilbene oxide was found to be selective with respect to the measured monooxygenase parameters when examined dose- as well as time-dependently. Preliminary experiments by Schmassmann *et al* also showed that there was no effect of *trans*-stilbene oxide treatment on the glutathione S-transferase activity of the cytoplasmic fraction.

The limits of the selectivity of the epoxide hydratase induction by *trans*-stilbene oxide were now investigated by treating rats with daily doses of 1 mmol *trans*-stilbene oxide per kilogram body weight for 3, 6, and 12 days (Schmassmann and Oesch, 1978). This experiment was intended to show whether a higher induction of epoxide hydratase could be achieved by repeated administration of *trans*-stilbene oxide and whether after such an extreme exposure to *trans*-stilbene oxide any gross pathological changes or a decrease in the body weight gain could be observed. Epoxide hydratase activity increased during the first 6 days of treatment to about 300% of controls, but no further increase occurred over the next 6 days, instead a slight decrease was found after 12 days when compared to the maximal induction after 6 days (Table 7). Apart from the substrates styrene oxide and benzo[*a*]pyrene 4,5-oxide, in this experiment epoxide hydratase activity was also measured with 3-methylcholanthrene 11,12-oxide as substrate. The high correlation of the increases (percentage of controls) of epoxide hydratase activity, when determined with three different substrates, suggests that the induced epoxide hydratase is the same protein as the enzyme in control animals.

As already seen in the dose–response curve, the parameters of the monooxygenase system were not significantly different from controls after 3 days of treatment, apart from an increase of the NADPH-cytochrome c reductase activity to 140% of controls. The augmentation of NADPH-cytochrome c

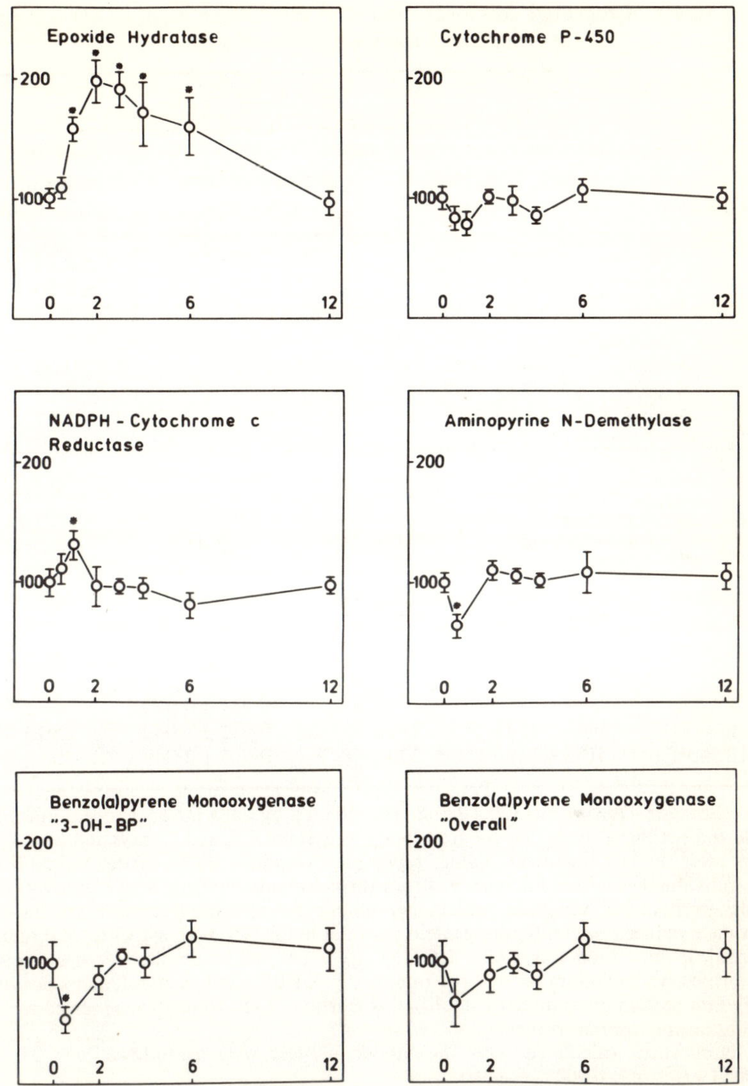

Figure 12 Time curves of liver epoxide hydratase activity and monooxygenase parameters after a single intraperitoneal treatment with *trans*-stilbene oxide. Rats were treated by a single intraperitoneal injection of 2·5 mmol *trans*-stilbene oxide per kg body weight. Activities or contents are expressed as percent of controls and represent the means ± S.D. Control activities expressed as nmol product per mg protein per min ± S.D. were: 7·10 ± 0·57 styrene glycol, 6·49 ± 0·81 benzo[a]pyrene-4,5-dihydrodiol, 371 ± 44 cytochrome c reductase, 3·88 ± 0·31 formaldehyde, and 0·334 ± 0·06 3-hydroxybenzo[a]pyrene. Control activity for the radiometric benzo-[a]pyrene monooxygenase was 5,490 ± 950 cpm per mg protein per min and cytochrome P-450 content in control was 0·815 ± 0·081 mmol per mg protein. *$p < 0.025$ as compared to controls. From Schmassmann and Oesch (1978)

Table 7 Effect of repeated administration of *trans*-stilbene oxide (TSO) on epoxide hydratase and monooxygenase system

| Treatment* | | Epoxide hydratase | | |
		Styrene oxide	Benzo[a]pyrene 4,5-oxide	3-Methyl-cholanthrene 11,12-oxide
TSO	3 days	14·85 ± 1·75 + +	15·78 ± 2·42 + +	2·56 ± 0.17 + + +
TSO	6 days	21·43 ± 1·51 + + +	20·37 + 2·28 + + +	2·87 ± 0·50 + +
TSO	12 days	18·20 ± 2·30 + + +	16·62 ± 0·65 + + +	2·57 ± 0·42 + +
Oil	3 days	6·42 ± 0·92	6·74 ± 0·99	1·08 ± 0·09
Oil	6 days	6·43 ± 1·07	6·61 ± 0·78	1·01 ± 0·13
Oil	12 days	6·52 ± 0·17	6·14 ± 0.83	1·15 ± 0·07

| Treatment | | Benzo[a]pyrene monooxygenase | | Cytochrome P-450 | NADPH–cytochrome c reductase |
		'Overall'	'3-OH-BP'		
TSO	3 days	5980 ± 1908	231 ± 79	0·825 ± 0·042	348 ± 7 +
TSO	6 days	7655 ± 2116	323 ± 70	1·045 ± 0·009 + +	368 ± 20 +
TSO	12 days	13504 ± 4014 +	434 ± 48	1·095 ± 0·098 +	391 ± 52
Oil	3 days	5141 ± 757	260 ± 45	0·811 ± 0·026	249 ± 49
Oil	6 days	4950 ± 1848	298 ± 52	0·835 ± 0·042	280 ± 48
Oil	12 days	5185 ± 1150	330 ± 48	0·807 ± 0·049	308 ± 34

* Male Sprague–Dawley rats (200–280 g) were treated by daily intraperitoneal injections of 1 mmole *trans*-stilbene oxide per kilogram body weight for 3, 6, and 12 days and were killed at 24 hours after the last treatment. Values represent the means ± S.D. of determinations performed individually on liver microsomes from three animals. Enzyme activities are expressed as nmoles product per milligram protein per minute for epoxide hydratase and as nmoles cytochrome c reduced per milligram protein per minute for NADPH–cytochrome c reductase. The benzo[a]pyrene monooxygenase activities are expressed as pmoles 3-hydroxybenzo[a]-pyrene formed per milligram protein per minute ('3-OH-BP') and as cpm (counts per minute) per milligram protein per minute ('overall'). Cytochrome P-450 content is expressed as nmoles per milligram microsomal protein.

The significances calculated with the Student's t-test were as follows: $p < 0.025$ (+), $p < 0.005$ (+ +), $p < 0.0005$ (+ + +).

reductase activity was not dependent on the duration of treatment and remained at about 130% of controls after 6 and 12 days respectively. However, the cytochrome P-450 content was clearly elevated after 6 and 12 days. The benzo[a]-pyrene monooxygenase activity determined fluorimetrically ('3-OH-BP') was still unchanged after 6 days but a tendency for it to be induced after repeated treatment with *trans*-stilbene oxide became apparent after 12 days. Although large interindividual variations were seen in the radiometric assay with benzo-[a]pyrene ('overall'), an increase of the monooxygenase activity after repeated administration of *trans*-stilbene oxide was most readily observed with this method. The increase of components of the monooxygenase system under these extreme conditions may be explained either by an (albeit low) affinity of *trans*-stilbene oxide to a receptor responsible for the induction of one or more cytochrome P-450 species, or by a secondary effect such as the release of an endogenous inducer of cytochrome P-450 after burdening the animal with repeated rather high doses of *trans*-stilbene oxide. However, no overt toxic effects were noticed and this treatment seemed to be tolerated by the animals quite well. Moreover, no gross lesions were observed on pathological examination. During this experiment the body weight gain of the rats was also followed, but no difference between control and *trans*-stilbene oxide-treated rats was noticed.

Thus the maximal induction of epoxide hydratase which can be reached by treatment with *trans*-stilbene oxide—at least for the rat strain used—ranges between 300% and 350% of controls. By repeated administration of high doses of *trans*-stilbene oxide, this induction of epoxide hydratase is not increased further but an induction of the monooxygenase system can be provoked. This induction of the monooxygenase system may be caused by an indirect effect of *trans*-stilbene oxide, mediated by release of an endogenous inducer.

Mechanism of Epoxide Hydratase Induction by *Trans*-Stilbene Oxide

When liver microsomes from control rats were incubated together with various amounts of liver microsomes from *trans*-stilbene oxide-treated rats, epoxide hydratase activities corresponding to the sum of the two components were always observed, indicating that the higher enzyme activity after treatment with *trans*-stilbene oxide is due to the presence of higher amounts of enzyme protein rather than to an activation of epoxide hydratase by *trans*-stilbene oxide or its metabolites.

The relatively rapid increase of epoxide hydratase activity after a single dose of *trans*-stilbene oxide allowed examination of whether this increase is dependent on RNA and protein synthesis. A rapid increase of enzyme activity after application of the inducer was needed, since the rats on treatment with the dosage schedule used for actinomycin D and cycloheximide would not have survived much longer than 24 hours or 48 hours respectively (Schmassmann and Oesch, 1978). Treatment with 1 mg cycloheximide or actinomycin D per kilogram body weight at 0·5 hours before application of a single dose of 2·5 mmol *trans*-stilbene oxide per kilogram body weight and repeated treatment with these protein and RNA syntheses inhibitors at intervals of 12 hours clearly prevented the induction of liver epoxide hydratase activity by *trans*-stilbene oxide (figure 13). Whereas in the experiment with cycloheximide the rats were killed at 48 hours after treatment with *trans*-stilbene oxide, the high toxicity of actinomycin D allowed treatment for only 24 hours. This is the reason for the less pronounced increase by *trans*-stilbene oxide in the experiment in which actinomycin D was used.

SDS–gel electrophoresis data also indicate that *trans*-stilbene oxide treatment results not only in higher epoxide hydratase activity but also in higher amounts of enzyme protein.

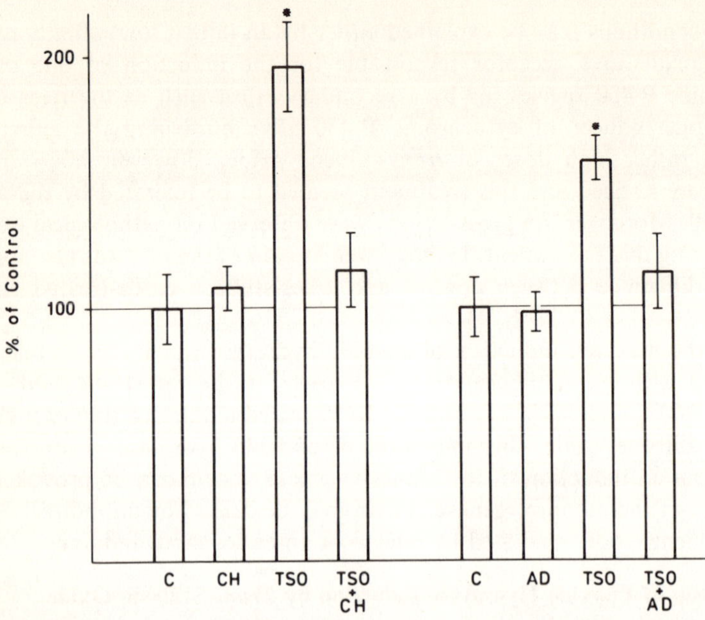

Figure 13 Effect of cycloheximide (CH) and actinomycin D (AD) on the induction of epoxide hydratase by *trans*-stilbene oxide (TSO). Where indicated TSO animals were treated by a single intraperitoneal injection of 2·5 mmol TSO per kg body weight. In a first experiment one group received 1 mg CH per kg body weight alone and another group was treated with the same dose half an hour before TSO was given. CH was injected at intervals of 12 hours. The animals were killed 48 hours after TSO treatment. In a second experiment animals received actinomycin D instead of CH. The same dose schedule was followed but the animals were killed 24 hours after TSO treatment. Bars represent the means of enzyme activities $\pm$ S.D. $*p < 0.01$ as compared to control (C) and TSO+AD or TSO+CH. From Schassmann and Oesch (1978)

Conclusions

Trans-stilbene oxide was demonstrated to be a potent and selective inducer of rat liver epoxide hydratase activity with respect to five monooxygenase parameters over a broad range of doses and when followed over the whole induction time-course of epoxide hydratase. Although high doses of *trans*-stilbene oxide did inhibit aminopyrine N-demethylase and the benzo[a]pyrene monooxygenase activities, no inhibition of these enzyme activities was observed when liver microsomes of controls and of rats which were treated with *trans*-stilbene oxide doses just sufficient to produce maximal induction of epoxide hydratase were incubated together, indicating that the selectivity of the epoxide hydratase induction was genuine and not an apparent selectivity caused by an inhibition of the monoxygenase activities by *trans*-stilbene oxide present in the microsomes. Moreover, the total cytochrome P-450 content and the difference spectrum of the reduced cytochrome P-450 CO-complex was not changed. It seems rather unlikely, but cannot be excluded, that upon treatment with *trans*-stilbene oxide the composition of the multitude of cytochrome P-450 forms might have changed in a way not leading to a different gel electrophoretic pattern and not leading to changes in monooxygenase activities for benzo[*a*]pyrene and aminopyrine as substrates but to different properties with respect to other substrates of the monooxygenase system. The *trans*-stilbene oxide-induced increase of epoxide hydratase activity was shown to be dependent on RNA and protein synthesis. SDS–gel electrophoresis showed an increased intensity of the band which co-migrated with the epoxide hydratase standard. Preincubation of control micro-somes with microsomes from *trans*-stilbene oxide-treated rats did not lead to an elevation of epoxide hydratase activity in the control microsomes. All of this indicates that the augmentation of the epoxide hydratase activity in rat liver after treatment with *trans*-stilbene oxide is due to higher amounts of enzyme protein and not only to an activation of the enzyme by *trans*-stilbene oxide or metabolites derived from it. The substrate specificity of the induced epoxide hydratase with respect to the three structurally widely different substrates was very similar to that of epoxide hydratase from untreated rats suggesting that the induced enzyme is the same or at least a functionally similar protein as the one in control rats.

Selective induction of epoxide hydratase has been found so far only in rat liver. This obviously limits its range of application. Nevertheless, selective induction of epoxide hydratase in rat liver should prove to be a useful tool to elucidate the role of epoxide hydratase in the overall biotransformation of poly-cyclic hydrocarbons leading to mutagenic and carcinogenic metabolites in *in vitro* model systems. Most of all, it shows that a selective induction of epoxide hydratase is intrinsically possible, thus providing the basis for further investi-gations to find a selective epoxide hydratase inducer for more typical target organs of polycyclic hydrocarbon-induced carcinogenesis such as skin and lung. Selective induction of epoxide hydratase should allow a direct study of the role of epoxide hydratase in the mechanism of tumour formation caused by compounds metabolized via epoxides which are substrates of the enzyme. If these studies are going to show that epoxide hydratase—despite its dual role—acts as a predominantly inactivating enzyme, selective epoxide hydratase inducers may even have practical importance in the prevention of tumour formation caused by polycyclic hydrocarbons or other compounds which are activated via epoxides.

DISTRIBUTION OF EPOXIDE HYDRATASE THROUGHOUT THE ANIMAL KINGDOM BUT IN DIFFERENT FORMS

Modulations of epoxide hydratase activity (such as selective induction) should be accompanied by investigations into whether the enzyme serves an endogenous role, in order to judge what the consequences of modulations of this enzyme activity would be with respect to its endogenous function. To gain an idea of the most promising direction which investigations of the enzyme's endogenous role might take, the occurrence of the enzyme in various organs was studied.

Using a recently developed highly sensitive assay with [³H]-benzo[*a*]pyrene 4,5-oxide as substrate, epoxide hydratase appeared ubiquitous, which suggests an important role of the enzyme. It was shown to be present in all 26 organs and tissues of the rat investigated (Oesch *et al*, 1977b) whereas in earlier studies with a less sensitive assay, epoxide hydratase activity was detected in rat liver and kidney but not in organs such as muscle, spleen, heart, and brain (Oesch *et al*, 1971a, 1973b). Although the enzyme activity in some organs was very low, it could always be precisely determined (Oesch *et al*, 1977b).

In whole blood no activity could be detected, indicating that the low enzyme activity in some organs is not due to blood components present in the tissues. However, in isolated monocytes or lymphocytes (stimulated or unstimulated) epoxide hydratase activity could be measured.

The highest epoxide hydratase activities were found in liver, testis, kidney, ovary, and lung (Table 8). The expectation that organs which come most

Table 8 Ubiquity of epoxide hydratase in organs of the rat*

Organ	Epoxide hydratase activity†	Organ	Epoxide hydratase activity†
Liver	6391 ± 636 (*n* = 8)	Caecum	80
Testis	1339 ± 245 (*n* = 6)	Colon	54, 60
Kidney	705 ± 118 (*n* = 8)	Epidermis	129, 156
Lung	362 ± 46 (*n* = 10)	Cutis	57, 66
Adrenal gland	196, 322	Subcutis	82, 115
Fat (kidney)	179, 249, 367	Submaxillary gland	240, 293
Bladder	90	Spleen	125, 155
Prostate gland	41, 52, 72	Thymus	111
Trachea	166	Brain	104
Tongue	59	Heart	20
Oesophagus	87	Triceps muscle	8, 9
Membranous stomach	37, 49	Blood	not detectable
Glandular stomach	59, 90	Ovary	556
Small intestine	95, 125, 158		

* The organs were taken from male Sprague–Dawley rats (220–280 g) except for the ovary which was taken from a 270 g female Sprague–Dawley rat.

† Specific activities are expressed as pmoles benzo[*a*]pyrene 4,5-dihydrodiol formed per milligram protein per minute. Values represent either means of the stated number of experiments (*n*) ± S.D. or single values representing means of three determinations at three different protein concentrations.

directly in contact with environmental compounds would, as a consequence of induction by such compounds or under evolutionary pressure, possess especially high epoxide hydratase activities was not confirmed. Thus the specific activities in skin, trachea, lung, tongue, oesophagus, membranous stomach, glandular stomach, small intestine, caecum, and colon were all considerably lower than those of such internal organs as liver, testis, and ovary, and of a similar order of magnitude to the remaining tissues. Also, the specific activities in the three layers of skin, epidermis, cutis, and subcutis were not very different from each other.

Of special interest is the high epoxide hydratase activity in testis and ovaries. In male NMRI mice (Oesch *et al*, 1977b) the specific epoxide hydratase activity in the testis was highest of all organs investigated, i.e. higher than in liver (2,200 versus 900 pmol benzo[*a*]pyrene 4,5-dihydrodiol produced per milligram protein per minute). Such activity may be taken to indicate an endogenous function of this enzyme in the testis, or else a protective function against mutagenic epoxides in this germinative gland.

In the mouse (NMRI) the distribution pattern was quantitatively quite different from that in the rat (Sprague–Dawley). The specific activities in the rat were in the order liver > testis > kidney > lung > intestine ≅ skin. In the mouse the order was testis > liver > lung > skin > kidney > intestine (Oesch *et al*, 1977b).

In organs possessing sufficiently high enzyme levels for accurate determination by the less sensitive assay with [^{3}H]styrene oxide as substrate (Oesch *et al*, 1971a) (rat liver, kidney, lung, and testis), epoxide hydratase activity was also measured with this substrate. In these organs the ratios of the specific activities for the two substrates were very similar (Oesch *et al*, 1977b). This supports the assumption that in these organs a single enzyme (or a group of functionally similar enzymes) is responsible for the hydration of both substrates—as was shown by several methods for the rat liver (Oesch and Bentley, 1976).

Does the same also hold for epoxide hydratase in different species? Can the measurement of epoxide hydratase with a given substrate for which an assay procedure exists be used to judge the capability of different species to hydrate epoxides metabolically produced from new compounds? In an earlier study (Oesch, 1974) epoxide hydratase preparations partially purified from liver microsomes of rat, guinea-pig, and man were compared. Inhibition of the hydration of styrene oxide by other epoxides was determined and some of the potential inhibitors were also assayed as substrates. Most of the potential inhibitors used were derivatives of propene oxide or styrene oxide. The enzymes of the three species were found to be similar with respect to the following criteria: monosubstituted oxiranes with a lipophilic substituent larger than an ethyl group (isopropyl, *t*-butyl, *n*-hexyl, phenyl) readily interacted as substrates or inhibitors whereas those with a small substituent (methyl, ethyl, vinyl) were inactive, probably reflecting greater affinity of the former epoxides owing to lipophilic binding sites near the active site of the enzyme. In a series of oxiranes having a lipophilic substituent of sufficient size (styrene oxides), monosubstituted as well as 1,1- and *cis*-1,2-disubstituted oxiranes readily served as substrates or inhibitors of the enzyme, but not the *trans*-1,2-disubstituted, tri- or tetra-substituted oxiranes. *Trans*-substitution at the oxirane ring apparently prevents access of the oxirane ring to the active site by steric hindrance. However, several quantitative differences were observed. Thus it was concluded that the epoxide hydratases from the three species were quite similar but not identical with each other. Studies with epoxide hydratase from guinea-pigs or rats therefore appear to be significant with respect to man. In addition, knowledge of structural requirements for epoxides to serve as substrates for human epoxide hydratase may prove useful for drug design. Compounds which need aromatic or olefinic moieties for their desired effect would not be expected to lead to accumulation of epoxides if their structure was such as to allow for a metabolically produced epoxide to be rapidly consumed by epoxide hydratase.

If the ubiquity of epoxide hydratase in rat organs were indeed due to a vital role of the enzyme, it may also be ubiquitously distributed throughout the animal kingdom. Although the enzyme appeared to be quite similar in the three mammalian species discussed above, rat, guinea-pig, and man, different epoxide hydratase forms may have appeared during evolution. In order to increase the likelihood of detecting different enzyme forms by differences in substrate preferences, three structurally widely different epoxides were used, styrene 7,8-oxide, benzo[a]pyrene 4,5-oxide, and HEOM (1,2,3,4,9,9-hexachloro-6,7-epoxy-1,4,4a,5,6,7,8,8a-octahydro-1,4-methanonaphthalene). Epoxide hydratase activity was measured in the liver microsomes of a range of vertebrate species including many non-mammalian species. A general trend of increasing epoxide hydratase activity was found, following the sequence from fish and amphibia, birds, rodents to the larger mammals.

All these substrates were enzymically hydrated by epoxide hydratase from all

Table 9 Epoxide hydratase activity towards three different substrates in liver microsomes from various animal species

	Epoxide hydratase substrates*		
	Styrene oxide	Benzo[a]-pyrene 4,5-oxide	HEOM
Trout (male and female)	2·7	0·6	0·08
Toad (male and female)	0·98	0·97	0·3
Quail (male)	8·9	0·2	0·40
Pigeon (male)	3·0	0·94	0·31
Mouse† (male)	0·73–1·3	1·5–2·1	0·87–1·1
Rat (male)	6·4	6·1	3·0
Guinea pig (male)	12	18	15
Rabbit (male)	10	16	82
Cat (female)	1·5	4·8	1·7
Pig (female)	6·8	6·9	30

* Incubations were performed on pooled samples of microsomes from four to six animals (except for cat and pig) at 37 °C (except for quail and pigeon, 42 °C, and trout and toad, 26 °C). In all cases linearity of product formation with respect to protein concentration and incubation time was assured. Epoxide hydratase activities are expressed as nmoles product per milligram protein per minute.

† The following mouse strains were used: C_3H/HeJ, A/J, $C_3HeB/FeJ \times A/J$, C57BL/6J, C_3HeB/FeJ, C57BL/6J $\times$ C_3HeB/FeJ.

species investigated (Walker *et al*, 1978) in line with the broad substrate specificity of the more thoroughly investigated rat enzyme (Oesch, 1974; Bentley *et al*, 1976; Oesch and Bentley, 1976; Lu *et al*, 1977; Oesch *et al*, 1977a). However, the preferences towards the individual substrates were very different in the liver microsomal preparations from different species or phylogenetic groups of species, providing evidence for the existence of different epoxide hydratase forms. Although it is not known whether the observed differences are due to different enzyme proteins or to differences in the membrane around the enzyme, these differences are important, because they make the enzyme functionally different in these different species.

The preferences towards one or a combination of two of the three substrates used were not very marked (differences between substrates from 1·0-fold to 2·3-fold) in liver microsomes from the three rodents investigated, the mouse, the rat, and the guinea-pig. But styrene oxide was hydrated at considerably higher rates than the other two substrates by liver microsomes from the birds and fish investigated (Japanese quail, pigeon, trout) the differences ranging from 3·2-fold to 45-fold. HEOM was hydrated at much higher rates than the other two substrates by liver microsomes from pig and rabbit (differences between 4·4-fold and 8·2-fold). The cat was the only species investigated whose liver microsomes hydrated benzo[*a*]pyrene 4,5-oxide at a clearly higher rate than the other two substrates. The liver microsomes of the only amphibian investigated (*Xenopus*) hydrated styrene oxide and benzo[*a*]pyrene 4,5-oxide at a similar rate which was considerably faster than that for HEOM (Table 9).

In the species where several strains were studied, the mouse, the same substrate preference (benzo[*a*]pyrene 4,5-oxide) was observed in all strains (C$_3$H/HeJ, A/J, C$_3$HeB/FeJ × A/J, C57BL/6J, C$_3$HeB/FeJ, C57BL/6J × C$_3$HeB/FeJ). In the species where several organs were investigated, the rabbit, the same substrate preference (HEOM) was found for all organs (liver, testis, kidney, lung) (Table 10). In the species where induction by *trans*-stilbene oxide

Table 10 Epoxide hydratase activity towards three different substrates in microsomes from various organs of the rabbit

	Epoxide hydratase substrates*		
	Styrene oxide	Benzo[*a*]-pyrene 4,5-oxide	HEOM
Liver	10	16	85
Testis	6·1	2·4	56
Lung	1·9	1·3	11
Kidney	0·32	1·7	42

* Assays were performed on pooled samples of microsomes from four rabbits (except for the liver assay when the microsomes from each animal were assayed individually, variation ±5% SEM). Epoxide hydratase activities are given as nmoles product formed per milligram protein per minute.

was studied, the rat, the increase in hydration rates was similar with respect to all three substrates indicating that, in contrast to what was observed between species or groups of species, the induced and non-induced forms of the enzyme are similar or identical.

CONCLUSIONS

Epoxide hydratase catalyses the transformation of epoxides to dihydrodiols. Epoxides are metabolically formed from many foreign compounds possessing olefinic or aromatic moieties. Epoxides are electrophilically reactive to varying degrees and can therefore irreversibly bind to nucleophilic moieties of cellular macromolecules thereby disturbing the normal biochemistry of a cell. This can lead to cell death, mutation, or transformation to a cancer cell. The dihydrodiols produced by the action of epoxide hydratase can sometimes be further epoxidized at other parts of the molecule. In some cases, the resulting dihydrodiol-epoxides are of special reactivity and high mutagenic and carcinogenic activity. Thus, epoxide hydratase plays a dual role, inactivating monofunctional epoxides and providing precursor molecules for dihydrodiol-epoxide biosynthesis.

In order to gain better insight into the true role of epoxide hydratase, the enzyme has been purified from rat liver microsomes to apparent homogeneity. A preparation was obtained which was homogeneous by gel electrophoretical, analytical, ultracentrifugal, and immunological criteria as well as according to the results of the analysis of the C-terminal and N-terminal amino acid of the enzyme. The pure enzyme has a minimum molecular weight of 49,000 and in agreement with its hydrophobic character, a high tendency to form very high molecular weight aggregates. Amino acid analysis showed that a very high percentage (56%) of hydrophobic amino acid residues was present. The pH optimum of the enzyme with styrene oxide as substrate is between pH 8·9 and 9·4 depending on the buffer used. The ionic strength has no effect on the catalytic activity. The maximal turnover rate is 40 molecules styrene oxide per molecule epoxide hydratase per minute. The homogeneous enzyme has a broad specificity for substrate epoxides, including epoxides derived from carcinogenic polycyclic hydrocarbons. No indication was obtained for an additional enzyme hydrating styrene oxide or benzo[a]pyrene 4,5-oxide in branching-off fractions during purification, the potencies of inhibitors remained similar for both substrates throughout purification, and antibodies raised against the homogeneous enzyme added to the crudest soluble preparation, the solubilized microsomes, precipitated the entire activity hydrating styrene oxide or benzo[a]pyrene 4,5-oxide. These observations taken together strongly suggest that a single enzyme in microsomal membranes is hydrating styrene oxide and benzo[a]pyrene 4,5-oxide and that this is the purified enzyme.

The homogeneous epoxide hydratase has been used to probe the importance of epoxides among possibly other metabolites of aromatic compounds and the role of epoxide hydratase in the control of reactive metabolites. One of the model substrates used was benzo[a]pyrene. Depending on the monooxygenase forms present and on the concentration of benzo[a]pyrene, epoxide hydratase played fundamentally different roles which were reflected by the effect of pure epoxide hydratase on the mutagenicity of metabolically activated benzo[a]pyrene: the enzyme had a protective function during activation by liver microsomes from untreated mice but a potentiating action during activation by microsomes from 3-methylcholanthrene-treated animals. The former effect was independent of the benzo[a]pyrene concentration while the latter was observable only at sufficiently low concentrations of benzo[a]pyrene allowing for extensive further oxidative metabolism of benzo[a]pyrene metabolites. With compounds not possessing an angular benzo-ring prone to metabolic formation of highly reactive dihydrodiol-epoxides, the complication with a potentiating action of epoxide hydratase is not to be expected. Thus, epoxide hydratase is expected to play a purely protective role with respect to epoxides metabolically produced from the great majority of pharmaceutical and other industrial compounds produced for human use. Although catalytically very efficient, the cytoplasmic glutathione S-transferases play, due to their subcellular localization, a minor role in the inactivation of epoxides derived from large lipophilic compounds. It was shown with such a lipophilic compound as a model substance, and with liver enzyme-mediated bacterial mutagenesis as biological endpoint, that species and strain differences in epoxide hydratase and monooxygenases are reflected in vast differences in mutagenicity of the same compound —which varied from a degree which could easily be overlooked to extremely potent. In order to investigate whether the differences in enzyme activities were causally linked to the observed differences in mutagenicity, the enzyme activities were modulated by inhibition and induction. These manipulations were always accompanied by the corresponding changes in mutagenicity. It was concluded that species such as mice which possess high monooxygenase activity but very low epoxide hydratase activity are much more susceptible than man to those toxic effects which are mediated by such epoxides which are substrates of epoxide hydratase. In this regard, it is especially noteworthy that mice possess a much lower hepatic epoxide hydratase activity than man.

Since all these arguments are based on *in vitro* systems and bacterial mutagenicity, a selective inducer of epoxide hydratase has been sought to provide a tool for probing the true role of the enzyme in the whole animal, and, if this induction should turn out to be predominantly protective, it might be used in certain human situations in order to afford protection. Good substrates of the enzyme proved to be poor inducers. Since a receptor for induction may be specific for epoxides without sharing other preferences with the catalytically active site of the enzyme, poor substrates were also tested. One of these, *trans*-stilbene oxide, turned out to induce epoxide hydratase selectively without inducing cytochrome P-450 levels or monooxygenase activity with benzo[a]pyrene or aminopyrine as substrate. It seems unlikely that monooxygenase activities towards other substrates may have been increased for the following reasons:

1. The two substrates chosen are known to be preferential substrates of different

monooxygenase forms. Moreover, the different monooxygenase forms iso-lated so far have proved to be of very broad specificity and there is not one substrate known to be excluded by a monooxygenase form.
2. The gel electrophoretic pattern of the various cytochrome P-450 forms appeared unchanged after *trans*-stilbene oxide treatment while the epoxide hydratase band was strongly increased. The possibility cannot be ruled out that an increase in monooxygenase activity towards a substrate not tested may have taken place.

The induction of epoxide hydratase activity by *trans*-stilbene oxide was shown to be dependent on RNA and protein synthesis (by the use of actino-mycin D and cycloheximide), not to be accompanied by a diffusible activator (by mixing experiments), and to result in higher amounts of enzyme protein (by SDS–gel electrophoresis).

Modulations of epoxide hydratase activity call for information on the endo-genous role of the enzyme to be able to predict whether serious disturbances might occur as a consequence of such modulations. As a first step, the occur-rence of the enzyme in microsomes from different organs and species has been investigated. The enzyme appears ubiquitous in the organs and species investi-gated, suggesting a vital role of the enzyme. Very high activities are found in testes and ovaries suggesting a role in steroid metabolism, or occurrence as a result of evolutionary pressure as a protection for the gonads. As far as investi-gated, the enzyme appears to be qualitatively similar (similar substrate prefer-ences) in different organs of the same species although specific activities can be different by three orders of magnitude. The enzyme appears also to be qualita-tively similar (similar substrate preferences) in different strains of the same species or in different phylogenetically closely related species (e.g. in all rodents investigated), but not in phylogenetically more remote species. Thus vastly different substrate preferences were observed between amphibians, birds, rodents, larger mammals (pig and rabbit), and cat (which was different from the other larger mammals). Hence functionally different epoxide hydratase forms must exist in these phylogenetically different groups. It is not known whether these functional differences are the results of different enzyme proteins or different membrane environments.

ACKNOWLEDGEMENTS

The author thanks his collaborators for their dedicated work quoted in this review and the Council for Tobacco Research (grant 1097) for financial support.

REFERENCES

Alvares, A. P., Bickers, D. R. and Kappas, A. (1973), *Proc. Nat. Acad. Sci. US*, **70**, 1321.
Ames, B. N., Durston, W. E., Yamasaki, E. and Lee, F. D. (1973), *Proc. Nat. Acad. Sci. US*, **70**, 2281.

Ames, B. N., McCann, J. and Yamasaki, E. (1975), *Mutat. Res.*, **31**, 347.

Arias, I. M. and Jakoby, W. B. (ed.) (1976), *Glutathione: metabolism and function*, Raven, New York.

Bentley, P. and Oesch, F. (1975), *FEBS Lett.*, **59**, 291.

Bentley, P., Oesch, F. and Glatt, H. R. (1977), *Arch. Toxicol.*, **39**, 65.

Bentley, P., Oesch, F. and Tsugita, A. (1975), *FEBS Lett.*, **59**, 296.

Bentley, P., Schmassmann, H. U., Sims, P. and Oesch, F. (1976), *Eur. J. Biochem.*, **69**, 97.

Booth, J., Boyland, E., Sato, T. and Sims, P. (1960), *Biochem. J.*, **77**, 182.

Brodie, B. B., Reid, W. D., Cho, A. K., Sipes, G., Krishna, G. and Gillette, J. R. (1971) *Proc. Nat. Acad. Sci. US*, **68**, 160.

Conney. A. H. (1967), *Pharmacol. Rev.*, **19**, 317.

Conney, A. H., Lu, A. Y., Levin, W., Somogyi, A., West, S., Jacobsson, M., Ryan, D. and Kuntzman, R. (1973), *Drug Metab. Disp.*, **1**, 199.

Cook, J. W., Hewett, C. L. and Hieger, I. (1933), *J. Chem. Soc.*, p. 395.

Daly, J. W., Jerina, D. M. and Witkop, B. (1972), *Experientia*, **28**, 1129.

Er-el, Z., Zaidenzaig, Y. and Shaltiel, S. (1972), *Biochem. Biophys. Res. Commun.*, **49**, 383.

Glatt, H. R. (1976), *Ph.D. thesis*, University of Basel.

Glatt, H. R. and Oesch, F. (1976), *Mutat. Res.*, **36**. 379.

Glatt, H. R. and Oesch, F. (1977), *Arch. Toxicol.*, **39**, 87.

Haugen, D. A., Van der Hoeven, T. A. and Coon, M. J. (1975), *J. Biol. Chem.*, **250**, 3567.

Heidelberger, C. (1975), *Ann. Rev. Biochem.*, **44**, 79.

Holder, G., Yagi, H., Dansette, P., Jerina, D. M., Levin, W., Lu, A. Y. H. and Conney, A. H. (1974), *Proc. Nat. Acad. Sci. US*, **71**, 4356.

Huberman, E., Sachs, L., Yang, S. K. and Gelboin, H. V. (1976), *Proc. Nat. Acad. Sci. US*, **73**, 607.

Jerina, D. M. and Daly, J. W. (1974), *Science*, **185**, 573.

Jerina, D. M. and Daly, J. W. (1977), in Parke, D. V. and Smith, R. L. (eds), *Drug metabolism—from microbe to man*, p. 15, Taylor and Francis, London.

Jerina, D. M., Daly, J. W. and Witkop, B. (1968), *J. Amer. Chem. Soc.*, **90**, 6525.

Jerina, D. M., Daly, J. W., Witkop, B., Zalzman-Nirenberg, P. and Udenfriend, S. (1970), *Biochemistry*, **9**, 147.

Jerina, D. M., Yagi, H. and Daly, J. W. (1973), *Heterocycles*, **1**, 267.

Kennaway, E. L. (1930), *Biochem. J.*, **24**, 497.

Knowles, R. G. and Burchell, B. (1977), *Biochem. J.*, **163**, 381.

Levin, W., Wood, A. W., Yagi, H., Dansette, P. M., Jerina, D. M. and Conney, A. H. (1976a), *Proc. Nat. Acad. Sci. US*, **73**, 243.

Levin, W., Wood, A. W., Yagi, H., Jerina, D. M. and Conney, A. H. (1976b), *Proc. Nat. Acad. Sci. US*, **73**, 3867.

Levin, W., Wood, A. W., Lu, A. Y. H., Ryan, D., West, S. and Conney, A. H. (1977), *Drug metabolism concepts*, p. 99, ACS Symposium Series No. 44.

Lu, A. Y. H., Jerina, D. M. and Levin, W. (1977), *J. Biol. Chem.*, **252**, 3715.

Lu, A. Y. H., Kuntzman, R., West, S., Jacobson, M. and Conney, A. H. (1972), *J. Biol. Chem.*, **247**, 1727.

Lu, A. Y. H., Ryan, D., Jerina, D. M., Daly, J. W. and Levin, W. (1975), *J. Biol. Chem.*, **250**, 8283.

Miller, E. C. and Miller, J. A. (1974), in Busch, H. (ed.), *Molecular biology of cancer*, p. 377, Academic, New York.

Nebert, D. W., Heiders, J. K., Strobel, H. W. and Coon, M. J. (1973), *J. Biol. Chem.*, **248**, 7631.

Nebert, D. W., Robinson, J. R., Niwa, A., Kumaki, K. and Poland A. P. (1975), *J. Cell. Physiol.*, **85**, 393.

Nemoto, N., Gelboin, H., Habig, W., Ketley, J. and Jakoby, W. B. (1975), *Nature*, **255**, 512.

Neville, D. M. (1971), *J. Biol. Chem.*, **246**, 6328.

Newbold, R. F. and Brookes, P. (1976), *Nature*, **261**, 52.

Oesch, F. (1973), *Xenobiotica*, **3**, 305.

Oesch, F. (1974), *Biochem. J.*, **139**, 77.

Oesch, F. (1976), *J. Biol. Chem.*, **251**, 79.

Oesch, F. (1977), *Arzneim.-Forsch.*, **27**, 1832.

Oesch, F. and Bentley, P. (1976), *Nature*, **259**, 53.

Oesch, F. and Daly, J. (1971), *Biochim. Biophys. Acta*, **227**, 692.

Oesch, F. and Glatt, H. R. (1976), in Montesano, R., Bartsch, H. and Tomatis, L. (eds), *Tests in chemical carcinogenesis*, p. 255, IARC Scientific Publications No. 12, International Agency for Research on Cancer, Lyon.

Oesch, F., Jerina, D. M. and Daly, J. (1971a), *Biochim. Biophys. Acta*, **227**, 685.

Oesch, F., Kaubisch, N., Jerina, D. M. and Daly, J. (1971b), *Biochemistry*, **10**, 4858.

Oesch, F., Jerina, D. M., Daly, J. and Rice, J. (1973a), *Chem.-Biol. Interact.*, **6**, 189.

Oesch, F., Morris, N., Daly, J., Gielen, J. and Nebert, D. (1973b), *Mol. Pharmacol.*, **9**, 692.

Oesch, F., Thoenen, H. and Fahrländer, H. with the technical assistance of K. Suda (1974), *Biochem. Pharmacol.*, **23**, 1307.

Oesch, F., Bentley, P. and Glatt, H. R. (1976), *Int. J. Cancer*, **18**, 448.

Oesch, F., Bentley, P. and Glatt, H. R. (1977a) in Jollow, D. J., Kocsis, J. J., Snyder, R, and Vainio, H. (eds.). *Biological reactive intermediates: formation, toxicity and inactivation*, p. 181, Plenum, New York.

Oesch, F., Glatt, H. R. and Schmassmann, H. U. (1977b), *Biochem. Pharmacol.*, **26**, 603.

Oesch, F., Raphael, D., Schwind, H. and Glatt, H. R. (1977c), *Arch. Toxicol.*, **39**, 97.

Rasmussen, R. E. and Wang, I. Y. (1974), *Cancer Res.*, **34**, 2290.

Remmer, H. (1972), *Eur. J. Clin. Pharmacol.*, **5**, 116.

Ryan, D. E., Thomas, P. E. and Levin, W. (1977), *Mol. Pharmacol.*, **13**, 521.

Schmassmann, H. U. and Oesch, F. (1978), *Mol. Pharmacol.*, **14**, 834.

Schmassmann, H. U., Sparrow, A., Platt, K. and Oesch, F. (1978), *Biochem. Pharmacol.*, **27**, 2237.

Sims, P. and Grover, P. L. (1974), *Adv. Cancer Res.*, **20**, 165.

Sims, P., Grover, P. L., Swaisland, A., Pal, K. and Hewer, A. (1974), *Nature*, **252**, 326.

Thakker, D. R., Yagi, H., Lu, A. Y. H., Levin, W., Conney, A. H. and Jerina, D. M. (1976), *Proc. Nat. Acad. Sci. US*, **73**, 3381.

Ullrich, V., Weber, P. and Wollenberg, P. (1975), *Biochem. Biophys. Res. Commun.*, **64**, 808.

Vainio, H. and Parkki, M. G. (1976), *Toxicology*, **5**, 279.

Vesell, E. S., Lang, C. M., White, W. J., Passananti, G. T., Hill, R. N., Clemens, T. L., Kiu, D. K. and Johnson, D. (1976), *Fed. Proc.*, **35**, 1125.

Walker, C. H., Bentley, P. and Oesch, F. (1978), *Biochim. Biophys. Acta*, **539**, 427.

Weber, K. and Osborn, M. (1969), *J. Biol. Chem.*, **244**, 4406.

Wiebel, F. J., Selkirk, J. K., Gelboin, H. V., Haugen, D. A., Van der Hoeven, T. A. and Coon, M. J. (1975), *Proc. Nat. Acad. Sci. US*, **72**, 3917.

Wislocki, P. G., Wood, A. W., Chang, R. L., Levin, W., Yagi, H., Hernandez, O., Dansette, P. M., Jerina, D. M. and Conney, A. H. (1976a), *Cancer Res.*, **36**, 3350.

Wislocki, P. G., Wood, A. W., Chang, R. L., Levin, W., Yagi, H., Hernandez, O., Jerina, D. M. and Conney, A. H. (1976b), *Biochem. Biophys. Res. Commun.*, **68**, 1006.

Wood, A. W., Goode, R. L., Chang, R. L., Levin, W., Conney, A. H., Yagi, H., Dansette, P. M. and Jerina, D. M. (1975), *Proc. Nat. Acad. Sci. US*, **72**, 3176.
Wood, A. W., Levin, W., Lu, A. Y. H., Yagi, H., Hernandez, O., Jerina, D. M. and Conney, A. H. (1976a), *J. Biol. Chem.*, **251**, 4882.
Wood, A. W., Wislocki, P. G., Chang, R. L., Levin, W., Lu, A. Y. H., Yagi, H., Hernandez, O., Jerina, D. M. and Conney, A. H. (1976b), *Cancer Res.*, **36**, 3358.

CHAPTER 6

The applications of nuclear magnetic resonance spectroscopy in drug metabolism

I. C. Calder

INTRODUCTION

Nuclear magnetic resonance (n.m.r.) spectroscopy is a technique which provides information about the environment of the nuclei of the atoms in a molecule. Both hydrogen and carbon atoms can be easily studied for structure determination of the molecule and for non-bonded interactions with other molecules. From the spectra, the chemical type of the atoms can be determined and their relationship to other hydrogen and carbon atoms ascertained. As a result, the technique of n.m.r. is a powerful tool for structural determination; it is somewhat limited by a lack of sensitivity and therefore is not often used as a quantitative analytical tool.

During metabolism studies of a new drug, an important task is to determine the structure of metabolites when they have been separated. Mass spectrometry provides a very sensitive means of determining the molecular weight and elemental composition of metabolites, and frequently the fragmentation pattern may provide further structural information. However, once sufficient compound has been isolated, n.m.r. spectroscopy provides the best means of obtaining detailed information from which a structure can be assigned. Furthermore, n.m.r. does not involve destruction of the compound which can then be used for other physicochemical measurements. Ultimately, however, the only proof of structure is to synthesize the compound and compare it directly with the metabolite.

The principal application of n.m.r. has been in the use of proton (^{1}H) spectra to determine the structure of isolated metabolites. Recent developments in carbon (^{13}C) n.m.r. spectroscopy have meant that the technique has been used extensively for the determination of the structure of complex molecules. Its potential in drug metabolism has not yet been fully realized but it shows great promise for the characterization of drug metabolites.

The applications of n.m.r. in drug metabolism have been reviewed (Case, 1973). The improvements in sensitivity in both ^{1}H- and ^{13}C-spectra have meant a significant increase in the applications and many more papers describing the use of n.m.r. in this area can be expected during the next few years. The purpose of this review is to discuss the sort of information which can be obtained from an n.m.r. spectrum and how it can be utilized to assign a structure to a metabolite. In most cases the structure of the administered drug is known, and a metabolite will usually result from one of the common biotransformation reactions, often an oxidation process. Thus particular changes in the spectra which might be expected from one or more of these reactions can be sought. In this review, the applications are arbitrarily discussed together with some of the possible metabolic reactions; in many cases though, more than one type of reaction occurs. Finally, the metabolites of phenacetin are discussed as an example where many metabolic paths operate, and the sort of ^{13}C-n.m.r. spectra which the metabolites exhibit.

PRINCIPLES OF NUCLEAR MAGNETIC RESONANCE

The basic principles of n.m.r. are treated in a wide variety of elementary spectroscopy texts such as those by Silverstein *et al* (1974) and Williams and Fleming (1966). For a more advanced treatment of the principles and applications of ^{1}H-n.m.r. and ^{13}C-n.m.r. spectroscopy, the texts of Jackman and Sternhell (1969) and of Stothers (1972) should be consulted.

The nuclei of all atoms carry a positive charge and the nuclei of some isotopes possess a mechanical spin. In these isotopes the spinning charge produces a magnetic dipole along the axis. This may be described in terms of a spin quantum number, I, which may have values of $0, \frac{1}{2}, 1, \frac{3}{2}, \ldots$. Only nuclei which have a spin give rise to n.m.r. spectra, so elements with $I = 0$ such as ^{12}C and ^{16}O cannot be studied. ^{1}H, ^{3}H, ^{13}C, ^{19}F, and ^{31}P, for which $I = \frac{1}{2}$, have a symmetrical charge distribution and are the simplest type of nuclei to study by n.m.r. spectroscopy. Nuclei which have I values of 1 or greater such as ^{2}H and

^{14}N have an asymmetrical charge distribution resulting in a quadrupole moment which makes their study by n.m.r. spectroscopy difficult.

The following discussion is confined to nuclei for which $I = \frac{1}{2}$, in particular to ^{1}H and ^{13}C, although the same principles apply to all nuclei for which $I = \frac{1}{2}$.

In an applied magnetic field, an atomic nucleus can adopt $(2I+1)$ orientations. Thus for $I = \frac{1}{2}$, there are two orientations, which can be visualized best if the nucleus is considered as a tiny bar magnet. The two orientations then are a high-energy state where the nuclear field is aligned against the applied field and a low-energy state where the nuclear field is aligned with the applied field. The larger the applied field the greater the difference there will be between the high-energy and the low-energy states.

In common with the other forms of absorption spectroscopy it is possible for the nucleus in the low-energy state to absorb energy in the form of a quantum of electromagnetic radiation and to be excited to the high-energy state. The frequency of the radiation, ν, required for excitation of the nucleus is related to the applied field strength, H_0, by the relationship:

$$\nu = \gamma H_0/2\pi$$

where γ is the gyromagnetic ratio. γ has a characteristic value for each nucleus and hence determines the frequency at a given field strength at which each nucleus will absorb energy and exhibit nuclear magnetic resonance. At a magnetic field strength, H_0, of 14,092 gauss, the ^1H-nucleus absorbs energy at 60 megahertz (MHz) and the ^{13}C-nucleus at 15·08 MHz, both of which lie in the radio-frequency range of the electromagnetic spectrum.

Under the conditions of the n.m.r. experiment only a small excess of the total population of nuclei are in the low-energy state. Under conditions of resonance this small excess of nuclei absorb energy and are excited into the high-energy state. They then lose the additional energy to their environment by spin-lattice relaxation. This process allows a continuous absorption of energy and the conditions for nuclear magnetic resonance can be created.

The simplest experimental equipment is shown schematically in figure 1. The nuclear magnetic resonance spectrometer has either a permanent magnet or an electromagnet which provides the external magnetic field, H_0. The sample is contained in a tube which can be spun to help increase the homogeneity of the applied field. The electromagnetic radiation required for the nuclear excitation is provided by a radiofrequency (r.f.) transmitter which can provide a variable frequency. Resonance is detected by a radiofrequency receiver which measures the amount of absorption of the radiofrequency energy, and this is then displayed on a precalibrated chart.

Two methods of determining spectra are available. The first, known as continuous wave n.m.r., involves continuously varying the irradiating frequency and measuring the absorption at each frequency. Under these conditions each different nucleus undergoes resonance in turn and the sweep time to record the spectrum is relatively long, 250–500 seconds. This method is used by most small proton n.m.r. spectrometers and requires relatively large samples of 10–100 mg.

The second, method, known as Fourier transform n.m.r., involves irradiating the sample with a short intense pulse of radiofrequency radiation which covers the entire frequency range in which absorption occurs. All the nuclei which can undergo resonance will be excited and, after the irradiation pulse is complete,

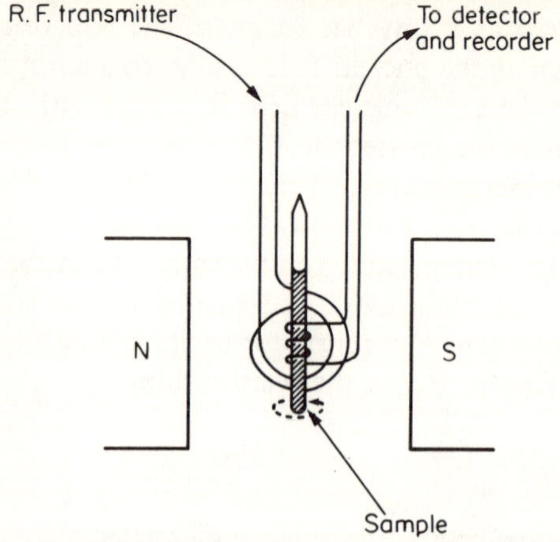

Figure 1   Schematic diagram of an n.m.r. spectrometer

they will return to the low-energy state after losing the absorbed energy. The loss of the energy gives rise to a signal which can be recorded. This signal then undergoes a mathematical Fourier transformation in order to generate the normal n.m.r. spectrum. Since only 1–2 seconds are required for a scan, the spectrum can be scanned repeatedly and a large increase in sensitivity can be gained by averaging the spectra obtained. This method is used for recording ^{13}C-spectra and proton spectra where only a small amount of material is available (0·1–1·0 mg for ^{1}H and 15–100 mg for ^{13}C). However, since a computer and more sophisticated equipment are required, these instruments are much more expensive and hence less widely used.

While the size of the sample varies considerably depending on the type of spectra required and instrument used, pure samples are required for good spectra. The sample is dissolved in 0·5–1·5 ml of solvent and the spectrum recorded. For ^{1}H-n.m.r. spectra this is normally a solvent without protons such as CCl_4, $CDCl_3$, D_2O, or other deuterated solvents where the hydrogen atoms are replaced with deuterium. In the case of deuterated solvents a residual proton peak may appear in the spectrum. For ^{13}C-n.m.r. spectra, deuterated solvents are also frequently used.

There are a number of differences in the types of spectra which can be obtained for the different nuclei. However, the basic principle governing the concepts of chemical shift and coupling constants are common to all nuclei and will be considered as general phenomena. The individual characteristics of ^{1}H- and ^{13}C-spectra will then be considered.

Chemical Shift

Each nucleus undergoes resonance at a characteristic frequency, at a given field strength which is dependent upon the environment of the nucleus. The chemical shift (δ) of a nucleus is defined as the difference between the absorption frequency of the nucleus and the absorption frequency of a reference nucleus. Chemical shifts are best expressed in dimensionless units (δ) so that the values are independent of the applied field strength. The chemical shift (δ) is defined as:

$$\delta = \frac{(\nu_s - \nu_{\text{ref}}) \times 10^6}{\nu_{\text{inst}}}$$

where ν_s and ν_{ref} are the resonance frequencies of the sample and reference respectively and ν_{inst} the operating frequency of the instrument. Thus δ units are expressed in parts per million (ppm). A positive value of δ indicates a resonance peak at higher frequency from the reference sample, and the sample nucleus may then also be referred to as being deshielded or at lower field.

The main factor determining the chemical shift of a nucleus is the electron density of its surrounding electrons. Under the influence of the applied magnetic field these electrons undergo an induced circulation which will generate their own magnetic field that will be opposite in direction to the applied field (figure 2). The field strength which the nucleus experiences will then be the sum of the

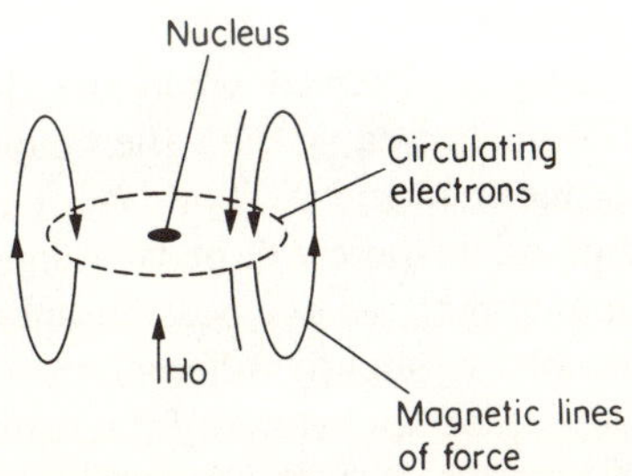

Figure 2 Shielding of nucleus by circulating electrons

applied field H_0 and the induced field. Since the induced field is proportional to the electron density and opposes the applied field, the lower the electron density around the nucleus the further downfield the resonance will occur. Thus a fairly good correlation of chemical shifts with the electronic effects of substituents can be observed, particularly in ^{13}C-n.m.r. spectra.

A second effect is due to anisotropic shielding, that is deshielding by electrons remote from the nucleus. In this case the applied field produces a circulation of electrons in a group of atoms. This ring current generates an induced field which is dependent on the orientation of the nucleus with respect to the group. For example, the nuclei outside an aromatic ring are found at lower field and those in the ring are found at higher field (figure 3). This effect is much more pronounced in proton n.m.r. spectra.

Other factors such as solvent and other molecules in solution may also affect the chemical shift. One particularly useful development in this area has been the use of shift reagents (Ramey *et al*, 1975; Saunders, 1977). In this case a small amount of a paramagnetic species such as $Eu(dpm)_3$, (tris-(di[pivaloyl]-methanato)europium) is added to the n.m.r. sample. This reagent causes changes in the chemical shifts of the nuclei which are dependent on the interaction of

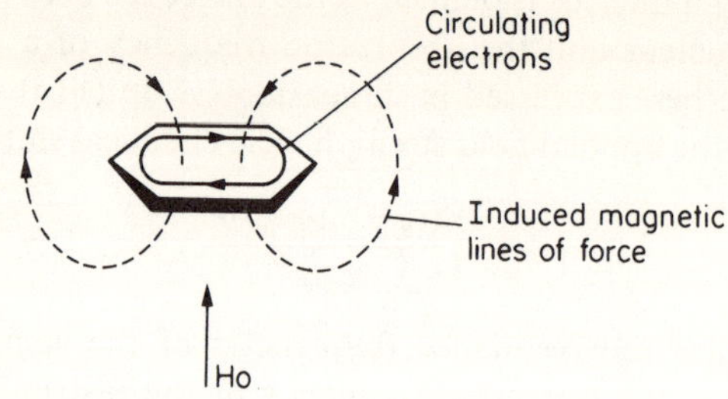

Figure 3 Anisotropic shielding in aromatic molecules

the molecule being studied with the reagent. The net result is to spread out the spectrum over a greater range and hence facilitate its analysis.

Spin–Spin Coupling

Nuclei which have $I = \frac{1}{2}$ may also interact with one another through the bonding electrons to produce fine structure in the n.m.r. spectrum. This interaction is known as spin–spin coupling and provides further information about the environment of the nucleus.

Simple spin–spin coupling is observed when the chemical shift difference, $\Delta\nu$, between the nuclei is much greater than the coupling constant. Consider the simplest case of two nuclei A and X (both $I = \frac{1}{2}$). Since A and X exert a magnetic influence on each other there will be two slightly different resonances for the A nucleus, corresponding to the two possible spin states of the X nucleus. Conversely, there will also be two slightly different resonances for the X nucleus corresponding to the two possible spin states of the A nucleus. The result is that instead of the A and X resonances each appearing as single peaks they will appear as double peaks. The separation, measured in Hz, between each pair of peaks is dependent on the degree of interaction between A and X and is known as the coupling constant, J_{AX}. The measured intensity of each of the peaks will be the same.

If more than one nucleus of either type is involved then all possible spin combinations must be considered. In an AX_2 system for example, there will be three possible spin combinations for the X nuclei which can be represented diagramatically as in figure 4, the small arrows representing the alignment of the nuclear spins with respect to the applied field, H_0. Since the two opposed spins are equivalent, the intensity in the central peak of the triplet is twice that of the other two peaks. For three X nuclei there will be four possible spin combinations, which will result in four resonance peaks of relative intensity $1 : 3 : 3 : 1$. The ^{13}C-spectrum of ethanol in figure 5(c) shows the splitting of the ^{13}C-signals resulting from coupling to the two and three hydrogens directly bound to the carbon atoms.

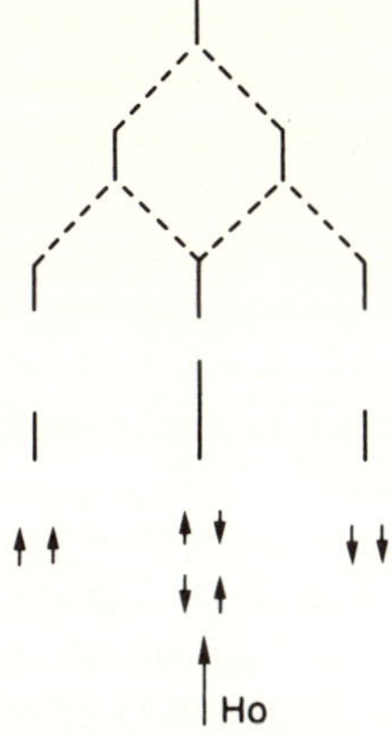

Figure 4   Three spin states for two nuclei

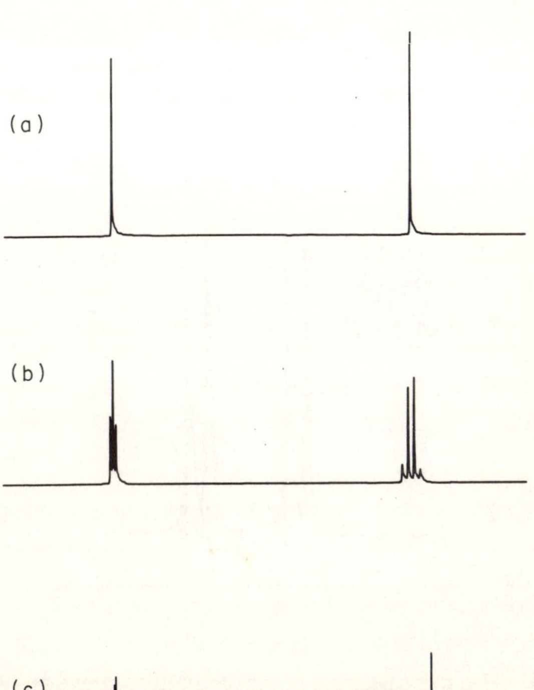

Figure 5 ^{13}C-n.m.r. spectrum of ethanol. (a) With broad band decoupling showing complete decoupling of all protons. (b) With off-resonance decoupling showing partial coupling. (c) With no decoupling showing full coupling.

Additional small splitting is visible on each multiplet due to coupling of each carbon atom with protons attached to the adjacent carbon atoms. The values of the coupling constants are for the methylene $^1J_{\mathrm{CH}} = 141\cdot6$ Hz and $^2J_{\mathrm{CH}} = 4\cdot9$ Hz and for the methyl $^1J_{\mathrm{CH}} = 125\cdot0$ and $^2J_{\mathrm{CH}} = 2\cdot0$ Hz (the superscript number refers to the number of bonds through which the nuclei are coupled).

If the chemical shift difference is comparable or less than the coupling constants then complex spectra are obtained. The simple spin–spin coupling rules above do not apply and deviations in the intensities of the resonance signals and their chemical shifts occur.

A nomenclature system has been developed for the designation of nuclei in an n.m.r. spectrum. When the chemical shift difference, $\Delta\nu$, is much greater than the coupling constant, J, then the nuclei are denoted by letters widely separated in the alphabet, e.g. AX and AMX; in these cases the spectra will show simple spin–spin coupling. When $\Delta\nu$ is comparable or less than J, then letters close together in the alphabet are used, e.g. AB and ABC. When more than one nucleus of the same magnetic type is present then a subscript is used to indicate the number of nuclei of that type, e.g. A_3X, A_3B_2, etc. Problems frequently arise in determining if nuclei are of the same magnetic type since chemically equivalent nuclei are not necessarily magnetically equivalent.

This is best illustrated with an example such as a *para*-disubstituted benzene (figure 6). The protons H-2 and H-6 are chemically equivalent but not magnetically equivalent since $J_{23} \neq J_{63}$ and $J_{65} \neq J_{63}$. As a result the spectrum is not

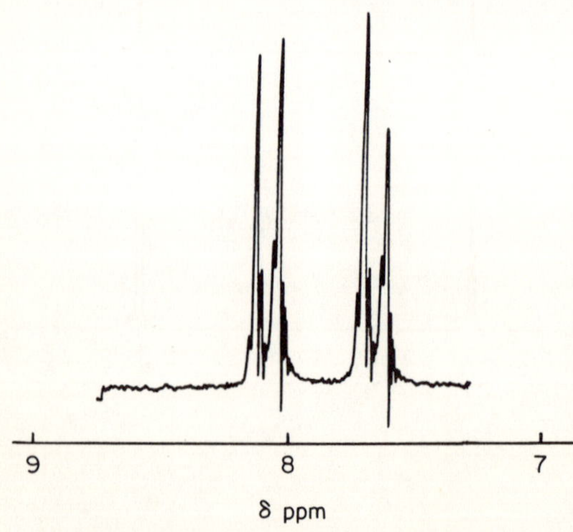

Figure 6 ^{1}H-n.m.r. spectrum of *p*-bromonitrobenzene at 100 MHz

of the A_2B_2 type but should be specified as AA′BB′. The literature has many similar examples of the wrong use of the designation and care should be taken to ensure that the correct spin system has been specified.

Spin–spin decoupling is a technique whereby the coupling between nuclei can be removed. The technique involves strongly irradiating one of the sets of nuclei at their resonance frequency while observing the non-irradiated nuclei.

The result is that the observed nuclei do not show any coupling to the irradiated nuclei. Either one specific resonance can be selected to detect which of the other nuclei are coupled to the nuclei concerned or, alternatively, a broad band of radiation which covers a group of resonances can be used. A common example of the latter type is where all ^{1}H-resonances of a compound are irradiated, thereby decoupling them from all the ^{13}C-nuclei; the ^{13}C-spectrum so obtained shows no ^{13}C–^{1}H-coupling and all the resonances appear as single peaks (figure 5a).

^{1}H-n.m.r.

Most n.m.r. research to date has been concerned with proton magnetic resonance and thus many of the examples of structure determination in drug metabolism have used this technique.

The range of chemical shifts in ^{1}H-n.m.r. cover about 10 ppm downfield from tetramethylsilane (TMS) which is usually used as the reference compound and for which δ_{TMS} is arbitrarily assigned a value of zero. The chemical shifts of saturated hydrocarbons are governed by the electronegativity of the atoms effecting the electron density at the proton. However, the dominant effect in determining the chemical shift of the proton is the anisotropic shielding of double bonds and aromatic rings. The general regions in which protons resonate are fairly broad and care must be taken in assigning chemical type. With suitable model compounds it is an easy task to identify biotransformations which have occurred to a particular compound. Some typical chemical shift values and ranges are shown in Table 1.

Table 1   Proton chemical shifts of some different types of protons (ppm from TMS)

Compound class	δ
Alkanes	0–2
α-Substituted alkanes	1·5–5
α-Disubstituted alkanes	2·5–7
Acetylene	2–3
Alkenes	4–7·5
Aromatic	6–9
Aldehydic	9–10·5
Carboxylic acids	10–13

Under normal conditions the size of the resonance signal in ^{1}H-n.m.r. spectra is dependent on the number of protons giving rise to the signal. ^{1}H-n.m.r. spectra frequently have superimposed a line representing the integrated areas of the peaks, from which can be assessed the relative number of protons in each signal or group of signals. It cannot be used to measure the absolute number of hydrogen atoms but only their ratio in different environments. With the molecular formulae determined from the mass spectrum, this procedure can be very useful.

More detailed information about the structure can be obtained from the spin–spin coupling observed between hydrogens. The coupling constants in aliphatic systems are 12–16 Hz between hydrogens on the same carbon, 7–9 Hz between hydrogens on adjacent carbons, and ~ 0 Hz over any greater distance. From the splitting pattern it is often easy to determine the position of a substituent in an aliphatic system. When the molecule is rigid, as in cyclic systems, the coupling constants for hydrogens on adjacent carbons vary over 0–9 Hz depending on the dihedral angle between the protons. From an analysis of the various coupling constants, the stereochemistry of a molecule can often be determined. In unsaturated systems a greater variation in coupling constants is observed. Frequently the stereochemistry of double bonds and the substitution pattern in aromatic compounds can be determined. Table 2 shows some of the typical coupling constants.

Table 2 Proton coupling constants (Hz)

System	J	System	J
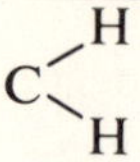 $\mathrm{C}\!\!<^{\mathrm{H}}_{\mathrm{H}}$	12–16	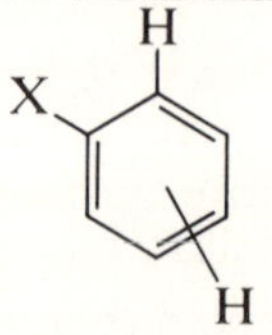 aromatic (X-substituted)	o- 7–10 m- 2–3
CH—CH	6–8		p- 0–1
CH—C—CH	0		
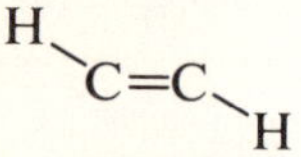 H,C=C,H (cis/trans)	11–18	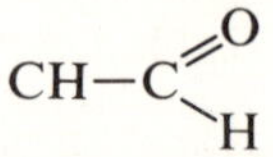 $\mathrm{CH}\!-\!\mathrm{C}{\displaystyle\mathop{}^{\mathrm{O}}_{\mathrm{H}}}$	2–4
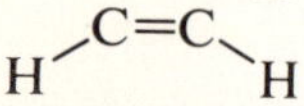 H,C=C,H	6–12	CH—C=C—H	2–3
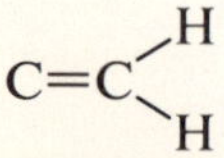 C=C$<^{\mathrm{H}}_{\mathrm{H}}$	0–2		

^{13}C-n.m.r.

Recent advances in instrumentation have made ^{13}C-n.m.r. spectra much easier to obtain, despite the low natural abundance of ^{13}C (1·1 %) and a relative sensitivity of only 1 % compared to ^{1}H. Spectra are recorded with Fourier transform pulsed spectrometers and are usually the average of at least 500 scans for samples of 200 mg.

Owing to the low sensitivity, most ^{13}C-n.m.r. spectra are recorded using broad band (noise) decoupling of all the protons in the molecule. Under these conditions all the protons are irradiated and hence no coupling between the ^{13}C-atoms and the protons is observed. Since also only 1 % of the carbon atoms in the molecule are ^{13}C, the adjacent carbon atoms will most likely be ^{12}C ($I = 0$), and no coupling of the ^{13}C-nuclei to other ^{13}C-nuclei will occur. Hence all the ^{13}C-resonances will appear as single resonance peaks. Figure 5(a) shows the normal ^{13}C-spectrum which is obtained for ethanol with noise decoupling.

Resonances for all carbon atoms can be observed, and unless they are equivalent it is rare for two nuclei to have the same chemical shifts. This means ^{13}C-spectra can be used to determine the number of different types of carbon atoms present in the molecule. Care must be taken, for the area of the resonances is determined by the relaxation times of the nuclei and under normal (fast) pulsing conditions is not proportional to the number of carbon atoms. The size of the peaks under the conditions that most spectra are recorded varies according to whether or not there are hydrogen atoms attached directly to the carbon atom. Thus, quaternary carbons, e.g. a carbonyl or the carbon of an aromatic ring

Table 3   Ranges for ^{13}C-chemical shifts observed in organic molecules (ppm from TMS)

Compound class	δ
Alkanes	20–45
Acetylene	40–100
Alkenes	100–165
Nitriles	110–125
Aromatic	110–150
Aldehydes	190–205
Ketones	195–210
Carboxylic acids	165–180
Esters	160–175
Amides	160–175

bearing a substituent, will show the smallest signals in the spectrum. The signals from carbon atoms with hydrogens attached will be considerably larger than the quaternary carbon signal, but the size is not directly proportional to the number of hydrogens.

The chemical shifts of ^{13}C vary over about 200 ppm, a much greater range than ^{1}H (Table 3). The shifts are basically determined by the electron density at the carbon atom, anisotropic shielding having little effect. As a result it is much easier to predict ^{13}C-chemical shifts, on the basis of the substituent present, than it is to predict ^{1}H-shifts. The observed shift can often be used to determine the type of substituent present. In fact, the effect of substituents is additive so that it is possible, by the use of model compounds, to predict accurately the chemical shift of a ^{13}C in a multiple substituted compound. This is particularly useful in determining the position of substitution in an aromatic ring, particularly a hydroxyl group. Some substituent parameters for aromatic systems are shown in Table 4.

The normal directly bound carbon–hydrogen coupling constant is found in the range 100–200 Hz. While this spin–spin coupling is not observed in most ^{13}C-spectra, an experimental technique, known as off-resonance decoupling, is commonly used where only partial coupling is observed. Under these conditions the normal spin–spin multiplicity is observed, but the size of the splittings is much smaller than the coupling constants (figure 5b). From this type of spectrum the number of protons bound to any carbon can be easily determined and hence

Table 4 Aryl carbon substituent effects* in monosubstituted benzenes relative to benzene, $\delta 128.7$

Substituent	Position			
	C_1	o-	m-	p-
—OH	$+26.9$	-12.6	$+1.8$	-7.9
—OCH$_3$	$+30.2$	-15.5	0.0	-8.9
—OCOCH$_3$	$+23.0$	-6.4	$+1.3$	-2.3
—NH$_2$	$+19.2$	-12.2	$+1.3$	-9.5
—N(CH$_3$)$_2$	$+22.6$	-15.6	$+1.0$	-11.5
—NHCOCH$_3$	$+11.1$	-9.9	$+0.2$	-5.6
—SH†	$+2.2$	$+0.5$	$+0.7$	-3.1
—SCH$_3$‡	$+9.9$	-1.9	$+0.1$	-3.1
—SOCH$_3$	$+17.6$	-5.1	$+0.7$	$+2.3$
—SO$_2$CH$_3$‡	$+12.3$	-1.5	$+0.6$	$+4.8$
—F	$+35.1$	-14.1	$+1.6$	-4.4
—Cl	$+6.4$	$+0.2$	$+1.0$	-2.0
—NO$_2$	$+19.6$	-5.3	$+0.8$	$+6.0$
—C$_6$H$_5$	$+13.0$	-1.1	$+0.5$	-1.0
CH$_3$	$+9.1$	-1.1	$+0.5$	-1.0
CH$_2$OH	$+12.3$	-1.4	-1.4	-1.4
CHO	$+9.0$	$+1.2$	$+1.2$	$+6.0$
COOCH$_3$	$+1.3$	-0.5	-0.5	$+3.5$

* From Stothers (1972) unless indicated.
† Kelly (1977).
‡ Buchanan *et al* (1974).

the latter can be characterized as being quaternary, methine, methylene, or methyl.

With the Fourier transform spectrometer it is easy to determine relaxation times for the individual nuclei. This allows a wide variety of interactions between molecules to be studied which are difficult with the continuous wave spectrometer. Typically drug–enzyme interactions can be investigated.

^{3}H-n.m.r.

Although the ^{3}H-nucleus has $I = \frac{1}{2}$, the natural abundance is zero, so that ^{3}H-resonances cannot be observed in normal molecules. However, it is common practice in drug metabolism to produce ^{3}H-labelled compounds for tracer studies so ^{3}H-compounds are available for n.m.r. work. About 20μCi of the ^{3}H-compound are required to observe ^{3}H-resonances.

For most ^{3}H-labelled compounds the level of ^{3}H is low, so the spectra are recorded with a Fourier transform spectrometer under conditions where the ^{1}H-coupling is removed by noise decoupling; the ^{3}H-resonances therefore appear as single peaks. The range of values and the factors governing the chemical shifts are similar to those for ^{1}H.

In most cases the structure of the ^{3}H-compound and the position of the ^{3}H-label in the molecule are known. ^{3}H-n.m.r. is finding greatest application in the study of interactions between small organic molecules and large biological polymers, proteins, and enzymes. The advantage of using ^{3}H lies in the fact that water can be used as the solvent and protons in the biological molecule do not interfere with the experiment. For further details see the papers by Elvidge *et al* (Al-Rawi *et al*, 1976 and references cited therein).

APPLICATIONS

Aromatic Oxidation

Ring hydroxylation of compounds containing aromatic rings is a metabolic reaction which commonly occurs. The ^{1}H-n.m.r. spectra of many substituted benzenes often show either a single broad resonance peak or complex multiplets which cannot be analysed. If the spectra are amenable to analysis then it is often possible to assign unambiguously the position of the new hydroxyl group or at least reduce the number of possible positions. If ^{13}C-spectra are available then due to the additivity of substituents, and in particular the large substituent effect of oxygen, it should be possible to determine the structure of the metabolite directly from the spectra.

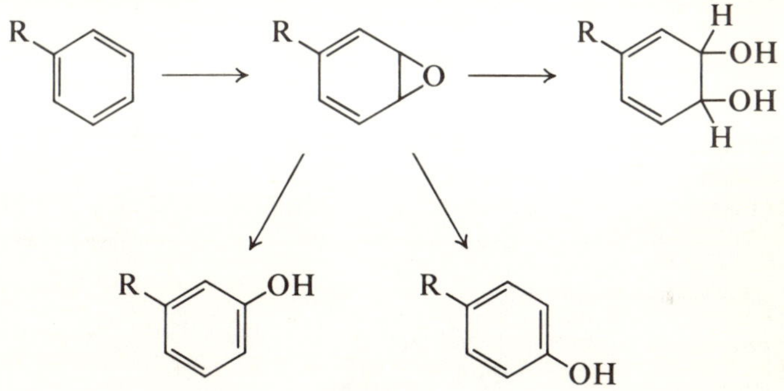

Scheme 1

Ring hydroxylation proceeds *via* a variety of routes and may involve an arene oxide, direct hydroxylation, or rearrangement of an N-hydroxy derivative. The arene oxide undergoes isomerization to the phenol or hydration to yield the dihydrodiol which possibly could lose water to form also an aromatic phenol (Scheme 1). In some cases where the loss of resonance stabilization is relatively

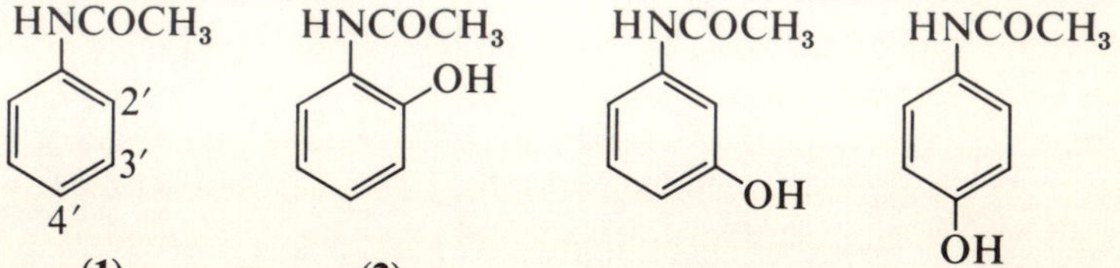

low such as with the polycyclic aromatic hydrocarbons, the arene oxides or the dihydrodiol intermediates may also be isolated. For simple phenyl derivatives, however, the loss of resonance energy is too great and these latter metabolites are rarely isolated.

316

In most cases a number of isomeric hydroxy compounds are possible but not
all of these will be produced. It is desirable then to determine which of these is
formed. In the case of the monosubstituted benzene derivative, acetanilide (1),
all the possible isomers have been observed as metabolites. The ^{1}H- and ^{13}C-
spectra of each of the isomers have been recorded and the aromatic portions
are reproduced in figure 7, as a set of typical spectra which might be observed.
It is noticeable that the ^{13}C-signals for carbons which bear hydrogens were
much more intense than those with substituents, considerably aiding in the
assignments. The carbon bearing the oxygen was the furthest downfield in each
case.

Table 5 ^{13}C-Chemical shifts of hydroxy-substituted acetanilides

Compound	CH_3	C-1	C-2	C-3
Acetanilide	24·1	139·3	119·5	128·5
2-OH-acetanilide	23·6	126·5	148·1	117·0
3-OH-acetanilide	24·2	140·0	107·2	157·5
4-OH-acetanilide	23·7	131·0	121·0	114·9

Compound	C-4	C-5	C-6	C=O
Acetanilide	123·1	128·5	119·5	168·5
2-OH-acetanilide	125·1	119·4	122·1	169·6
3-OH-acetanilide	110·6	129·2	111·1	169·0
4-OH-acetanilide	153·3	114·9	121·0	167·6

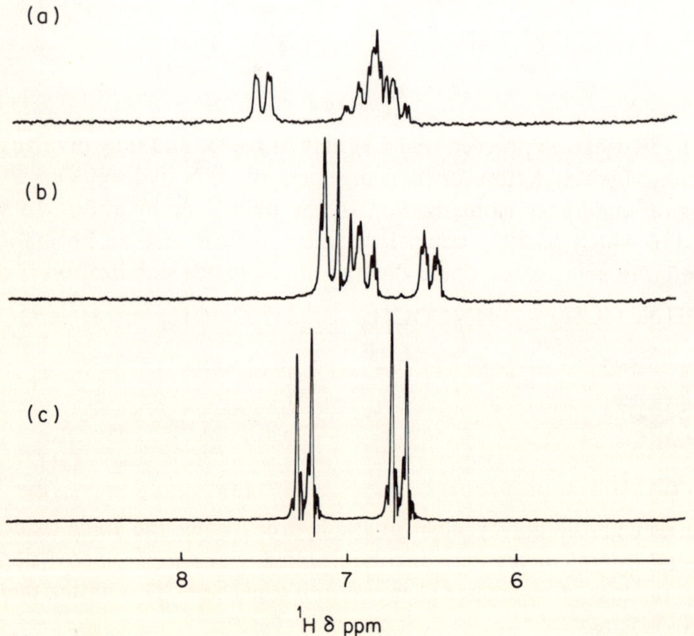

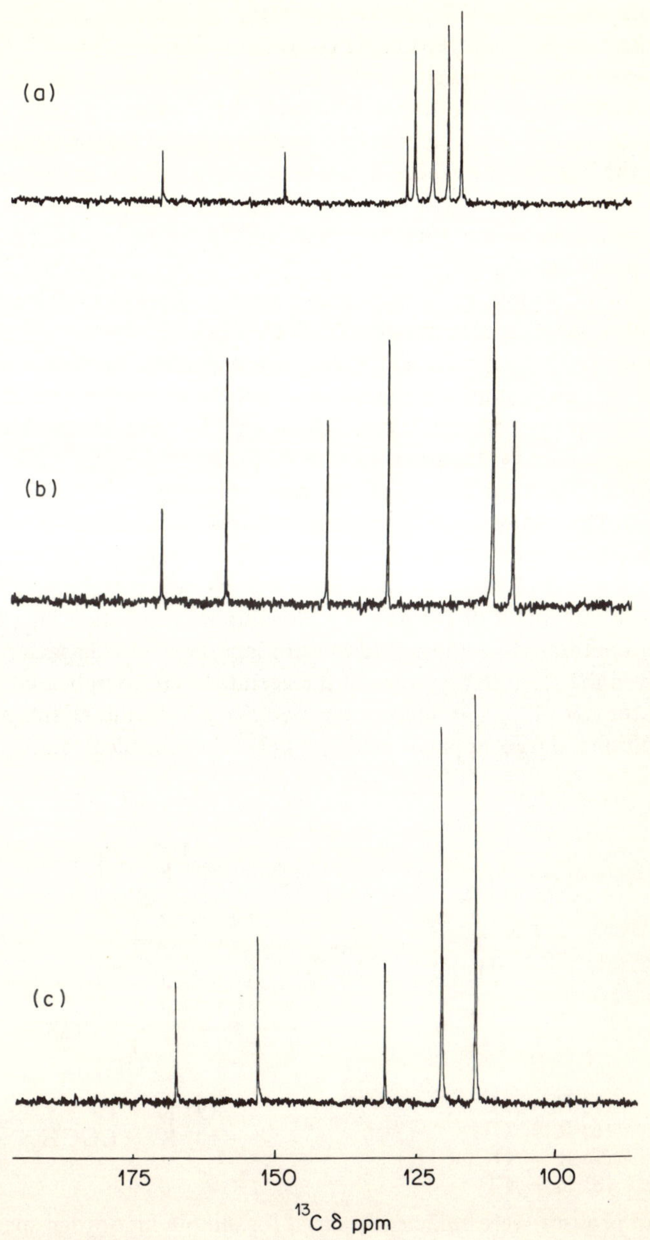

Figure 7 ^{1}H- and ^{13}C-spectra of (a) *ortho*, (b) *meta-*, and (c) *para*-hydroxyacetanilide

318

The 4′-hydroxy compound (4) showed the simplest spectra with an AA′XX′ system in the ¹H-spectrum and four resonance signals in the ¹³C-spectrum. These simple spectra result from the symmetry of the molecule, the 2′ and 6′ as well as the 3′ and 5′ positions being equivalent. The 2′- (2) and 3′ (3) isomers could not easily be distinguished by their proton spectra as the spectra were complex. It is sometimes possible to recognize the 2′-proton in the 3′-isomer by the absence of a large coupling. The ¹³C-spectra allowed easy assignment of the isomers on the basis of the expected substituent effect of the oxygen atom; thus the carbon bearing the nitrogen was shifted upfield by 13 ppm in the 2′-isomer, downfield by 1 ppm in the 3′-isomer, and upfield by 8 ppm in the 4′-isomer, relative to acetanilide.

Metabolism of simple monosubstituted phenyl derivatives frequently produces the *para*-substituted compound, which can often be recognized by the characteristic AA′XX′ or AA′BB′ type proton spectra. In these spectra the presence of the lower intensity inner lines in the spectrum is characteristic of the *para*-disubstituted benzene rings; these can be seen in the spectrum of 4′-hydroxyacetanilide (4) (figure 7).

The study of the metabolism of the chlorobiphenyls by Safe *et al* (1974, 1975a, b, 1976) provides a nice example of the application of ¹H-n.m.r. spectroscopy to the structure determination of metabolites resulting from ring hydroxylation. The simplest of these, 4-chlorobiphenyl (5), was metabolized by pigs to give 4′-chlorobiphenyl-4-ol (6) and 4′-chlorobiphenyl-3,4-diol (9) (Safe *et al*, 1975a). The compounds in these studies were separated and characterized as the acetates. Even the ¹H-n.m.r. spectra of the acetates were complicated and it was found that the use of 220 Hz spectra was necessary to facilitate analysis. Under these conditions (large applied field, 50 kG), the chemical shift differences

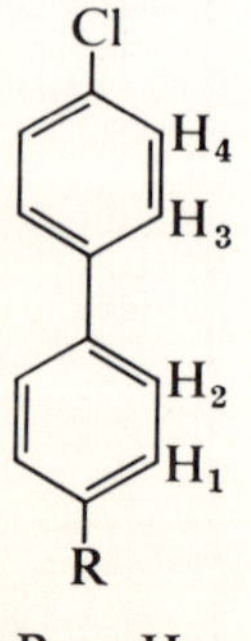

(5) R = H
(6) R = OH
(7) R = OCOCH₃
(8) R = Cl

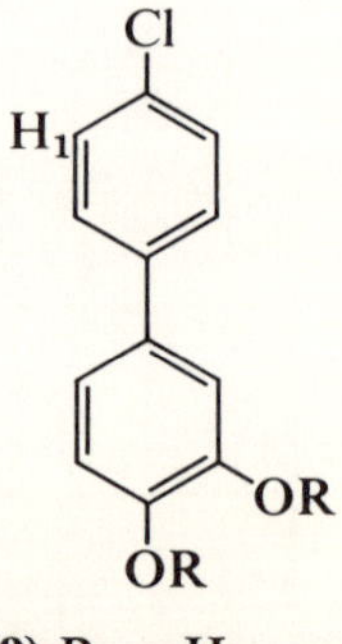

(9) R = H
(10) R = COCH₃

between the protons were sufficiently large for simple first-order spectra to be observed. Thus the spectrum of the acetate (7) showed two *para*-substituted benzene rings in which each of resonances could be easily picked out and assigned thus: δ 7·15 (*d, J* = 8·2 Hz), 7·42 (*d, J* = 8·2 Hz), 7·48 (*d, J* = 8·2 Hz), and 7·55 ppm (*d, J* = 8·2 Hz) assigned to H₁, H₄, H₃, and H₂ respectively. The spectrum of the diacetate (10) of the diol (9) showed an AA′BB′ system δ 7·46 and 7·39 ($J = 8·2$ Hz) and an ABX pattern δ 7·41 ($d, d, J = 8·3, 2·2$ Hz), 7·36 ($d, J = 2·2$ Hz) and 7·25 ppm ($d, J = 8·3$ Hz). On this basis the structure (9) can be reasonably assigned to the second metabolite.

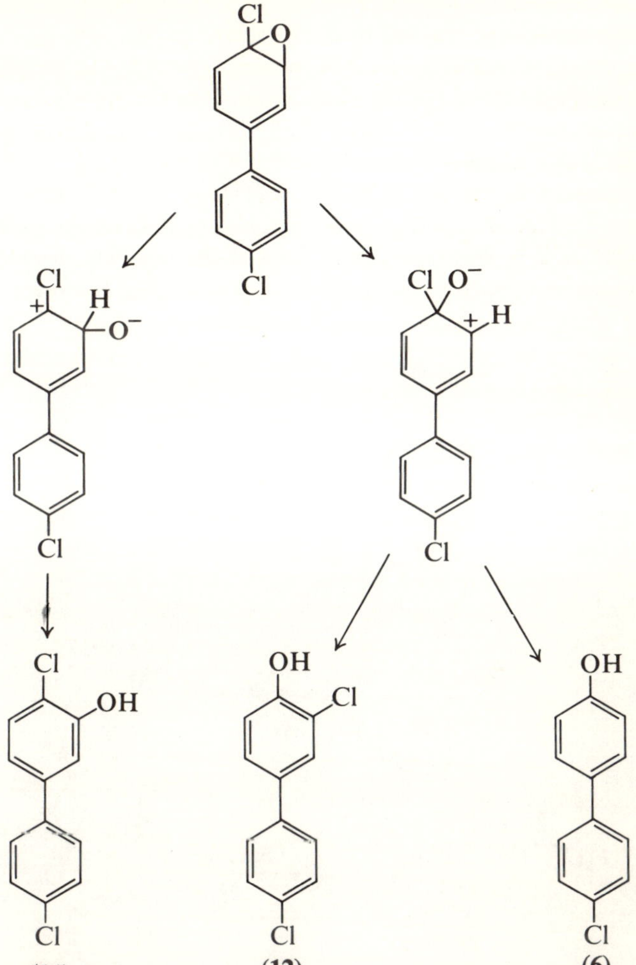

Scheme 2

The same workers have examined the metabolism of a variety of halogenated and hydroxylated biphenyls. However, the metabolism of 4,4′-dichlorobiphenyl (8) is one of considerable interest as it involves three metabolites which are representative of three different routes of biotransformation of an intermediate arene oxide (Safe *et al*, 1976). In addition to the ring hydroxylated compound, 4,4′dichlorobiphenyl-3-ol (11), the substituted compound 4′-chlorobiphenyl-4-ol (6) and the rearranged compound 3,4′-dichlorobiphenyl-4-ol (12) were observed. These result from the alternative ways in which the arene oxide can be opened and the subsequent reactions, often known as the NIH shift (Scheme 2). For a detailed discussion of those reactions see Daly and Jerina (1972) and Jerina and Daly (1974). While 4'-chlorobiphenyl-4-ol (6) can be easily identified and tentative structures assigned to the two alternative hydroxydichlorobiphenyls, to distinguish between the latter is a significant problem. Both would be expected to have similar mass spectra and their ^{1}H-n.m.r. spectra will show an AA'BB' pattern for the disubstituted ring and an ABX pattern for the trisubstituted ring. The spectra observed for the phenols were for the 4,4'-dichloro-3-ol (11): δ 7·05 (1H, q, $J = 8·5$ and 2·2 Hz), 7·21 (1H, d, $J = 2·2$ Hz), 7·36 (1H, d, $J = 8·5$ Hz), 7·38 (2H, d, $J = 8·5$ Hz) and 7·47 ppm (2H, d, $J = 8·5$ Hz), and for 3,4'-dichlorobiphenyl-4-ol (12) δ 7·09 (1H, d, $J = 8·5$ Hz), 7·37 (1H, q, $J = 8·5$ and 2·2 Hz), 7·39 (2H, d, $J = 8·5$ Hz), 7·45 (2H, d, $J = 8·5$ Hz) and 7·52 ppm (1H, d, $J = 2·2$ Hz). On the basis of the highfield doublet, the latter compound can be tentatively assigned to structure (12). However, the assignments were confirmed by unambiguous synthesis.

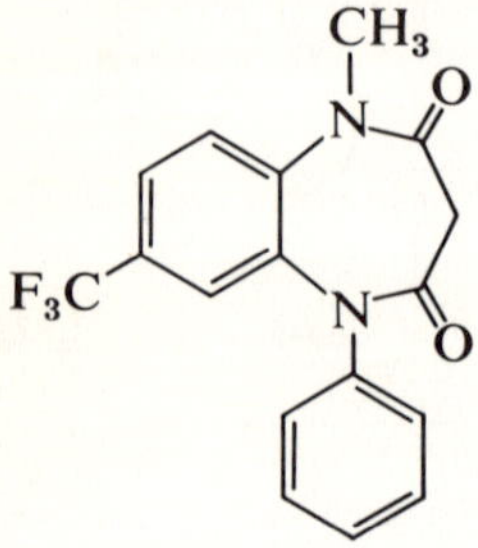

(13)

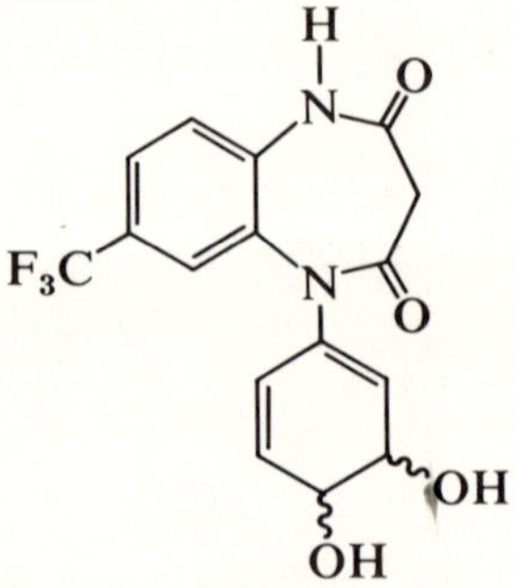

(14)

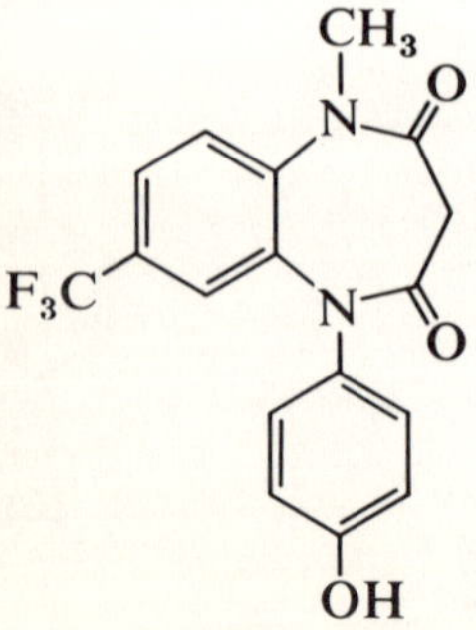

(15)

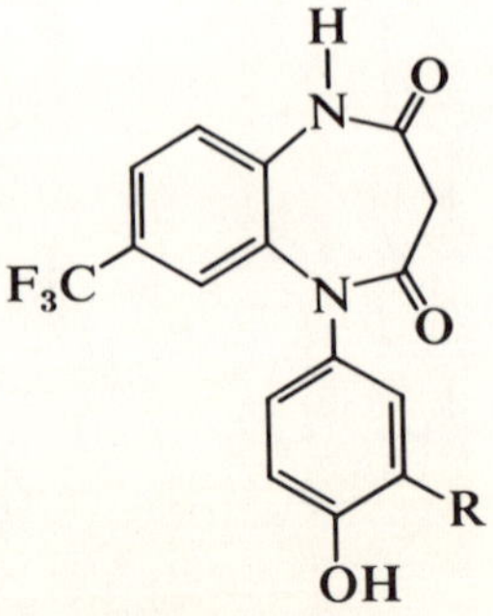

(16) R = H
(17) R = OH
(18) R = OCH$_3$

The metabolism of the 1,5-benzodiazepine, triflubazam (13), by man is a typical example where the *para*-hydroxylation of a phenyl ring is an important reaction (Alton *et al*, 1975). The metabolism involved the loss of the N-methyl group and oxidation, presumably via the arene oxide. In this case about 20% of the dihydrodiol compound (14) was isolated. The structure was formulated on the basis of the mass spectrum and further confirmed by the proton n.m.r. spectrum which showed resonance peaks described as characteristic of the dihydrodiol at δ 3·48 (*s*, 2H), δ 5·6–6·17 (*m*, 3H) and δ 7·5–7·7 ppm (*m*, 3H). Presumably the peaks at δ 5·6–6·17 are the olefinic protons, but unfortunately the full spectral data were not given nor was the spectrum reproduced. The major metabolite was the 4′-hydroxy derivative (**16**) which had also lost the N-methyl group. Some 4′-hydroxylated material retaining the N-methyl (**15**) was also obtained. Other metabolites identified included those which resulted from dehydrogenation of the dihydrodiol, for example the 3′,4′-dihydroxy-(**17**) and the 4′-hydroxy-3′-methoxy-(**18**) compounds. Authentic samples of all the metabolites except the dihydrodiol were available and spectra were used to confirm the identities of the compounds isolated.

Since loss of water can occur from the dihydroxy-dihydro compound to give two different phenols with the hydroxyl group either *meta* or *para* to the substituent, the position of hydroxyl cannot be assumed to be *para*. In many cases a mixture of both isomers is formed; thus metabolism of the 6-phenylbenzodiazepine (**19**) has been shown to give the 4′-hydroxy derivatives in man and in rats (Kanai, 1974). However, in dogs the 3′-hydroxy compound was also produced. Both phenyl hydroxylations were accompanied by some oxidation in the triazine and diazepine rings and a large number of metabolites were observed. Only the two metabolites with 4′-hydroxyl substituents, e.g. (**20**),

(19) R = H
(20) R = OH

(21)

were isolated in sufficient yield for the proton n.m.r. spectra to be recorded. The spectra showed the expected patterns for the aromatic protons. All the metabolites were identified by comparison with authentic samples. The spectra from the *meta*-substituted compounds would be expected to be much more complex than those from the *para*-isomers and may be difficult to distinguish from the unsymmetrically substituted *ortho*-isomer.

Hydroxylation of unsymmetrically *ortho*- and *meta*-disubstituted benzenes can possibly occur in four positions. In man, two major urinary metabolites resulted from administration of viloxazine (**21**) (Case and Reeves, 1975). Each had one hydroxyl group; the proton n.m.r. spectrum of the major isomer showed the hydroxyl to be at position 4 or 5, by a characteristic ABC type spectrum where $J_{AB} = 8$ Hz, $J_{BC} = 3$ Hz, and $J_{AC} = 0$ Hz. The choice between the two alternatives could not be made on the basis of the chemical shifts and final identification was made by comparison with authentic samples of both possible isomers. The major isomer was found to have the hydroxyl located at the 5-position.

The substituted flufenamate (22) has two disubstituted benzene rings, either of which could be hydroxylated. In most species studied (Kodama *et al*, 1975), oxidation of the aliphatic hydroxyl to a carboxylic acid (23) was the major biotransformation although in guinea-pigs the major metabolite was a ring hydroxylated compound. Analysis of the proton n.m.r. spectrum of the administered drug allowed assignment of the aromatic proton resonances. The spectrum of the hydroxylated metabolite showed the protons of the trifluoromethyl substituted ring to be unchanged, and the collapse of the triplet due to H-6 or H-7; thus hydroxylation must have occurred in the quinazoline ring system. H-5 was assigned to the highfield resonance due to the effect of the phenyl ring; thus an analysis of the spectrum placed the hydroxy at C-6 where $J_{78} = 8$ Hz and $J_{57} = 2$ Hz, the metabolite being (24).

1,2,3-Trisubstituted benzenes such as lidocaine (25) and mepivacaine (26) are much simpler systems to assign the position of a new hydroxyl substituent. When the hydroxyl is *para* to the nitrogen, a singlet will be observed for the

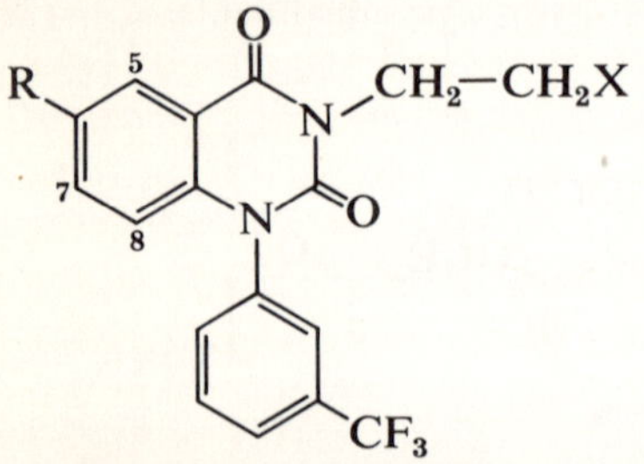

(22) R = H, X = OH
(23) R = H, CH$_2$X = COOH
(24) R = OH, X = OH

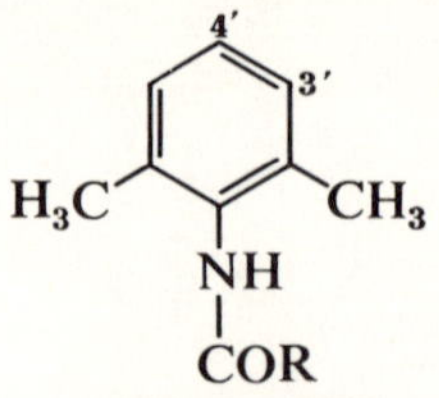

(25) R = (C$_2$H$_5$)$_2$NCH$_2$-
(26) R = 2-(N-methylpiperidinyl)-
(27) R = 2-(N-butylpiperidinyl)-

aromatic protons and when *meta*, an AB doublet ($J \simeq 8$ Hz). The spectra have been used to determine the structures of the 3′- and 4′-hydroxy metabolites of lidocaine and mepivacaine (Thomas and Meffin, 1972) and the 3′-hydroxy metabolite of bupivacaine (27) (Goehl *et al*, 1973).

The Fourier transform n.m.r. spectra of the trifluoroacetyl derivatives of two metabolites of (28) were obtained using 2 µg for ^{1}H-spectra and 2 mg for ^{13}C-spectra (Scott *et al*, 1973). The ^{1}H-spectra showed only one aromatic methyl group in (29) and the presence of a CH$_2$ adjacent to an oxygen atom (δ 4·68), with the remainder of the spectrum similar to that of (28). In contrast, the aromatic A$_2$B spectral splitting pattern of (28) was replaced by a two proton singlet in (30). Thus the ^{1}H-spectra allowed assignment of a structure to both metabolites. The ^{13}C-spectra could then be predicted by applying the known substituent effects to the spectrum of (28). The spectra observed for both metabolites were consistent with those expected, thus proving the structures. At the low concentrations used, the quartet due to the carbon of the CF_3 group, expected to be a quartet due to the coupling with fluorine ($I = \frac{1}{2}$), was not observed. Most of the other resonances were observed demonstrating the power of the Fourier transform technique for obtaining spectra on small quantities of

(28) R = H, R' = H
(29) R = OH, R' = H
(30) R = H, R' = OH

metabolites. As a further confirmation of the structures the spectra were recorded without proton decoupling. Under these conditions all the peaks could be unequivocally assigned from the coupling observed to the protons.

Aliphatic Oxidation

The first step in the metabolic oxidation of aliphatic groups results in the formation of alcohols. These are characterized in ^{1}H-n.m.r. spectra by the loss of the initial alkyl group resonance and the appearance at lower field of a signal with one less proton. Analysis of the splitting pattern can often allow assignment of the position of the hydroxyl in an alkyl chain with a number of carbon atoms. The observation of the resonance of the hydroxyl proton is dependent on the solvent. In dimethylsulphoxide-d$_6$ the exchange reaction is slowed down and coupling may be observed. In most solvents the exchange results in broad signals and the resonance is not of much diagnostic value. The ^{13}C-n.m.r. spectrum will show the hydroxylated carbon shifted downfield by about 50–60 ppm.

Further oxidation may occur either enzymatically or non-enzymatically to give carboxylic acids from primary alcohols or ketones from secondary alcohols. In the case of hydroxylation on a carbon α- to a hetero-atom, the alkyl group may be lost completely; this is the mechanism for dealkylation of many amines and ethers. Examples of the latter reactions are considered under dealkylation reactions.

In (31) there is a methyl group and an n-propyl group which can be hydroxylated. Deacetylation to (33) was the major biotransformation route, and was accompanied by hydroxylation of the methyl and the α-carbon of the propyl group. Thus various amounts of the hydroxylated metabolites (32), (34), and (35) as well as other metabolites were found, the relative amounts being dependent on the species of animal (Case *et al*, 1972). Dogs were much better at hydroxylating the side-chain than the other species studied. The hydroxylated compounds were readily characterized by their mass and ^{1}H-n.m.r. spectra.

The aromatic methyl (δ 2·3) in (33) showed the characteristic broadening due to small coupling to the *ortho*-ring proton ($J \simeq 2$ Hz), and on hydroxylation (35) shifted downfield to δ 4·45 as a two proton singlet. On the other hand, hydroxylation of the α-proton in the propyl group to (34) showed a downfield shift of a triplet ($J = 7$ Hz) from δ 3·05 to δ 4·92 with a reduction in the coupling ($J = 6$ Hz). The position of hydroxyl groups on side-chains are on the whole easy to determine by ^{1}H-n.m.r.

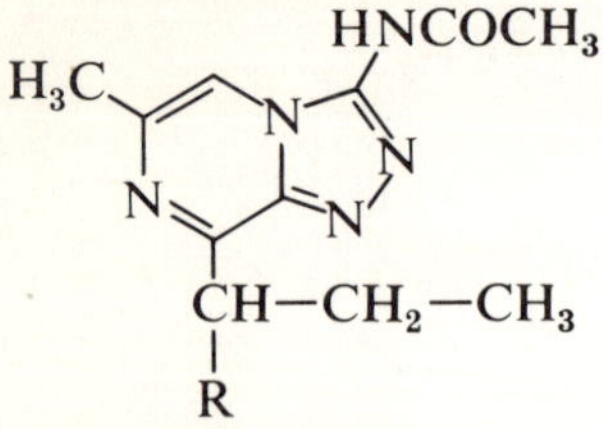

(31) R = H
(32) R = OH

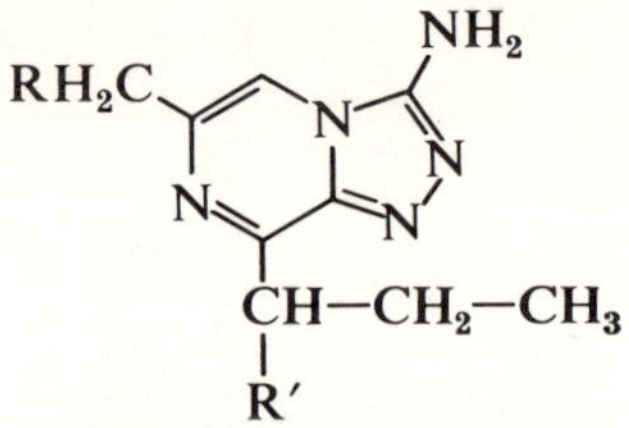

(33) R = H, R′ = H
(34) R = H, R′ = OH
(35) R = OH, R′ = H

Most of the metabolites of γ-phenylpropyl carbamate (36) were acidic; however, the neutral fraction contained a mixture of carbamates which led to a disparity between g.l.c. and colorimetric methods for the analyses of (36) (Farrier, 1975). The main neutral carbamate was identified as (37) resulting from hydroxylation on the benzylic carbon. The spectrum (figure 8) showed a much more complex pattern than might be expected and is worth close examination.

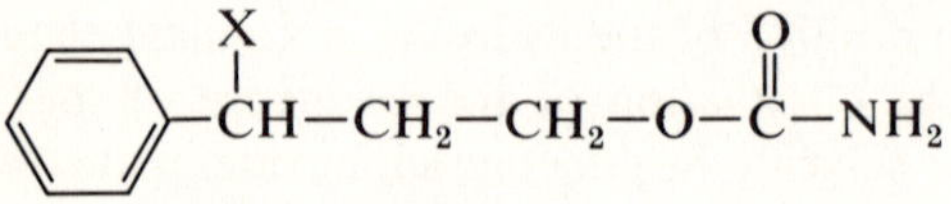

(36) X = H
(37) X = OH

Firstly, the hydrogen on the benzylic carbon bearing the oxygen showed a triplet, each line being further split into doublets. This coupling was usually not observed unless the spectrum was recorded in DMSO-d$_6$, and required the presence of strong hydrogen bonding as is indicated in figure 8. The hydroxyl also occurred as a doublet. This coupling was readily removed by exchange with a little D$_2$O and the spectrum then showed a triplet for the hydrogen on the γ-carbon and the removal of the signal due to the hydroxyl. Secondly, the signal from the methylene protons (C-1) adjacent to the carbamate group was very complex. The substitution of a hydroxyl on the benzylic methylene resulted in an asymmetric carbon atom. The two enantiomers (*R* and *S* forms) did not have different spectra but rather the asymmetry caused the hydrogens of nearby methylene groups to become non-equivalent. In this case the two hydrogens on C-1 were non-equivalent and the coupling between them produced an AB quartet ($J \simeq 16$ Hz). In this case also, each of the four lines of the AB quartet could be further split into a quartet by the adjacent methylene and a total of

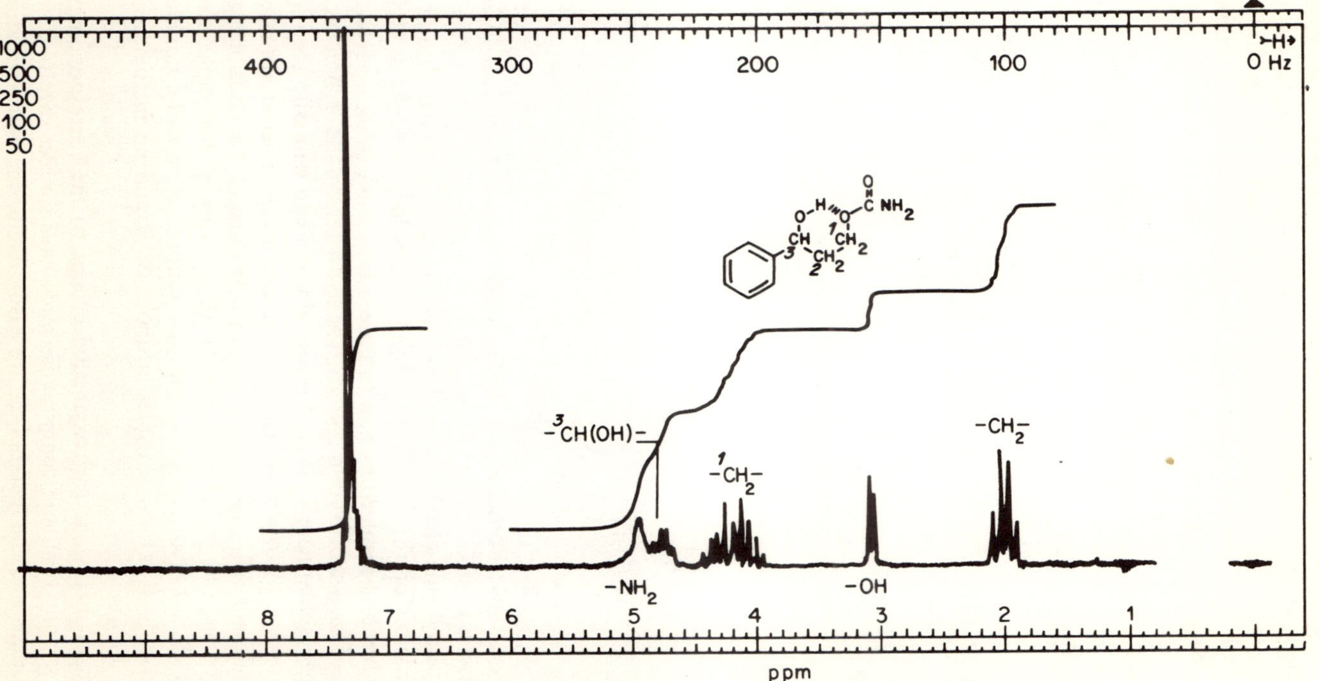

Figure 8 ¹H-n.m.r. spectrum of 3-hydroxyphenprobamate (reproduced with permission, Farrier, 1975)

16 lines could be observed, although they are not all detected. Surprisingly the two hydrogens of the C-2 methylene were equivalent and a quartet was observed; thus part of the spectrum was somewhat simpler than might have been expected.

Because of the psychotomimetic properties of cannabis the metabolism of cannabinols has been studied extensively. The metabolism of Δ^9-tetrahydrocannabinol (**38**) was first reported to involve hydroxylation of the C-9 methyl, and the structure of the product was proved by synthesis and its ^{1}H-n.m.r. spectrum (Wall *et al*, 1970; Ben-Zvi *et al*, 1970). Subsequent studies of Δ^9-tetrahydrocannabinol (**38**) (Widman *et al*, 1975), Δ^8-tetrahydrocannabinol (Binder *et al*, 1974), cannabidiol (**39**) (Martin *et al*, 1976), and cannabinol (**40**)

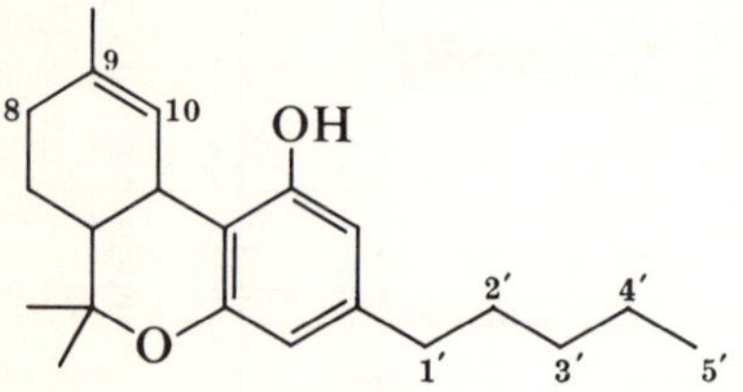

(**38**)

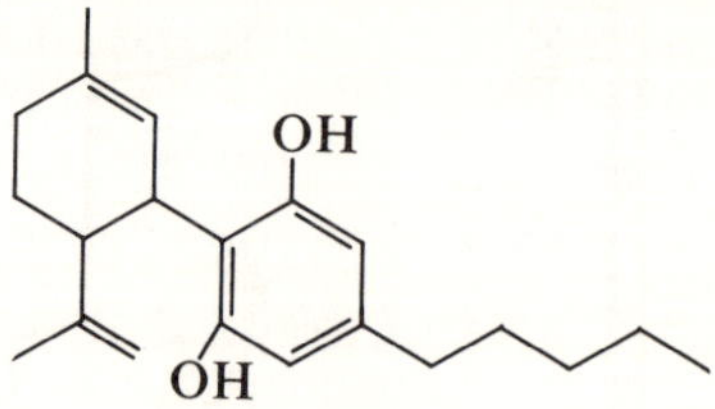

(**39**)

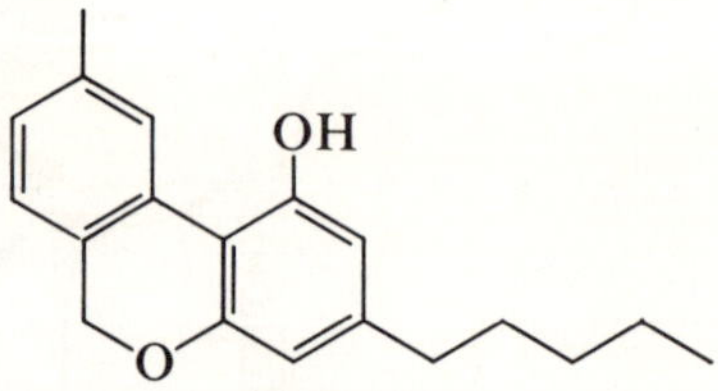

(**40**)

(Petrzilka *et al*, 1969; Fonseka and Widman, 1977) have confirmed hydroxylation at the methyl at C-9, and subsequent hydroxylation at all possible positions in the pentyl side-chain occurred as well as some hydroxylation at C-8. The determination of the structures of the metabolites presents a complex problem which is best resolved by n.m.r., since it is possible to pick out features characteristic of each substitution pattern. The hydrogen on the carbon carrying the new oxygen substituent is moved downfield and can be easily seen in the spectrum. Thus a 1'-hydroxyl was characterized by a 1H triplet at about δ 4·5; a 2'-hydroxyl by an ABX pattern for the 1'-methylene and a multiplet about δ 3·8; a 3'-hydroxyl by a 2H pentuplet at about δ 3·8 and a triplet for the methyl at δ 0·95; a 4'-hydroxyl by a multiplet at about δ 3·6 and a doublet for the methyl; a 5'-hydroxyl by a triplet at about δ 3·7 and no methyl at δ 0·9 (Binder *et al*, 1974).

Metabolism of methyl or hydroxymethyl groups to the corresponding carboxylic acids usually results in compounds which have simpler spectra than the parent compounds and the metabolites are easily identified. Thus oxidation of the methyl group of (**41**) to the acid (**42**) resulted in the loss of the methyl group (δ 2·45) and a downfield shift of the protons *ortho* to the methyl in the aromatic ring from δ 7·27 to δ 7·76 (Sumner *et al*, 1975). Where the oxidized group is part of an alkyl chain, then as well as a downfield shift of the adjacent group, there will be a simplification of the coupling pattern. The spectrum of the acid (44) derived from the alcohol (43) showed such a simplification (DiCuollo *et al*, 1973). Thus triplets were observed for both the methylenes in (44) presumably $J = 7$ Hz, since all the couplings reported seemed to be double the expected value.

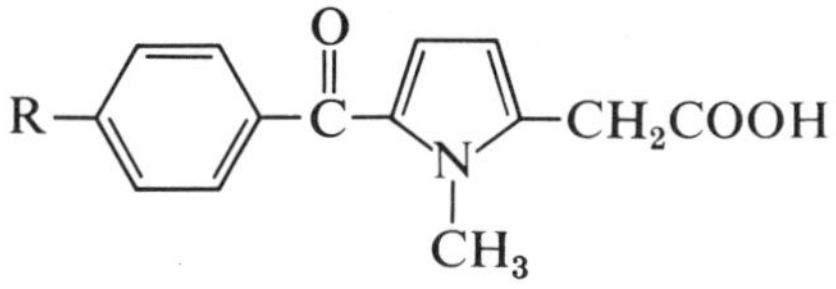

$$R\!-\!\!\underset{}{\bigcirc}\!\!-\!\!\overset{\overset{\text{O}}{\|}}{\text{C}}\!-\!\underset{\underset{\text{CH}_3}{|}}{\underset{\text{N}}{\bigcirc}}\!-\!\text{CH}_2\text{COOH}$$

(41) R = CH₃
(42) R = COOH

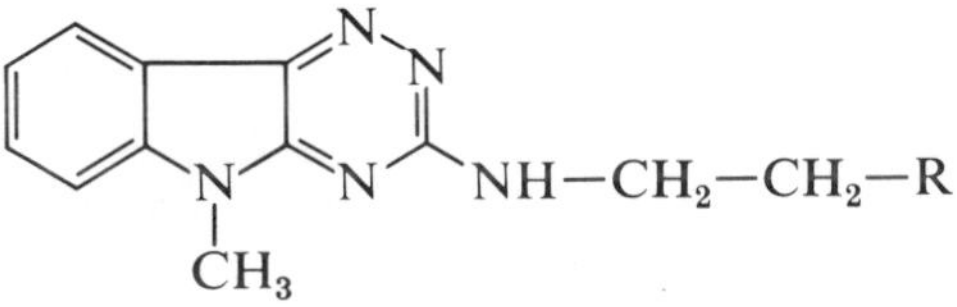

(43) R = CH₂OH
(44) R = COOH

An interesting sequence of reactions was proposed to account for the oxidative metabolism of the anticoagulant (45) by rat liver microsomes which were found to produce one principal metabolite (Thonart *et al*, 1977). The metabolism was postulated to proceed via tautomerism of the 4-hydroxycoumarin moiety to a 2-hydroxychromone and the decarboxylation of the 2-hydroxychromone structure with simultaneous oxidation of the carbon in the 3-position to the α-diketone (46). The metabolite formed was thought to be a 1 : 1 mixture of the two enols (47) and (48), the structures of which were assigned on the basis of their u.v., i.r., mass, and n.m.r. spectra. It seems unlikely that five- and six-membered enol structures such as (47) and (48) would contribute equally to a tautomeric mixture and the authors did not give any basis for their assignments from the n.m.r. spectrum. It is difficult in this sort of situation to assign resonances to specific isomers unless they can be separated, and an alternative structure might account better for the spectra observed. Two carbonyls were observed in the i.r. spectrum, so that only one is required in each isomer. The hydroxyl resonances were found at δ 6·38 and δ 6·67 whereas the hydroxyl in *o*-hydroxyacetophenone was found at δ 12 and enols such as acetylacetone at around δ 15–16. This would suggest that the two compounds did not contain two strongly hydrogen bonded enols but rather some other sort of hydroxyls. Perhaps the two possible isomeric forms of the cyclic five-membered ring compound (49) could account better for the spectra, as presumably an *RS* mixture of stereoisomers at C-9 was used.

Oxidation of cyclic saturated systems with the introduction of a hydroxyl group leads to compounds which often have complex ¹H-n.m.r. spectra. This is due to the fact that the protons of methylene groups will not be equivalent and hence complex coupling patterns will be observed. Also, the rings are often conformationally unstable and a number of isomers may contribute to the spectrum. On the other hand, detailed analyses of the spectrum may allow the determination of the stereochemistry of the system, as the coupling constants are dependent on the dihedral angle between the protons. Even the ring hydroxy

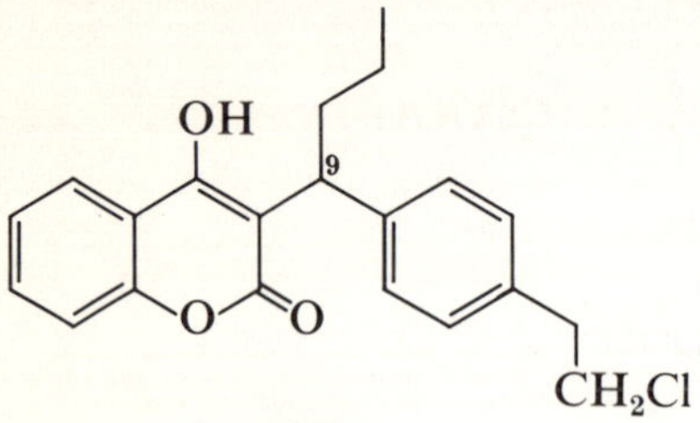

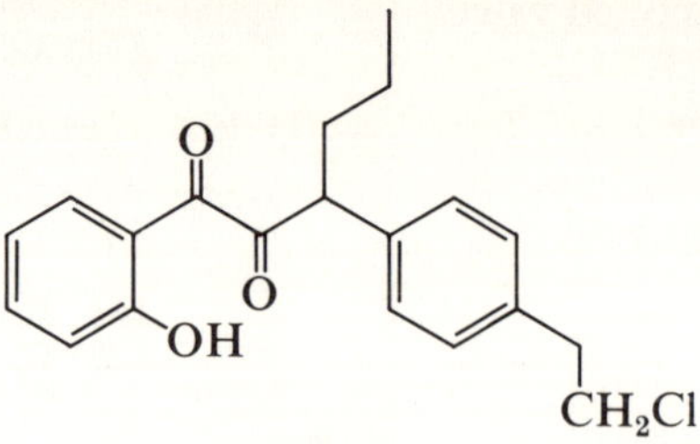

derivative (51) of the glutarimide (50) showed a complex spectrum, despite the fact that there are only two methylene groups in the parent compound. The hydroxy compound showed a quartet which was attributed to the X region of an ABX system, but the remainder of the spectrum was not analysed. From the chemical shifts and the other spectroscopic data the structure (51) was proposed for the metabolite (Ambre and Fischer, 1974).

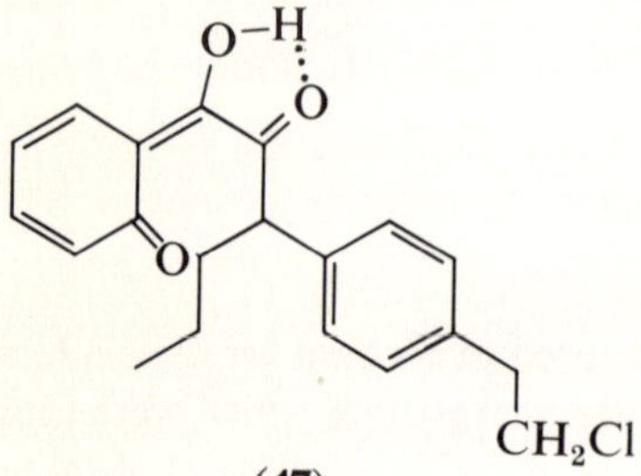

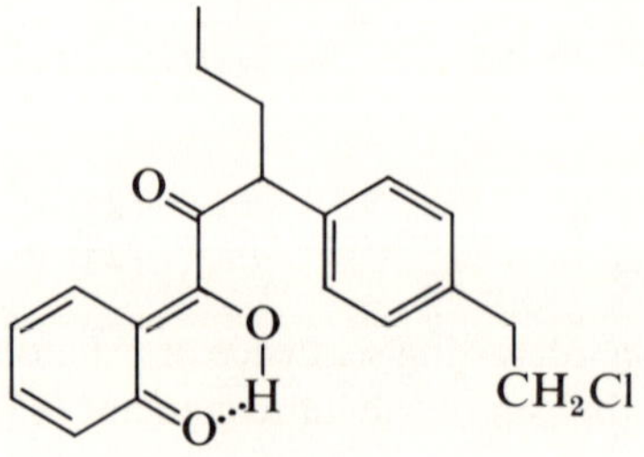

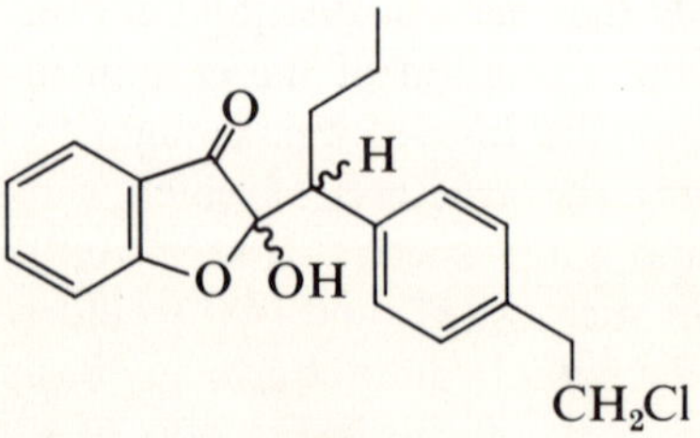

In a much more complex situation, bucloxic acid (52) was converted to a number of metabolites (Gros *et al*, 1974). The side-chain was degraded to an acetic acid residue and the cyclohexane ring was hydroxylated to (53). The phenyl ring was found to be equatorial in all metabolites and the hydroxyl group was observed in both the axial and equatorial positions. The spectra were very complex and the assignments were made on the basis of spin decoupling and the use of europium shift reagents. The stereochemistry was assigned on the basis of the line width of the signal from the hydrogen adjacent to the phenyl and hydroxyl groups. Axial hydrogens would be expected to show broader signals than their equatorial counterparts, due to the larger axial–axial couplings as compared with axial–equatorial couplings. The spectra were not reproduced and only a qualitative description of the results was given.

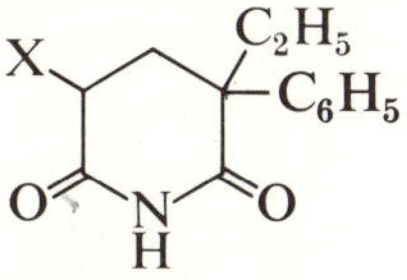

(50) X = H
(51) X = OH

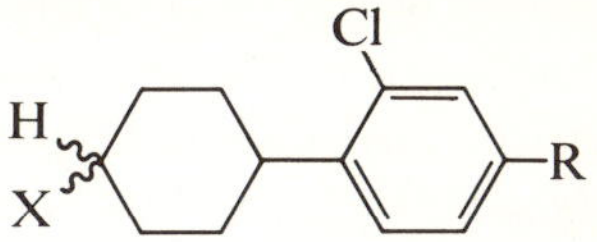

(52) X = H, R = $-\overset{O}{\overset{\|}{C}}-CH_2CH_2-COOH$
(53) X = OH, R = $-CH_2-COOH$

The macrolide antibiotic **(54)** was hydroxylated at position 14 and lost the ester function at position 3 (Inouye *et al*, 1972). The assignment of the position of hydroxylation to position 14 by ^{1}H-n.m.r. demonstrates the power of the technique. In a complex series of spin decoupling experiments most of the resonances could be assigned; in particular, those from the olefinic hydrogens could be observed as well as those at C-14 and C-15. The hydrogen at C-15 appeared as an octet due to coupling with the methyl hydrogens and the hydrogen adjacent to the new hydroxyl. This became a doublet when the methyl was

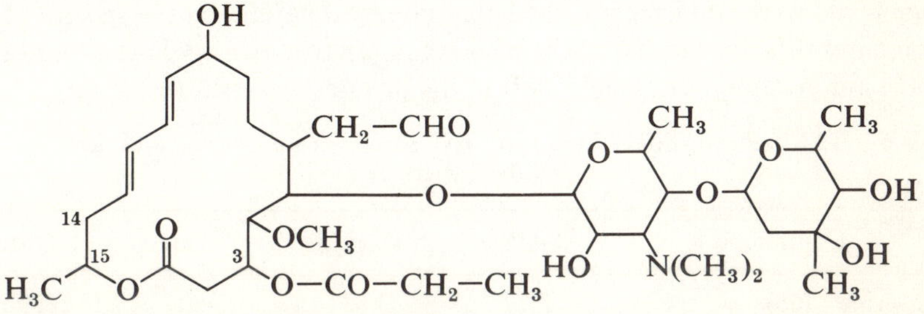

(54)

irradiated. When the hydrogen at C-14 was irradiated, the octet became a quartet and at the same time the quartet due to H-13 became a doublet. Thus the hydroxyl was assigned to C-14, which was consistent with the rest of the spectrum.

Dealkylation

Dealkylation reactions are the consequence of aliphatic hydroxylation at the carbon atom α to a hetero atom. After hydroxylation, the α-hydroxy compound is readily hydrolysed to the aldehyde and the free alcohol, thiol, or amine. This reaction will often occur spontaneously and the α-hydroxy compound cannot be isolated, although in some cases, where nitrogen is the hetero atom, both the α-hydroxy compound and the amine can be isolated by careful procedures.

When the group is lost, the n.m.r. spectrum will be much simpler; most of the spectrum will be the same as the administered drug with the absence of the peaks due to the lost alkyl group. A new signal due to the NH, OH, or SH may be visible, but not always as the signals can be broad because of exchange with other protons.

O-Demethylation is normally easily recognized, and the resultant products readily characterized. However, in molecules such as papaverine (**55**) which has several methoxyl groups, mono-O-demethylation can give rise to a number of different products and perhaps the best method to distinguish between them is ^{1}H-n.m.r. spectroscopy. Each of the methoxyl signals could be observed and have been assigned (Table 6, Brochmann-Hanssen and Hirai, 1968). The structure of (**56**) and (**59**)—obtained from microbial transformation (Rosazza

(**55**) R_1, R_2, R_3, R_4 = CH_3
(**56**) R_1 = H: R_2, R_3, R_4 = CH_3
(**57**) R_2 = H: R_1, R_3, R_4 = CH_3
(**58**) R_3 = H: R_1, R_2, R_4 = CH_3
(**59**) R_4 = H: R_1, R_2, R_3 = CH_3

et al, 1977)—and of (**57**) and (**59**)—from incubation with rat liver microsomes (Belpaire, *et al*, 1975)—were assigned on the basis of their n.m.r. spectra. The assignments were confirmed in the latter case by determining the spectra of the metabolites dissolved in base. The increase in electron density in the ring carrying the anion caused an upfield shift in the protons attached to the ring.

Table 6 ^{1}H-Chemical shifts of the methoxyl groups of papaverine and demethylated derivatives

Compound		3'-OMe	4'-OMe	7-OMe	6-OMe
Papaverine	(**55**)	3·77	3·82	3·90	3·99
	(**56**)	3·67	3·82	3·92	—
	(**57**)	3·72	3·77	—	4·02
	(**58**)	3·73	—	3·89	4·00
	(**59**)	—	3·82	3·90	3·99

Metabolism of the side-chain of the oxadiazole (**60**) showed the typical features expected for N-demethylation (Allen *et al*, 1971). The N-methyl group appeared as a singlet in the ^{1}H-n.m.r. spectrum at δ 3·10, which was at the same chemical shift as the methylene adjacent to the oxadiazole ring. Two main metabolites were isolated. The first showed no N-methyl group and a broad signal due to an NH at δ 6·0 as expected for the demethylated compound (**61**). The second was unstable, and when extracted under basic conditions also gave the demethylated compound (**61**). Treatment of a methanolic solution of the metabolite with HCl yielded the methoxymethyl compound (63) which was characterized by two new singlets replacing the N-methyl signal, one at δ 4·6 (2H), due to the methylene between the N and O, and one at δ 3·21 (3H) due to the O-methyl. The methoxymethyl compound (63) thus was derived by the acid catalysed methylation of the hydroxymethyl compound (62)

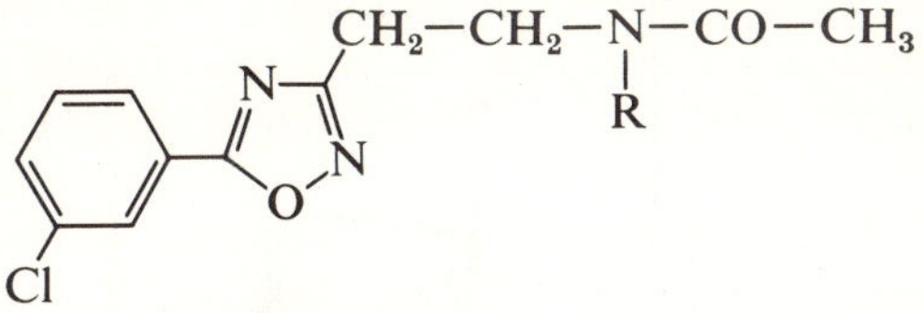

$$CH_2-CH_2-N-CO-CH_3$$

(60) R = CH_3
(61) R = H
(62) R = CH_2OH
(63) R = CH_2-O-CH_3

Metabolism of piromidic acid (64) produced some of the possible oxidative metabolites which can be formed from cyclic amines (Sekine *et al*, 1976). These are easily characterized by their ^{1}H-n.m.r. spectra. The first step involved the formation of the α-hydroxy compound (65) which showed an extremely complex series of signals from the pyrrolidine ring protons which were all non-equivalent (figure 9a). Ring opening to the aldehyde and oxidation to the carboxylic acid yielded the second metabolite (66) isolated. This provided a simpler spectrum than (65) as the hydrogens of each of the methylenes in the chain were now equivalent. The methylene adjacent to the carboxyl appeared as a triplet, δ 2·4; due to slow exchange in dimethylsulphoxide, the NH showed coupling

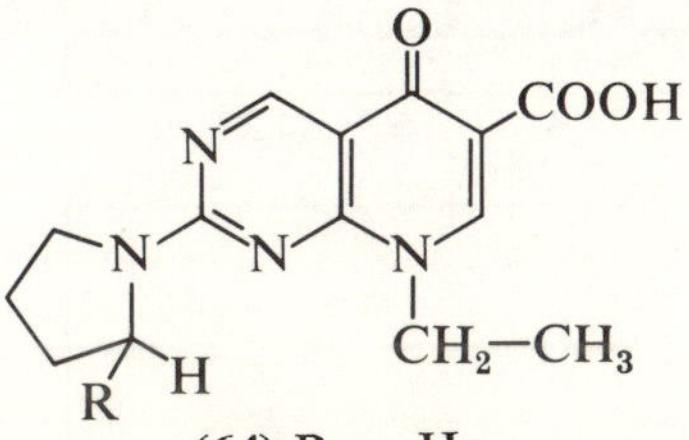

(64) R = H
(65) R = OH

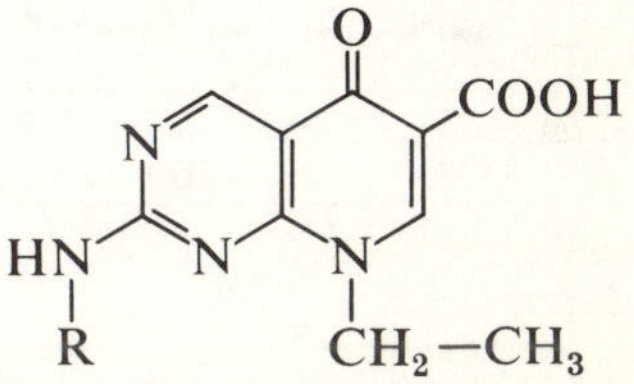

(66) R = $-CH_2-CH_2-CH_2-COOH$
(67) R = H

to the adjacent methylene, which occurred as a broadened quartet at δ 4·3, and the NH a broadened triplet at δ 8·8 (figure 9c). Formation of the third metabolite involved complete loss of the pyrrolidine ring (67). Its spectrum showed the protons of the remainder of the molecule together with an amino group at δ 7·9 (figure 9b).

The metabolism of debrisoquine sulphate (68) yielded two acidic metabolites resulting from ring opening and oxidation to the carboxylic acids (Allen *et al*, 1976). To facilitate identification, the $N-C{\stackrel{-N}{\scriptscriptstyle \searrow N}}$ groups were condensed with acetylacetone to form pyrimidines and the acids esterfied with diazomethane.

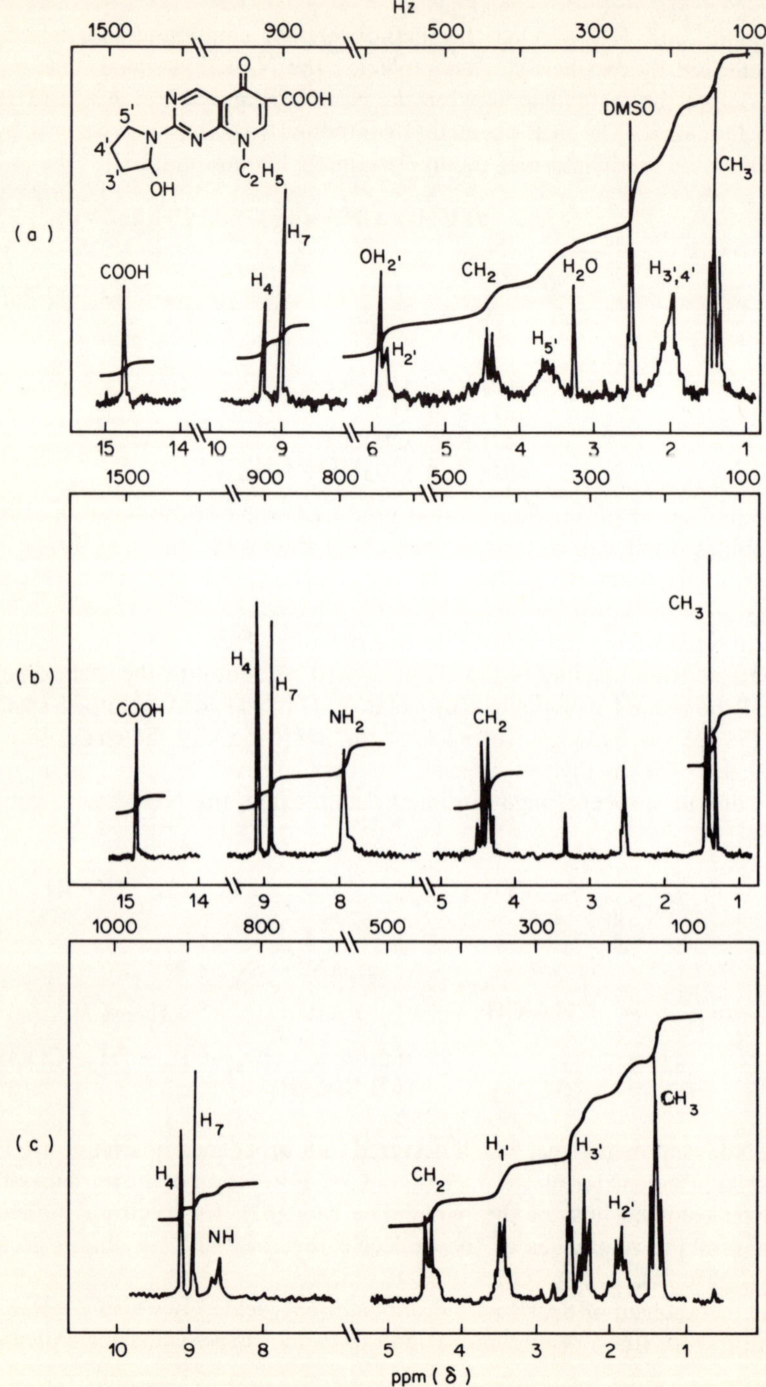

Figure 9 ^{1}H-n.m.r. spectra of metabolites of piromidic acid (a) **65**, (b) **(67)**, and (c) **(66)** (reproduced by permission, Sekine *et al*, 1976)

The two metabolites (69) and (70) formed by ring opening at positions 1 and 3 respectively could then be characterized from their ^{1}H-n.m.r. spectra. The former showed two triplets at δ 3·28 and δ 3·74, J = 7 Hz, whereas (70) showed two singlets at δ 3·82 and δ 4·68.

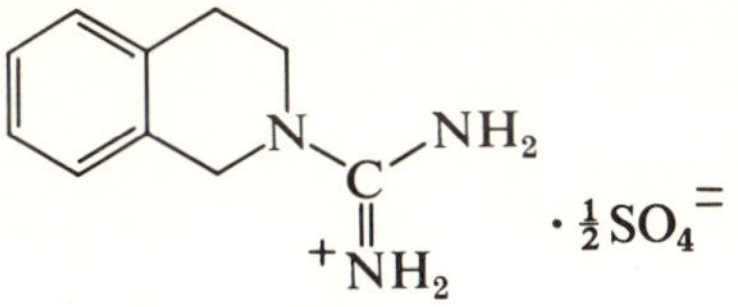

(68)

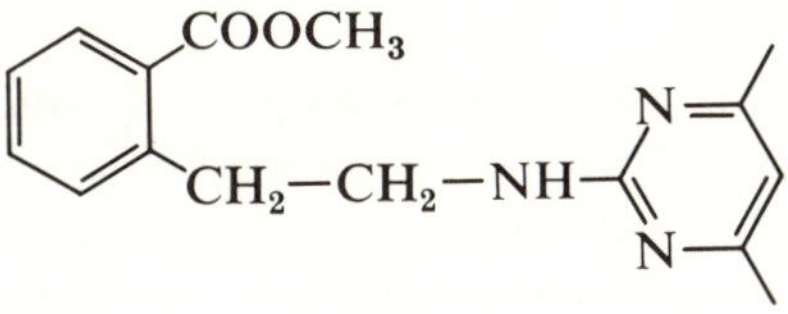

(69)

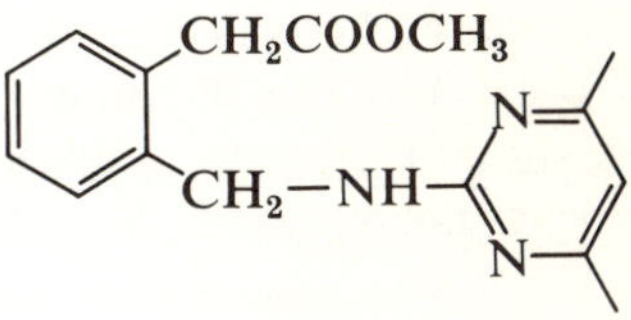

(70)

Methylation

Metabolic O-methylation is a common pathway for catechols where a monomethyl derivative is formed, and it also occurs occasionally with phenols. The methylation may occur subsequent to the introduction of the hydroxyl group, and the methoxyl group thus produced is characterized by a singlet (3H) at about δ 4·8, a region in ^{1}H-n.m.r. spectra which is usually relatively free of other resonances.

A good example of this type of reaction was seen in the metabolism of (71) (Zacchei et al, 1976; Zacchei and Wishousky, 1977). In this case both one (72)

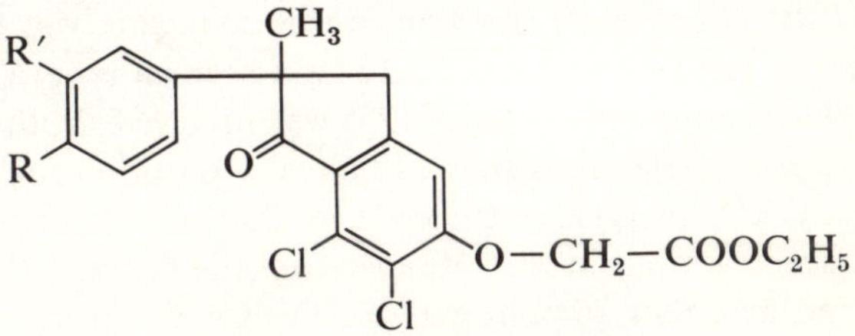

(71) R = H, R' = H
(72) R = OH, R' = H
(73) R = OCH$_3$, R' = H
(74) R = OH, R' = OH
(75) R = OH, R' = OCH$_3$
(76) R = OCH$_3$, R' = OH

and two hydroxyl (74) groups were introduced into the phenyl ring and in both cases monomethylated compounds were produced. Thus the 4-methoxy compound (73) and a methoxyhydroxy compound were obtained. The latter was probably (75) by analogy with other monomethylated catechols, but if it was formed from (72) then (76) is more likely; the final proof of structure must await synthesis.

Conjugation

A second step in biotransforming a drug into an easily excretable compound is usually conjugation which may involve a variety of pathways. Typically with phenols and alcohols, conjugation to form sulphates and glucuronides occurs, carboxylic acids form hippuric acids, and many compounds form sulphur conjugates with glutathione which are converted to cysteine conjugates and mercapturic acids. The structure of most of these conjugates is not established but rather it is preferred (because it is usually simpler) to remove the conjugating group and determine the structure of the unconjugated compound. As a result, there are very few examples of the application of n.m.r. to the determination of the structure of conjugates.

The structure elucidation of the major metabolite of isopropylantipyrine (77) (Tateishi and Shimizu, 1976a) is a particularly nice application of n.m.r. to conjugate analysis. The first step in the metabolism was N-demethylation to (78) which then underwent a conjugation reaction to yield the glucuronide.

(77) R = CH$_3$
(78) R = H

(79)

The presence of the glucuronide function in this conjugate was established by conventional means, but the conjugate could have been an N- or O-glucuronide, depending on which tautomeric form of (78) was involved. Both ^{1}H- and ^{13}C-n.m.r. spectra were used and both showed typical absorption for the isopropyl, methyl, and phenyl groups. The glucuronide residue provided complex absorptions in the ^{1}H-spectrum but in the ^{13}C-spectrum the furanosyl carbons could be easily observed at about 75 ppm and the O—C—O carbon at 106·1 ppm. The significant observation which allowed structure assignment was that the characteristic carbonyl group absorption observed at 163·4 ppm in (78) was absent in the conjugate; instead a new absorption was observed at 140·0 ppm, a shift of some 23 ppm to higher field. This difference must have been due to the formation of an enol tautomer as shown in (79), rather than the alternative N-glucuronide.

An interesting conjugate has been observed in the metabolism of 2-hydroxynicotinic acid (80) by dogs and rats. In this case an N-riboside was formed, rather than a glucuronide or other conjugates (Schwartz *et al*, 1973). The ^{1}H-spectrum of (81) determined in dimethylsulphoxide-d$_6$ showed a complex spectrum, partly due to the slow exchange of the hydroxyl protons and to the complex nature of the splitting pattern expected for the sugar residue. The spectrum was, however, sufficiently well resolved to allow a tentative structure assignment to the sugar residue: notably the three hydroxyls could be separately observed as well as the methylene and the anomeric proton. That the compound was the N-riboside rather than the alternative O-riboside was shown by examination of the u.v. spectrum, and the structure was confirmed by synthesis.

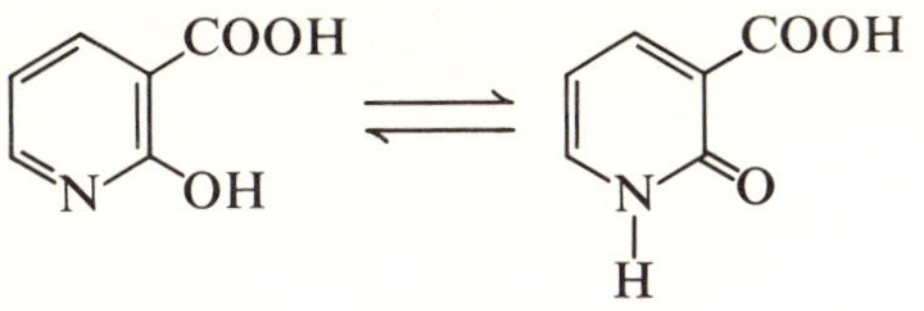

(80)

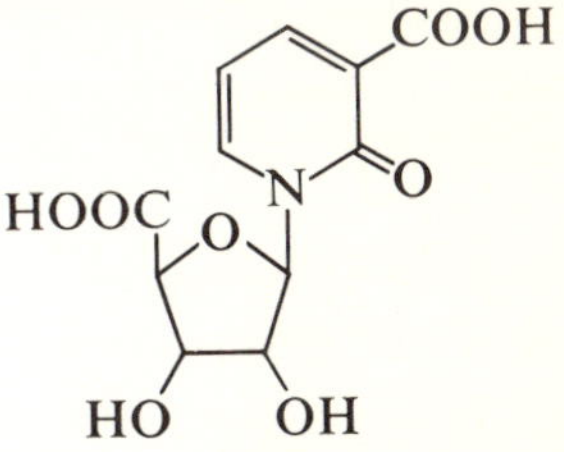

(81)

The simplest of the sulphur conjugates are those where a thiomethyl group is added to the drug. This may be further oxidized so that the sulphoxide and the sulphone as well as the thio compound are observed. The metabolism of bromazepam **(82)** resulted in the formation of all three compounds (Tateishi and Shimizu, 1976b).

In this case the ^{1}H-n.m.r. spectra allowed easy identification of the compounds. The proton adjacent to the nitrogen in a pyridine ring showed a characteristic downfield shift (relative to its phenyl counterpart) to about

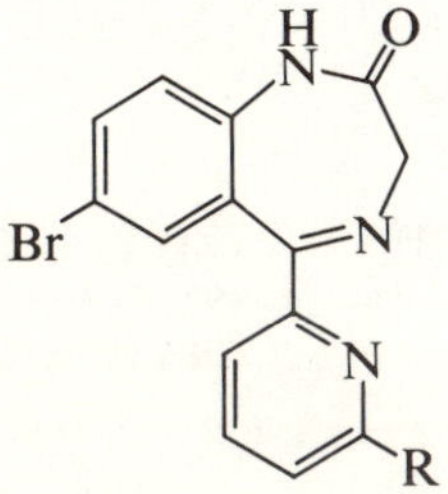

(82) R = H
(83) R = SCH$_3$
(84) R = SOCH$_3$
(85) R = SO$_2$CH$_3$

δ 8·6, and the coupling to the adjacent hydrogen (4–5 Hz) was smaller than normal *ortho*-couplings for aromatic systems. This signal was absent in all three metabolites and hence the substitution was assigned *ortho* to the nitrogen (6′-position). Each metabolite showed a new three proton singlet which could be assigned to the thiomethyl group, the chemical shift of the methyl being characteristic of the oxidation state of the sulphur atom. Thus the thiomethyl **(83)** singlet occurred at δ 2·36, the sulphoxide **(84)** at δ 2·8 and the sulphone **(85)** at δ 3·5. The sulphoxide could be further distinguished by the fact that due to the asymmetry of the sulphoxide group, the methylene hydrogens of the seven membered ring were non-equivalent and an AB quartet ($J = 11$ Hz) was observed in place of the singlet observed for the other compounds.

A number of other more complex sugar and sulphur conjugates have been characterized, but due to the lack of n.m.r. data these have not been considered here.

Phenacetin Metabolism

The metabolism of the analgesics phenacetin (**86**) and paracetamol (**87**) has been extensively studied. The principal metabolite of phenacetin is paracetamol, and a wide range of minor metabolites are also produced. Oxidation occurs at

$$HNCOCH_3 \qquad\qquad HNCOCH_3$$

$$OC_2H_5 \qquad\qquad OH$$
$$(\textbf{86}) \qquad\qquad (\textbf{87})$$

all possible positions of phenacetin; thus aromatic hydroxylation gave (**88**) (Buch *et al*, 1967) and (**92**) (Uehleke, 1969). Aliphatic hydroxylation of the methyl group (Kiese and Lenk, 1969) yielded (**94**) (Fischbach *et al*, 1977) while aliphatic hydroxylation on the methylene (**95**) led to loss of the ethyl group and formation of paracetamol (**87**), and N-hydroxylation gave (**97**) (Hinson and Mitchell, 1976). Further oxidation of (**90**) and (**94**) led to the corresponding

$$HNR \qquad\qquad HNCOCH_3 \qquad\qquad HNCOCH_3$$
$$OH$$

$$X$$
$$OC_2H_5 \qquad\qquad OC_2H_5 \qquad\qquad OR$$

(**88**) R = $COCH_3$ | (**92**) X = OH | (**94**) R = CH_2CH_2OH
(**89**) R = H | (**93**) X = SCH_3 | (**95**) R = $CHOH—CH_3$
(**90**) R = $COCH_2OH$ | | (**96**) R = CH_2COOH
(**91**) R = $COCO_2H$

$$HONCOCH_3 \qquad\qquad HNCOCH_3$$
$$SCH_3$$

$$OR \qquad\qquad OC_2H_5$$
$$(\textbf{97})\ R = C_2H_5 \qquad\qquad (\textbf{99})$$
$$(\textbf{98})\ R = H$$

carboxylic acids (**91**) and (**96**) (Dittman and Renner, 1977). Subsequent metabolism of the principal metabolite, paracetamol, also occurred to give the 3-hydroxy derivative (**100**) which can undergo a methylation reaction to the 3-methoxy derivative (**101**) (Andrews *et al*, 1976). A number of sulphur conjugates were also observed which all have a thio-group in the 3-position of

Table 7 ^{13}C-Chemical shifts of phenacetin metabolites

Compound		CH$_3$CH$_2$	CH$_3$CO	CH$_2$	C-1	C-2	C-3	C-4	C-5	C-6	C=O	XCH$_3$
Phenacetin	(86)	14·8	23·9	63·3	132·4	121·3	114·4	155·0	114·0	121·3	168·3	
N-OH	(97)	14·7	22·1	63·4	134·9	123·6	114·1	156·3	114·0	123·6	169·1	
2-OH	(88)	14·7	23·2	63·3	123·3	149·8	103·7	157·1	105·5	119·8	169·6	
3-OH	(92)	14·9	23·9	64·7	133·2	108·2	146·9	142·8	113·9	110·4	168·0	
N-COCH$_2$OH	(90)	14·7	62·1	63·3	131·2	121·2	114·3	155·0	114·3	121·2	170·3	
O-CH$_2$CO$_2$H	(96)	170·6	24·0	65·3	133·2	121·4	114·7	154·1			168·6	
2-SCH$_3$	(99)	14·8	23·3	63·3	128·6	134·6	110·9	156·8	113·1	127·2	168·8	15·5
3-SCH$_3$	(93)	14·8	23·9	64·4	133·2	117·6	127·4	151·3	111·7	117·0	168·2	14·3
p-Phenetidine	(103)	14·9		63·9	140·2	116·2	115·4	152·0	115·4	116·2		
p-Nitrosophenetrole	(104)	14·6		64·5	164·0	124·2	114·4	165·2	114·4	124·2		
4,4′-Diethoxyazoxybenzene	(107)	14·8		63·7	141·7	127·9	114·4	161·2	114·4	127·9		
				64·1	138·0	123·8	114·0	159·8	114·0	123·8		
Paracetamol	(87)		23·7		131·0	121·0	114·9	153·5	114·9	121·0	167·6	
N-OH	(98)		21·7		133·1	124·5	115·2	155·8	115·2	124·5	169·3	
3-OH	(100)		23·8		131·1	108·4	144·4	140·9	114·8	110·6	167·6	
3-OCH$_3$	(101)		23·8		131·6	105·3	147·4	142·8	115·1	112·5	168·3	55·7
3-SCH$_3$	(102)		23·8		131·4	118·4	123·8	150·1	114·0	117·5	167·6	14·7
p-Aminophenol	(105)				139·6	116·2	115·2	149·0	115·2	116·2		
Quinol	(106)				149·8	116·0	116·0	149·8	116·0	116·0		

paracetamol. The simplest of these was the thiomethyl compound (**102**) (Focella *et al*, 1972). These may have been formed via N-hydroxyparacetamol (**98**). A series of compounds were observed resulting from deacetylation to *p*-phenetidine (**103**) and subsequent oxidation reactions gave (**89**) and (**104**) (Uehleke, 1969) and (**107**) (Nery, 1971). *p*-Aminophenol (**105**) (Uehleke, 1969) and quinol (**106**) (Nery, 1971) have also been found in trace amounts.

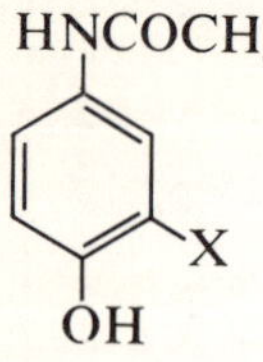

(**100**) X = OH
(**101**) X = OCH₃
(**102**) X = SCH₃

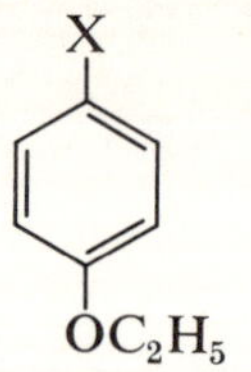

(**103**) X = NH₂
(**104**) X = NO

(**105**) X = NH₂
(**106**) X = OH

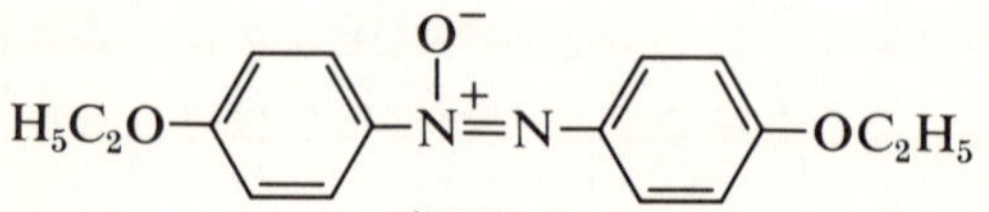

(**107**)

The identification of most of these metabolites is a relatively easy matter, particularly as authentic samples are readily available. However, the ^{13}C-n.m.r. spectra have been recorded and the data are shown in Table 7. These show the sort of changes which can be expected to occur, resulting from most of the possible metabolic reactions. The simplest spectra to interpret may result from loss of resonances following the removal of a group, e.g. (**87**) and (**103**), or the downfield shift of the carbon due to the introduction of a hydroxyl (**90**) or (**94**). Note that N-hydroxylation (**97**) had very little effect on the ^{13}C-spectrum whereas the more complex interpretations of the position of aryl substitution of a hydroxyl required detailed analysis of the spectra.

CONCLUSIONS

Nuclear magnetic resonance has developed rapidly over the last five years so that both ^{1}H- and ^{13}C-spectra are routinely available. The sensitivity of the instruments has improved dramatically so that it is possible to obtain a sufficient quantity of minor metabolites easily to determine their spectra. As a result, there will be increasing use of n.m.r. for the determination of the structure of metabolites and less reliance on deducing the structure from mass spectra alone.

An n.m.r. spectrum contains a large amount of information which can be used to determine a structure. All the signals in the spectrum must be accounted for in terms of the structure proposed. If all the peaks cannot be assigned then the structure should be reconsidered. Thus when n.m.r. is encountered for the first time by an investigator, it is advisable to seek the assistance of a person experienced in the interpretation of spectra so that the maximum amount of information can be obtained. Then care must be taken to ensure that the data reported can be accurately interpreted once published in scientific journals.

Undoubtedly then it can be expected that nuclear magnetic resonance spectroscopy will be used more extensively over the next decade when problems involving drug metabolism are encountered.

ACKNOWLEDGEMENT

I would like to express my appreciation to Dr D. P. Kelly for discussions on n.m.r. over the years and for reading the manuscript.

REFERENCES

Allen, J. G., Blackburn, M. J. and Caldwell, S. M. (1971), *Xenobiotica*, **1**, 3.

Allen, J. G., Brown, A. N. and Marten, T. R. (1976), *Xenobiotica*, **6**, 405.

Al-Rawi, J. M., Bloxsidge, J. P., Elvidge, J. A. and Jones, J. R. (1976), *Steroids*, **28**, 359.

Alton, K. B., Grimes, R. M., Shaw, C., Patrick, J. E. and McGuire, J. L. (1975), *Drug Metab. Disp.*, **3**, 352.

Ambre, J. J. and Fischer, L. J. (1974), *Drug Metab. Disp.*, **2**, 151.

Andrews, R. S., Bond, C. C., Burnett, J., Saunders, A. and Watson, K. (1976), *J. Int. Med. Res.*, **4**, Suppl. 4, 34.

Belpaire, F. M., Bogaert, M. G., Rosseel, M. T. and Anteunis, M. (1975), *Xenobiotica*, **5**, 413.

Ben-Zvi, Z., Mechoulam, R. and Burstein, S. (1970), *J. Amer. Chem. Soc.*, **92**, 3468.

Binder, M., Agurell, S., Leander, K. and Lindgren, J. (1974), *Helv. Chim. Acta*, **57**, 1626.

Brochmann-Hanssen, E. and Hirai, K. (1968), *J. Pharm. Sci.*, **57**, 940.

Buch, H., Pfleger, K., Rummel, W., Ullrich, V., Hey, D. and Staudinger, H. (1967), *Biochem. Pharmacol.*, **16**, 2247.

Buchanan, G. W., Reyes-Zamora, C. and Clarke, D. E. (1974), *Can. J. Chem.*, **52**, 3895.

Case, D. E. (1973), *Xenobiotica*, **3**, 451.

Case, D. E., McDonald, R. S. and Illston, H. (1972), *Xenobiotica*, **2**, 45.

Case, D. E. and Reeves, P. R. (1975), *Xenobiotica*, **5**, 113.

Daly, J. W. and Jerina, D. M. (1972), *Experientia*, **28**, 1129.

DiCuollo, C. J., Zarembo, J. E. and Pagano, J. F. (1973), *Xenobiotica*, **3**, 171.

Dittman, B. and Renner, G. (1977), *Arch. Pharmacol.*, **296**, 87.

Farrier, D. S. (1975), *Arzneim. Forsch.*, **25**, 813.

Fischbach, T., Lenk, W. and Sackerer, D. (1977), in Jollow, D. J., Kocsis, J. J., Snyder, R. and Vainio, H. (eds), *Biological reactive intermediates*, p. 380, Plenum, New York.

Focella, A., Heslin, P. and Teitel, S. (1972), *Can. J. Chem.*, **50**, 2025.

Fonseka, K. and Widman, M. (1977), *J. Pharm. Pharmacol.*, **29**, 12.

Goehl, T. J., Davenport, J. B. and Stanley, M. J. (1973), *Xenobiotica*, **3**, 761.

Gros, P. M., Davi, H. J., Chasseaud, L. F. and Hawkins, D. R. (1974), *Arzneim. Forsch.*, **24**, Suppl. 9A, 1385.

Hinson, J. A. and Mitchell, J. R. (1976), *Drug. Metab. Disp.*, **25**, 599.

Inouye, S., Shomura, T., Tsuruoka, T., Omoto, S., Niida, T. and Umemura, K. (1972), *Chem. Pharm. Bull.*, **20**, 2366.

Jackman, L. M. and Sternhell, S. (1969), *Applications of nuclear magnetic resonance spectroscopy in organic chemistry*, 2nd edn, Pergamon, Oxford.

Jerina, D. M. and Daly, J. W. (1974), *Science*, **185**, 573.

Kanai, Y., (1974), *Xenbiotica*, **44**, 441.

Kelly, D. P. (1977), personal communication.

Kiese, M. and Lenk, W. (1969), *Biochem. Pharmacol.*, **18**, 1325.

Kodama, R., Yano, T., Furukawa, K., Noda, K. and Ide, H. (1975), *Xenobiotica*, **5**, 39.

Martin, B., Agurell, S., Norquist, M. and Lindgren, J. (1976), *J. Pharm. Pharmacol.*, **28**, 603.

Nery, R. (1971), *Biochem. J.*, **122**, 317.

Petrzilka, T., Haefliger, W. and Sikemeiev, C. (1969), *Helv. Chim. Acta*, **52**, 1102.

Ramey, K. C., Lini, D. C. and Krow, G. (1975), in Mooney, E. F. (ed.), *Annual reports on n.m.r. spectroscopy*, vol. 6A, p. 147, Academic, London.

Rosazza, J. P., Kammer, M., Youel, L., Smith, R. V., Erhardt, P. W., Truong, D. H. and Leslie, S. W. (1977), *Xenobiotica*, **7**, 133.

Safe, S., Hutzinger, O. and Ecobichon, D. J. (1974), *Experientia*, **30**, 720.

Safe, S., Ruzo, L. O., Jones, D., Platonow, N. S. and Hutzinger, O. (1975a), *Can. J. Physiol. Pharmacol.*, **53**, 392.

Safe, S., Hutzinger, O., Ecobichon, D. J. and Grey, A. A. (1975b), *Can. J. Biochem.*, **53**, 415.

Safe, S., Jones, D. and Hutzinger, O. (1976), *J. Chem. Soc. Perkin I*, 357.

Saunders, J. K. M. (1977), *Chem. Soc. Rev.*, **6**, 467.

Schwartz, M. A., Kolis, S. J., Williams, T. H., Gabriel, T. F. and Toome, V. (1973), *Drug Metab. Disp.*, **1**, 557.

Scott, K. N., Couch, M. W., Wilder, B. J. and Williams, C. M. (1973), *Drug Metab. Disp.*, **1**, 506.

Sekine, Y., Miyamoto, M., Hashimoto, M. and Nakamura, K. (1976), *Xenobiotica*, **6**, 185.

Silverstein, R. M., Bassler, C. G. and Merrill, T. C. (1974), *Spectrometric identification of organic compounds*, 3rd edn, New York.

Stothers, J. B. (1972), *Carbon-13 n.m.r. spectroscopy*, Academic, New York.

Sumner, D. D., Dayton, P. G., Cucinell, S. A. and Plostnieks, J. (1975), *Drug Metab. Disp.*, **3**, 283.

Tateishi, M. and Shimizu, H. (1976a), *Xenobiotica*, **6**, 207.

Tateishi, M. and Shimizu, H. (1976b), *Xenobiotica*, **6**, 431.

Thomas, J. and Meffin, P. (1972), *J. Med. Chem.*, **15**, 1046.

Thonart, N., Vanhaelen, M. and Vanhaelen-Fastre, R. (1977), *J. Med. Chem.*, **20**, 604.

Uehleke, H. (1969), *Arch. Pharmacol.*, **264**, 434.

Wall, M. E., Brine, D. R., Brine, G. A., Pitt, C. G., Freudenthal, R. I. and Christiensen, H. D. (1970), *J. Amer. Chem. Soc.*, **92**, 2466.

Widman, M., Nordquist, M., Dollery, C. T. and Briant, R. H. (1975), *J. Pharm. Pharmacol.*, **27**, 842.

Williams, D. H. and Fleming, I. (1966), *Spectroscopic methods in organic chemistry*, McGraw-Hill, England.

Zacchei, A. G. and Wishousky, T. (1976), *J. Pharm. Sci.*, **65**, 1770.

Zacchei, A. G., Wishousky, T. I., Arison, B. H. and Fanelli, G. M. (1976), *Drug Metab. Disp.*, **4**, 479.

350

358

360

Contents—Volume 1

Contents—Volume 2

Contents—Volume 3